Psychosis and Schizophrenia in Hong Kong

Psychosis and Schizophrenia in Hong Kong

Navigating Clinical and Cultural Crossroads

Eric Yu Hai Chen
Yvonne Treffurth

Hong Kong University Press
The University of Hong Kong
Pok Fu Lam Road
Hong Kong
https://hkupress.hku.hk

© 2024 Hong Kong University Press

ISBN 978-988-8842-85-8 (*Hardback*)

All rights reserved. No portion of this publication may be reproduced or transmitted in any form or by any means, electronic or mechanical, including photocopying, recording, or any information storage or retrieval system, without prior permission in writing from the publisher.

British Library Cataloguing-in-Publication Data
A catalogue record for this book is available from the British Library.

Digitally printed

This work is dedicated to the patients and carers with whom we have had the privilege of sharing the journey of making sense of a condition that presents such a challenge to humanity and the medical sciences.

Contents

Foreword by Professor Sir Robin Murray	xi
Foreword by Professor William G. Honer	xiii
Preface	xv
Acknowledgements	xvii
About the Cover Design	xix
List of Abbreviations	xx
Introduction	**1**
Population Diversity in Psychotic Disorders	1
Population and Mental Health Service Contexts in Hong Kong	2
Psychosis Studies in the Hong Kong Population	4
Relevance of the Hong Kong Studies to Asia, China, and the West	4
The Boundary of Psychotic Disorders	5
Background: Key Questions Concerning Psychotic Disorders	5
Themes in Hong Kong	9
References	10

PART I: THE IMPACT OF PSYCHOSIS ON THE LIVES OF PATIENTS

1.	The Experience of Psychosis as One of the Most Devastating Illnesses	19
	The Subjective Illness Perspective in Psychotic Disorders	19
	The Subjective Experience of Psychosis in Hong Kong	21
	Reflections: The Subjective Experience of Psychosis and Its Clinical Implications	27
	References	29
2.	The Stigma of Psychosis: How It Affects Illness Outcome	34
	Background	34
	Studies on Stigma in Hong Kong	38
	Personal Reflections on Stigma	42
	References	45

viii • Contents

3. Quality of Life and Functional Outcomes in Psychotic Disorders as
Ultimate Intervention Targets 51
Background: Short- and Long-Term Functional Outcomes and
Quality of Life in Psychosis 51
The Outcome of Psychosis in Hong Kong 53
Reflections: The Importance of Context 56
References 57

PART II: EARLY INTERVENTION FOR PSYCHOSIS

4. Early Intervention in Psychosis: A Paradigm Shift 65
Background: Services for Psychotic Disorders in Hong Kong before
Early Intervention 65
Global Background and Historical Context of Early Intervention for
Psychosis 66
Early Intervention for Psychosis in Hong Kong 67
Reflections: Meeting the Local Needs of Psychosis Patients 71
References 72

5. The Naming of Psychosis: Concepts Matter in Community Education 76
Background: Renaming Schizophrenia in East Asia 76
Naming Psychosis in Hong Kong 78
The Naming of Clinical High-Risk States in Hong Kong 80
Reflections: The Evolution of Psychiatric Terminology 80
References 82

6. Delays in Help-Seeking: Duration of Untreated Psychosis and Its
Determinants 84
Background 84
Studies on the Duration of Untreated Psychosis in Hong Kong 87
Reflections: Can the Duration of Untreated Psychosis Be Shortened
Further? 90
References 91

7. Prevention Starts from Risk States: Risk States and Psychotic-Like
Experiences 95
Background: Psychotic-Like Experiences 95
Studies of Psychotic-Like Experiences in Hong Kong 96
Background: Clinical High-Risk Studies 96
Clinical High-Risk Studies in Hong Kong 98
Reflections and the Way Forward 101
References 102

Contents • ix

8. Can Early Intervention Improve Long-Term Outcomes? Evidence from
Hong Kong 107
    Background 107
    Outcomes of Early Intervention in Hong Kong 109
    Reflections: The Innovative Potential of Early Intervention
    Programmes 112
    References 115

PART III: PSYCHOPATHOLOGY AND CLINICAL PATHWAYS

9. Pharmacological Treatments: What They Can and Cannot Do 121
    Background 121
    Pharmacological Interventions for Psychosis in Hong Kong 123
    Reflections: Antipsychotic Prescribing in Context 127
    References 128

10. Relapse in Psychotic Disorders: Prediction, Prevention, and
Management 134
    Background 134
    Relapse in Psychotic Disorders in Hong Kong 136
    Reflections: The Importance of Maintenance Treatment in Relapse
    Prevention 142
    References 143

11. Treatment-Refractory States: An End-Game Scenario? 148
    Background 148
    Studies on Treatment-Refractory Psychosis in Hong Kong 151
    Reflections: The Challenges of Managing Treatment-Refractory Psychosis 154
    References 155

12. Ideas of Reference: Complexities in the Most Common Symptom in
Psychosis 159
    Background 159
    Ideas and Delusions of Reference in Psychosis in Hong Kong 161
    Reflections: The Unique Nature of Ideas and Delusions of Reference 164
    References 165

13. Mortality and Suicide: Silent Killers in Psychosis 168
    Background 168
    Suicide and Mortality in Hong Kong 170
    Suicide in Psychotic Disorders 173
    Suicide in Psychosis and Its Predictors in Hong Kong 173
    Mortality Other Than Suicide 174
    The Impact of Early Intervention on Suicide 174

x • Contents

Reflections: The Role of Early Intervention Programmes in Suicide
Prevention and Reducing Mortality   175
References   175

PART IV: NEUROCOGNITIVE DYSFUNCTIONS

14. Cognitive Dysfunctions: The Hidden Impediments of Psychosis   183
Background   183
Studies on Cognitive Functioning in Hong Kong   186
Reflections on Cognitive Deficits in Psychosis   189
References   191

15. Semantic Dysfunctions: The Central Role of Language Processes in
Psychosis   196
Background   196
Semantic Function Studies in Psychosis in Hong Kong   198
Reflections: The Central Role of Language Functions   203
References   205

16. Neurological Soft Signs: A Simple Enough Clinical Sign in Psychosis   210
Background   210
Studies on Neurological Soft Signs in Hong Kong and China   212
Reflections: Neurological Soft Signs as a Proxy Measure of Brain
Dysfunction   214
References   215

PART V: RECOVERY

17. Ways to Improve Cognition: Beyond Medications   221
Background   221
Studies on Interventions for Cognitive Dysfunction in Hong Kong   223
Reflections: The Emerging Evidence of Exercise Interventions
Supporting Cognitive Recovery   226
References   227

18. Remission and Recovery: The Journeys towards Getting Well   232
Background   232
Studies on Remission and Recovery in Hong Kong   234
Reflections: The Concepts of Remission and Recovery   237
References   240

Epilogue   243
Index   245

Foreword by Professor Sir Robin Murray

This book brings together an extensive body of work undertaken by the team led by Professor Eric Chen over the last 25 years. With the implementation of one of the most comprehensive early intervention programmes for psychosis in Asia in the late 1990s, the team's research has been driven by a desire to improve longitudinal outcomes in psychosis and enhance the lives of patients by offering culturally sensitive interventions. Readers across the world will be extremely impressed not only by the breadth of the research, covering the subjective experiences of patients, stigma, symptomatology, relapse, recovery, and innovative exercise interventions but also the team's reports of their meticulous long-term outcome studies.

The findings in Hong Kong, a major Asian city at the confluence between Western and Chinese influences, confirm universal aspects of psychosis but also reveal particular cultural facets such as the intense stigma associated with mental illness when compared to Western populations. Thus, the team's public awareness campaigns and introduction of the less stigmatising term *sijueshitiao* ('dysregulation of thought and perception') in the early 2000s to describe early psychosis have been pioneering and have prompted a wider debate on the naming of psychotic illnesses in many countries. Of note has also been the emphasis on phase-specific early intervention implemented across the city, which has undoubtedly contributed to its effectiveness despite the relatively low resources available to treat psychiatric disorders.

Professor Chen's particular interests have focused on the study of cognitive dysfunction and his work on semantic functional impairments has been innovative. Cognitive functioning as one of the major prognostic factors in psychosis has been a connecting theme in Hong Kong and has highlighted the importance of developing innovative interventions to ameliorate the potentially devastating effects of the disorder. The team has also conducted important work on the impact of early intervention as well as relapse prevention strategies on the long-term outcome of psychotic disorders.

This scholarly work also offers personal reflections on the extensive clinical and research programme undertaken in Hong Kong and, to my knowledge, is the first of its kind in Asia. It serves as a shining example of how similar initiatives might be implemented in low-resource settings across the Asian continent and in the Global South.

Professor Sir Robin Murray, FRS
Professor of Psychiatric Research
Institute of Psychiatry, Psychology and Neuroscience
King's College London

Foreword by Professor William G. Honer

Readers of *Psychosis and Schizophrenia in Hong Kong* will find a rich source of knowledge on these enigmatic disorders, derived in the main from the author's extensive experience with an early intervention programme. Considerable attention is paid throughout the text to context, ranging from a granular level in the interpretation of individual symptoms of psychotic disorders, to the structure of the early intervention service, and most broadly to the social environment in Hong Kong. Such careful descriptions will allow insights to be selectively applied to the care of individual patients, and the design and operation of services.

From 1999 to 2019, I visited Professor Chen's group regularly, travelling to Hong Kong most years. The integration of research with clinical care, and the application of research findings to result in changes in service delivery was quite remarkable. The reach of the early intervention service was population-wide, as I saw in visits from one end of Hong Kong to another. Ease of access, not only to care, but also to records of inpatient and outpatient visits (the latter including the early intervention teams) allowed longitudinal studies of remarkably large sample sizes with high retention rates. The near-equal gender representation, low prevalence of substance use, and access to social support, education and employment opportunities provide confidence that the findings reported here may represent the best-case scenario to assess the outcomes of early intervention services. The findings described herein are based on direct contact of patients with a highly motivated team of clinician–investigators, providing a complementary source of information to studies in other regions based primarily on administrative records. Readers can decide for themselves when and how to apply each type of information when making clinical decisions.

Professor Chen and Dr Treffurth provide readers with an opening that places the personal experiences of patients first and foremost. Then in each chapter that follows, they implement an approach of a focused review of the literature, setting the stage for an account of the findings of integrated care and research in Hong Kong, and closing with reflections on their 20 years of experience with the early intervention services. Returning to the theme of context, like other great urban centres, Hong Kong changed greatly during the period of time covered in the account provided here. Wise readers, who understand their local ecosystems as thoroughly as the authors understood Hong Kong, will see beyond local differences to the opportunities that shared understanding can provide.

As those in the field know, the hope and optimism of the early psychosis movement created great change in service delivery for youth worldwide, with measurable benefits. Yet still, the challenges of maintaining gains remain, particularly for patients with schizophrenia, the most serious of the psychotic disorders. The authors do not shy away from interpreting those findings from their studies that illustrate the work that still needs to be done. The book, *Psychosis and Schizophrenia in Hong Kong: Navigating Clinical and Cultural Crossroads*, adds to the value created in Hong Kong through the implementation of a 'think globally, act locally' strategy for clinical care and research. There may be no better source of inspiration for the work to come, to write the future of early psychosis intervention.

William G. Honer, MD, FRCPC, FCAHS
Professor, and Jack Bell Chair in Schizophrenia
University of British Columbia

Preface

The book brings together unique insights gained from a sustained period of a clinical research programme focusing on psychotic disorders carried out in Hong Kong over several decades. It offers a distinct perspective to complement findings observed in Western populations reported in most of the published manuscripts and standard textbooks regarding the nature and presentation of psychotic disorders. Culturally relevant issues such as societal responses to potentially serious and enduring mental illnesses and factors driving clinical care for psychotic disorders are also examined. In this respect, Hong Kong represents a contrasting reference as a major East Asian metropolitan population anchored in oriental traditions, yet enjoying a high degree of cultural diversity. In this context, Hong Kong has also served as a portal between China and many international networks. This opportunity is particularly poignant as the global scientific and clinical progress in psychotic disorders has served as a prime paradigm for the understanding of complex psychiatric disorders. A predominantly Western perspective has driven, but at times also impeded, progress in understanding and treating the enigmatic disorder that many researchers and clinicians have grappled with in lifelong struggles. The Hippocratic aphorism 'Ars longa, vita brevis, occasio praeceps, experimentum periculosum, iudicium difficile' ('life is short, the art [of medicine] long, opportunity fleeting, experiment treacherous, judgement difficult') is especially applicable to psychosis research. Like in any long journey, the spectacles presented to the traveller on the way change as the path meanders through different landscapes. On this long and arduous adventure, there are opportune moments for looking back over the ground covered from a new height attained by sustained efforts.

Following initial work in the context of a World Health Organization international epidemiology project on schizophrenia in the 1980s, systematic research in psychotic disorders in Hong Kong started in the 1990s with investigations into neurocognitive dysfunctions in order to identify core brain system abnormalities that could be related to symptom dimensions in psychosis. This was followed by a series of studies examining first-episode psychosis and the longitudinal evolution of symptoms, cognition, functioning, and outcomes. These observational studies have been complemented by studying various possible methods to improve outcomes in psychotic disorders such as early intervention, case management, relapse prevention programmes, and psychological and exercise interventions.

Globally, research programmes in mental health have followed two approaches. The technical approach focuses on particular investigational methods such as brain imaging or genetics and applies these techniques to various psychiatric conditions. In contrast, a clinical approach concentrates on the condition itself and organises research questions around understanding the nature of the disorder and its treatments. The research team in Hong Kong has largely followed the clinical approach. Over the years, the team has been conducting research into improving outcomes for psychotic disorders and has been using a variety of approaches to address pertinent questions. This has enabled us to cover a large number of clinically relevant areas in the understanding and management of psychotic disorders as covered in this volume.

As the research team and research activities have grown over the years, the need for reflection and discussion has also increased. While the weekly research meetings in the psychosis team have served as a primary platform for discussion, they are still focused on the details of current projects. Thus, the need for a broader reflection on how local research themes developed in a wider context and over a longer period of time became apparent. An occasion for this reflection was also precipitated by when Yvonne joined the team from the UK. With her background in child psychiatry and psychotherapy, she was able to join our discussions with a broader perspective than our team of seasoned psychosis researchers. The book's topics have been developed from a series of thematic discussions in our team for nearly two years, forming the basic material covered in this work. We organised the content further so that each topic has an introduction of the global advances in psychosis and relevant clinical context, followed by a summary of key observations from our research in Hong Kong, and ending with a reflective summary of insights for future clinical and research directions.

We have attempted to gather our observations in a coherent fashion in the context of contemporary psychosis research and its application, rather than merely to present a collection of our published studies. This has prompted further reflections on some of our observations, particularly those that had not been the primary focus of our initial inquiry. With other more recently emerging information, this has offered novel perspectives and fuelled further directions in our research programme. Equally, we hope that readers will find thought-provoking material in the book and be inspired by innovative developments in the field with the ultimate goal of supporting patients to live productive and meaningful lives.

Acknowledgements

The information and insights summarised in this book would not have been possible without the many colleagues who have worked with the Psychosis Studies and Intervention (PSI) Team at the University of Hong Kong as well as our collaborators over the years. They include past and present colleagues, in particular my predecessors and mentors in this area of work, Professor Felice Lieh Mak and Professor Peter Lee. Key colleagues in the team included Dr Ronald Chen, Dr Agatha Wong, Dr Raymond Chan, Dr Christy Hui, Dr Gloria Wong, Dr Josephine Wong, Dr Cindy Chiu, Dr May Lam, Dr Sherry Chan, Dr Wing Chung Chang, Dr Edwin Hui, Professor Pak Sham, Dr Yi Nam Suen and Dr Stephanie Wong. Within the Department of Psychiatry at the University of Hong Kong, we have worked closely with Professor Pak Sham, Dr Siew E Chua, and Dr Grainne McAlanon.

We have been supported by many excellent research assistants, graduate students, postdoctoral fellows, and research assistant professors. Many of them have continued to work in the field. Indispensable to the work were many clinical colleagues who worked alongside us in developing various interventions and studies to improve outcomes of psychotic disorders in Hong Kong. These include Dr Se Fong Hung, Dr Dicky Chung, Dr Steve Tso, Dr Eric Cheung, Dr Chi Wing Law, Dr Jessica Wong, Dr Eric Yan, Dr Catherine Chong, Dr Eva Dunn, Dr Wai Nan Tang, Dr Wai Fat Chan, Dr Tak Lum Lo, Dr Alison Lo, Dr Ka Chi Yip, and Dr Frendi Li. Support from key collaborating non-profit organisations in the field has been vital to many of the pioneering early intervention projects, such as The New Life, The Mental Health Association, Caritas Social Service, the Baptist Oi Kwan Social Services and the Early Psychosis Foundation (EPISO). They have worked tirelessly to improve the care of people recovering from psychotic disorders. In particular, the EPISO is a small charity working creatively to reduce stigma, increase help-seeking, and improve family support for patients with psychotic disorders through exercise interventions. Equally vital has been the support of the Advisory Committee for Mental Health, which has been working to overcome the many barriers to facilitate mental health work in Hong Kong. The Jockey Club Charity Fund has played an essential role in providing support for some of the pilot projects.

xviii • Acknowledgements

While we used the work of the PSI team as an anchoring focus in the book, we are glad that we are not the only researchers in the locality. The Hong Kong Schizophrenia Research Society has been fostering a platform promoting multi-disciplinary research in psychosis. The PSI team is indeed privileged to have been working alongside, and sometimes in close collaboration with other colleagues in Hong Kong, the Asian region, and other parts of the world. We are indebted to the support of many international colleagues, among them Professors Robin Murray, Tim Crow, Eve Johnstone, German Berrios, Peter McKenna, Brita Elvavaag, Bill Honer, Peter Falkai, Peter Jones, Pat McGorry, Byron Good, Oliver Howes, Larry Seidman, Thara Rangaswamy, Siow Ann Chong, Swapna Varma, Chung Chul Young, Masafumi Mizuno, Mythily Subramanium, and Robert Miller.

Last but not least, this book and the insights we have gained over the years would not have been possible without the positive involvement of the many patients and carers who co-worked with us in the clinical programmes, community projects, and research studies.

About the Cover Design

We have used an artwork of the seascape in Hong Kong, together with a calligraphy inscription written by one of Professor Eric Chen's patients who has given generous permission to use her work on the cover of this book.

The inscription is based on an ancient Chinese expression that means 'Broad is the ocean and clear is the sky'. It denotes the broadened psychological space available if one is able to step back to take in a wider perspective, particularly in adversity.

List of Abbreviations

AED	accident and emergency department
AESOP	Aetiology and Ethnicity in Schizophrenia and Other Psychoses
ALFF	amplitude of low-frequency fluctuations
AMPA	α-amino-3-hydroxy-5-methyl-4-isoxazolepropionate
ARMS	at-risk mental states
BPRS	Brief Psychiatric Rating Scale
CAARMS	Comprehensive Assessment of 'At-Risk Mental State'
CAFE	Comparison of Antipsychotics in First Episode Psychosis
CapQOL	capacity to report subjective quality of life
CBT	cognitive-behavioural therapy
CBTp	cognitive-behavioural therapy for psychosis
CEDAR	Centre for Intervention Development and Advanced Research
CGI	Clinical Global Impressions
CHIME	connectedness, hope and optimism about the future, identity, meaning in life, and empowerment
CHR	clinical high-risk
CLANG	Clinical Language Disorder Rating Scale
CMS	cortical midline structures
CNI	Cambridge Neurological Inventory
CR-TRS	clozapine-resistant schizophrenia
CSPT	cortico-striato-pallido-thalamic
DMN	default mode network
DOR	delusions of reference
DUP	duration of untreated psychosis
EASY	Early Assessment Service for Young People
EI	early intervention

EPISO	Early Psychosis Foundation
EPPIC	Early Psychosis Prevention and Intervention Centre
EUFEST	European Union First Episode Schizophrenia Trial
FEP	first-episode psychosis
FGA	first-generation antipsychotic
fMRI	functional magnetic resonance imaging
FTD	formal thought disorder
GABA	γ-aminobutyric acid
HIIT	high-intensity interval training
HKMMS	Hong Kong Mental Morbidity Survey
HMPAO SPECT	hexamethylpropylene amine oxime single photon emission computed tomography
HSCT	Hayling Sentence Completion Test
I/DOR	ideas and delusions of reference
IOR	ideas of reference
IPSS	International Pilot Study of Schizophrenia
IRAOS	Interview for the Retrospective Assessment of the Onset of Schizophrenia
IRIS	Ideas of Reference Interview Scale
ISoS	International Study on Schizophrenia
JCEP	Jockey Club Early Psychosis Project
JSPN	Japanese Society of Psychiatry and Neurology
LAIA	long-acting injectable antipsychotic
L-FAI	Life Functioning Assessment Inventory
LSAS	Leibowitz Social Anxiety Scale
MSET	Modified Six Elements Test
NEMESIS	The Netherlands Mental Health Survey and Incidence Study
NFFMIJ	National Federation of Families with Mentally Ill in Japan
NGO	non-governmental organisations
NMDA	N-methyl-D-aspartate
NOS	Nottingham Onset Schedule
NSS	neurological soft signs
OA	oral antipsychotic
OCD	obsessive compulsive disorder
OECD	Organisation for Economic Co-operation and Development

PANSS	Positive and Negative Syndrome Scale
PIPE	Psychological Intervention Programme in Early Psychosis
PLE	psychotic-like experience
PRI	Psychosis Recovery Inventory
PSI	Psychosis Studies and Intervention
PSQ	Psychosis Screening Questionnaire
QoL	quality of life
RAISE	Recovery After an Initial Schizophrenia Episode
RCT	randomised controlled trial
RSWG	Remission in Schizophrenia Working Group
rTMS	repetitive transcranial magnetic stimulation
SAD	social anxiety disorder
SARS	severe acute respiratory syndrome
SC	standard care
SCI	subjective cognitive impairment
SEPS	Subjective Experiences of Psychosis Scale
SF-12	Short Form 12-Item Health Survey
SF-36	Short Form 36-Item Health Survey
SGA	second-generation antipsychotic
SIPS	Structured Interview for Psychosis Risk Syndromes
SOHO	Schizophrenia Outpatients Health Outcomes
SOPS	Scale of Psychosis-Risk Symptoms
SQoL	subjective quality of life
SRGP	self-referential gaze perception
tDCS	transcranial direct current stimulation
TLC	thought, language, and communication
ToM	theory of mind
TRP	treatment-resistant psychosis
TRRIP	Treatment Response and Resistance in Psychosis
TRS	treatment-resistant schizophrenia
UHR	ultra-high-risk
WCST	Wisconsin Card Sorting Test
WHO	World Health Organization

Introduction

Psychotic disorders are conditions in which some of the most profound mechanisms of the human mind are disrupted. They impair a person's ability to process and interpret information from the environment in order to constitute a continuous experience of reality and the self, resulting in spurious perceptions and aberrant representations of the outside world. These psychotic disturbances are clinically described as hallucinations, delusions, and disordered thinking (1). Psychotic disorders are often also associated with motivational and cognitive impairment with a long-term impact on the person's ability to function in their occupational and social roles (2). Despite treatment with antipsychotic medication, individuals with psychosis are prone to relapse. The psychotic state may become persistent or non-remitting over the course of the illness for some patients (3, 4). Psychotic disorders impact not only the individual but also their family and social relationships (5, 6). They carry a high global disease burden with devastating experiential and functional consequences (7).

Because of their putative impact on some of the most fundamental functions of the human mind, psychotic disorders have been studied intensely from multiple perspectives since their nosological recognition emerged at the turn of the twentieth century (1, 2, 8, 9, 10, 11, 12, 13, 14). The resulting research data have mostly been reported as individual studies. It has been challenging to integrate these data more systematically due to differences in populations, variable definitions, divergent outcome measures, high loss to follow-up and other factors. However, more recently international efforts have been made to agree on standardised definitions of clinically relevant concepts such as remission and it is hoped that these efforts will provide more coherent insights into the nature of this devastating illness (15).

Population Diversity in Psychotic Disorders

Recent data have revealed significant diversity of the disorder in different populations in terms of incidence rates, genetics, presentation, and outcome. However, most studies of psychotic disorders have been carried out in European and North

American populations (16, 17, 18). Studies on psychosis in non-Western populations are few and isolated (16). Although a variety of factors such as differences in study design and case ascertainment will affect incidence rates in different countries, it is likely that other factors, such as urbanicity, gender, migratory status, substance use rates and genetic risks, impact observed rates (16, 18). For example, it has been shown that common genetic variants that confer the risk of schizophrenia share similar effects in European and East Asian populations; but variants specific to Chinese Han ancestry have also been discovered, suggesting at least some genetic heterogeneity (19, 20).

Hong Kong has one of the highest population densities in the world and is highly urbanised; however, substance use rates are significantly lower in our clinic population compared to their Western counterparts (21, 22, 23). In addition, due to severe housing shortages, the majority of our patients reside with their families. Social isolation has been identified as an important factor in the recovery of psychosis sufferers (24). Although objectively, our patients are less isolated when compared to Western patient groups, outcomes are very similar to European and US samples. Findings indicate that the quality of relationships has a greater effect on the maintenance of recovery than the quantity of social interactions and that the concept of high-expressed emotions similarly applies in the Asian context (25). To ameliorate the potentially devastating effects of family discord on recovery, our service has increasingly focused on carer engagement and the use of a dialogical approach to support patients and their relatives in managing the complexities of having a psychotic disorder. Also, a wide range of health beliefs in Asian culture differ from those in the West, most notably the stigma associated with psychotic illness and mental disorders per se, not only affecting individuals but also whole families (26, 27). In Chinese culture, mental disorders are considered to bring shame and embarrassment to the family, potentially impacting carers' resilience and increasing familial stigma (28).

Accessing a coherent set of data on different aspects of psychotic disorders studied in the same population using similar approaches will be instrumental in helping gauge the extent of population diversity in aetiology, pathophysiology, clinical presentation, and treatment response. In addition, this will also aid the development of culturally sensitive treatment strategies (16).

Population and Mental Health Service Contexts in Hong Kong

The studies and observations in this book were undertaken in a context highly relevant to the future development of mental health services and research programmes in Asia, as well as metropolitan populations in which Asian communities may constitute a significant proportion of service users. Like many city populations in Asia, the communities in Hong Kong are largely affluent. However, income inequalities are vast, and mental health services are often disproportionately inadequate compared to other medical services. In the 1990s, Hong Kong had two to five psychiatrists per 100,000 people, a fraction of those in Organisation for Economic Cooperation and Development (OECD) countries. This relative shortage of medical professionals also extended to mental health nursing, clinical psychology, occupational therapy, and social services.

Hong Kong adopted a specialist training programme closely modelled on the UK system. Medical graduates who wish to practise psychiatry enter into a rotational training scheme lasting six years. Training positions were exclusively located in public hospitals with a cap on trainee numbers determined by the hospital authority. The public healthcare system was heavily focused on hospital inpatient units based upon regional clusters of hospitals giving rise to underfunded and crowded outpatient services with consultation times for psychosis patients averaging five to six minutes.

The emphasis on psychiatric inpatient care was partly historical. Mental health care in Hong Kong had pivoted on Castle Peak Hospital, a large psychiatric hospital, which opened its doors in the 1960s, catering to 3,000 to 4,000 patients, with many being long-stay patients. A second big psychiatric hospital was built in the 1980s. Subsequent developments saw the establishment of smaller psychiatric units in general hospitals. However, not all general hospitals have psychiatric departments, and some of the largest general hospitals in Hong Kong, including one major teaching hospital, still do not host psychiatric units. Apart from hospitals and their affiliated outpatient clinics, there is a substantial private sector consisting mainly of clinics. Around one-third of psychiatrists in Hong Kong work in private practice.

At the time of the initiation of the early intervention for psychosis programme, community services were almost non-existent, case management was not systematically adopted, and collaboration with non-governmental organisations funded by social services was minimal. Partly as a result of the high service load, mental health care was impoverished, with patient needs largely unmet apart from the assessment and medical treatment of core symptoms. Most patients with first-episode psychosis presented in crisis via accident and emergency and were admitted to inpatient units. After discharge, few community services were available other than brief outpatient reviews. Mental health service development was rarely based on data, and its evaluation was only taking place sporadically. The introduction of the early intervention for psychosis service provided a catalyst for the transformation of psychiatric care in general. The improvements were not only restricted to psychosis services but benefitted all mental health services. Nonetheless, there are still undeniable tensions between manpower and service quality.

The stigma around mental illness is severe in Asian communities. This is particularly the case for psychotic disorders. Patients with psychosis usually cannot

4 • *Psychosis and Schizophrenia in Hong Kong*

speak about their illness to anyone outside their immediate family and discrimination in the workplace is widespread. Worryingly, the fear of having a mental health record in the public health system still is a significant barrier to help-seeking.

Psychosis Studies in the Hong Kong Population

Hong Kong has an urban population sharing many characteristics with other major populations in East Asia, such as in Japan, Korea, China, Taiwan, and Singapore (29, 30). A sustained programme of research has been yielding data on psychotic disorder patients in Hong Kong for more than two decades. The programme has investigated psychotic disorders from a variety of perspectives, looking at aetiological factors, pathogenesis pathways, prodromal risk states, clinical presentation, different interventional approaches, early intervention systems, clinical course and outcomes, as well as social determinants of help-seeking behaviours and recovery. Most of the studies have been separately published in relevant journals, mostly as individual contributions towards the generic understanding of aspects of psychotic disorders. Here, we consider this information from a different perspective: as a coherent body of work undertaken in the same population of psychosis patients in a non-Western setting. Reflecting on the results of our work will provide a valuable overview of the contemporary understanding of psychotic disorders and offer thought-provoking insights into population diversities regarding clinical presentation and treatment approaches.

Relevance of the Hong Kong Studies to Asia, China, and the West

In many ways, mental health services in Hong Kong represent a system that has been developing along a pathway shared by many other metropolitan areas in Asia and China. In Mainland China, for example, the mental health workforce comprises even fewer psychiatrists and psychiatric nurses than in Hong Kong and although there have been community-based mental health initiatives in several large cities, most psychiatric care has been provided in long-stay inpatient facilities (31). With the introduction of the mental health services reform in 2004, a training programme was collaboratively developed by the Beijing University Institute of Mental Health, the University of Melbourne, and the Chinese University of Hong Kong. The programme has aimed to build a culturally sensitive skill set for the assessment and management of psychosis in the community. Despite many challenges, it has been widely adopted and has led to further important mental health policy reforms (31). Similarly, Singapore, Japan, and Korea have heavily relied on inpatient treatment of patients with mental disorders (32, 33, 34).

Hong Kong exemplifies a city that initially focused on economic development, which subsequently led to higher expectations of healthier lives for its citizens. As demands on mental health increase, the possibility of developing services that share a vision to support individuals with psychiatric difficulties to reach their full potential becomes a common goal for service providers. In this context, psychotic disorders pose a distinct challenge that requires taking into consideration their scientific understanding, available clinical evidence, and service provision. How professionals, service users, and other stakeholders contribute to a way forward based on the best possible data and the background of inadequate resources is a taxing problem that requires local solutions. This book would serve its purpose if it can contribute towards providing some insights and information for colleagues involved in similar developments, whether in China, Asia, or other parts of the world.

The Boundary of Psychotic Disorders

Ever since the evolution of a more explicit conceptualisation in the late nineteenth century, the diagnostic concepts of psychotic disorders have been under discussion and have been evolving (35). The latest position suggests that the category boundaries of psychotic disorders involve multiple dimensions, some of which may have fuzzy rather than discrete boundaries (36). Thus the matter of deciding on the scope of psychotic disorders is likely to be driven by historical as well as pragmatic clinical factors (37). In the studies we are reviewing, a consistent two-level pragmatic approach has been adopted, namely a broader category of psychotic disorders involving non-organic, non-affective psychotic disorders; and a narrower approach involving the schizophrenia prototype according to conventional diagnostic criteria. These boundaries have remained largely stable over the period of our studies.

Over the last 25 years, we have witnessed several developments in the management of psychotic disorders globally. First of all, there have been more public awareness and anti-stigma programmes in society (38). Secondly, early intervention services, comprising specialised teams providing case management for patients with psychosis, became available in many locations over the last two to three decades (39). Thirdly, pharmacological interventions have witnessed the advent of second-generation antipsychotics (40). Finally, recovery-focused service models in the rehabilitation of psychosis patients have been widely adopted (41). The significance of these changes for Hong Kong psychosis patients will be reviewed in our book.

Background: Key Questions Concerning Psychotic Disorders

Research themes on various aspects of psychotic disorders have been evolving over the past two decades. Appreciating the driving forces behind these developments and integrating the various research strands into a coherent account is instrumental to advancing our understanding of psychotic disorders.

Aetiological Risk Factors

Psychotic symptoms are encountered during episodes of acute psychotic states. The prototype of a psychotic disorder is schizophrenia. It was observed that apart from psychotic symptoms, schizophrenia is also accompanied to a varying degree by negative symptoms, and cognitive and functional impairments (1). There is a high degree of genetic heritability, but genetic determination is not complete; environmental and individual factors also play significant roles. It was difficult to identify a small number of relevant candidate genes until the emergence of large genetic consortiums, which have yielded data suggestive of a highly polygenic background in which hundreds of common genes, each with small effects, are likely to be involved (42, 43, 44). A smaller number of rare genes with large effects have been reported but are not typically found. It is increasingly recognised that a set of implicated genes is overlapping but is not identical in different ethnic groups (29).

Environmental factors affecting early brain development in foetal and perinatal periods, such as the effects of maternal viral infection and malnutrition, as well as obstetric complications at birth, contribute to a small but significant extent to the aetiology of psychotic disorders. The discovery of early insults on brain development contributing to the emergence of psychotic disorders later in life has led to the formulation of the neurodevelopmental theory of psychosis (45). It was postulated that key environmental aetiological factors impact the brain during early development and result in a vulnerable but latent state during childhood. The emergence of the illness during adolescence was considered an unfolding event during the last stages of brain maturation. This theory has implied that most of the neurocognitive dysfunction is already present before the onset of the illness, with little subsequent progression (46, 47). This view had driven research focusing on the first episode of psychosis and the clinical high-risk conditions before the onset of illness, rather than the subsequent course of the disorder, which was assumed to be relatively stable.

The identification of additional aetiological risk factors has challenged this view. Cannabis use in early adolescence was found to have a close relationship with the risk of subsequent psychosis (48). It is likely that the use of other psychoactive substances is also associated with heightened risk states (49). Moreover, growing up in an urban environment was found to have a close relationship with psychosis. Migration has been shown to increase the risk of psychosis in both the first and second generation, and epidemiological data suggests that minority group identity, as well as experiences of discrimination, may contribute to the risk as well (50, 51).

Further studies have suggested a role of early adverse life experiences, such as abuse during childhood, as well as being bullied at school, in the emergence of psychotic disorders later in life (52, 53). Studies have pointed towards psychosis being associated with multiple layers of possible aetiological factors that affect individuals to different extents in a given population, in a manner described by the stress-vulnerability model (54). Importantly, this research suggests that the underlying profile of contributing disease mechanisms may vary in different populations.

How these aetiological factors lead to the expression of clinical psychosis has been intensely studied using two main approaches. The first focuses on identifying the intermediate expression of the inherited genetic profile of the disorder. This has led to the recognition of the schizotypal spectrum, a diluted form of the schizophrenia phenotype. Also, efforts have been made to link neurocognitive markers to heritable entities in the endophenotype approach (55, 56). The second approach concentrates on identifying mechanistic pathways towards the expression of psychotic states by elucidating additional processes involved in converting stable heritable traits into florid psychotic states (57).

Researchers have also redirected their efforts from early attempts to identify the 'holy grail' of a single underlying neurocognitive mechanism that could explain all the psychotic symptoms, to investigating different permutations of networks with interacting sub-domains at the levels of brain networks and neurocognitive processes (58, 59).

The Multiple Dimensions of Psychosis

The current state of affairs compels the researcher to reflect on the different dimensions of psychosis and the old question of the boundary of 'the psychotic disorder'. In addition to the classic dopamine hypothesis, neuroanatomical and neurophysiological findings have revealed histological evidence for the involvement of oligodendrocytes and hippocampal dentate granule cells, as well as parvalbumin-positive γ-aminobutyric acid (GABA) inhibitory neurons in the cortex (60, 61, 62). Myelination defects have also been shown to be associated with psychotic disorders (63). Processes in the brain related to these findings are generic and widespread, such as perceptual binding, i.e., the process of merging individual pieces of sensory information into coherent representations, and neural synchronisation, excitatory and inhibitory control, contrast enhancement of representations, and memory processes (64, 65, 66). In terms of gross anatomical brain structure, there is a generalised reduction in cortical grey matter, with a specific reduction in the hippocampus, possibly being more prominent on the left side. In contrast to the neurodevelopmental thesis, brain volume reduction has been shown to be not static, but progressive with age. These progressive changes are possibly more rapid than age-related changes seen in a healthy control population (61, 67, 68).

Neurotransmitter changes involve dopaminergic transmission and it appears that presynaptic dopamine synthesis rather than post-synaptic receptor function is impaired. These findings have encouraged research into upstream cortical systems controlling dopaminergic pathways. Several functional cerebral systems and networks seem to be involved, such as the salient network, theta synchronisation, the supplementary motor cortex, and default mode network, in addition to the classic task-based deficits in executive, attentional, and memory functions (69, 70, 71, 72, 73, 74). Coherent with neuroanatomical findings, there appears to be widespread cognitive impairment that can be traced back to basic information processing in early sensory signals, such as the P100 event-related potential. However, more complex processes such as the integration of contextual information or social cognition are also likely to be affected by dysfunction in the aforementioned networks (2, 74, 75).

The presentation of the clinical high-risk state has received much attention, with data suggesting that there is a 10–20% risk of conversion to frank psychosis (76, 77). The risk appears to be dependent on the context of screening and case identification, with most patients developing mood or anxiety disorders rather than a psychotic illness in the longer term. The transdiagnostic nature of the clinical high-risk state and its emergence during adolescence has highlighted the importance of youth mental health. Transient psychotic experiences are not uncommon in adolescence and are also reported by patients with borderline personality traits and other non-psychotic conditions. Transient psychotic phenomena not only present a clinical dilemma for accurate assessment and treatment but also complicate the boundary of the psychosis state (78). Although it is conceivable that psychotic-like states in non-psychotic disorders may arise on the background of rather different aetiological pathways, they are clinically often very similar in form and content to psychotic states when isolated symptoms are considered.

Cognitive Dysfunction

Longitudinal studies involving individuals at genetic high-risk of psychosis have suggested that cognitive decline may precede the development of psychotic symptoms in schizophrenia by one to two years and that it is an inherent feature of the illness (79, 80). In addition, a significant proportion of patients experience an insidious onset resulting in a delay in help-seeking. Measurements of the duration of untreated psychosis (DUP) have confirmed that treatment is often delayed and that the delay leads to poorer outcomes (9, 81, 82). In addition, outcomes are negatively affected by comorbid substance use. This is a difficulty encountered in many Western populations, whereas psychosis is less commonly precipitated by substance use in East Asia (23, 77).

Early Intervention in Psychosis

Intervention studies have evolved with the emergence of new service models. Early intervention for psychosis has been a major theme, with studies confirming its efficacy during the first few years of the illness. Varying evidence has suggested a sustained improvement over the time course of a decade or more, thus supporting the critical period hypothesis (83, 84, 85, 86). Improvements in functional outcomes and reduced suicide rates have been convincingly demonstrated in patients receiving early intervention when compared to standard care (87).

Longitudinal studies have also revealed that the clinical course of the disorder may not be static and that there are later recoveries as well as later deterioration from around year five to year ten of the disorder (83, 84). Much less is currently known about the processes involved in determining long-term outcomes in the later stages of the illness.

Future directions in key interventions will lie in the strengthening of relapse prevention and the management of treatment-refractory psychosis (88, 89). In addition, pharmacological interventions have been shown to be less effective for cognitive and functional outcomes (90, 91). In contrast, cognitive remediation, exercise interventions, and neurostimulation have been found to hold some promise in enhancing cognitive and functional outcomes (92, 93, 94). However, it will require additional adjustments to enable patients to overcome amotivational states in order to make full use of these interventions.

Informal family support is likely to be more prominent in Asian cultures. However, close attention needs to be paid to the quality of family relationships and individual family culture. Cultural factors likely influence attitudes towards mental illness and this should be borne in mind in order to harness effective carer involvement (95).

Themes in Hong Kong

Apart from focusing on the classic symptomatic presentations, the Psychosis Studies and Intervention (PSI) team at the University of Hong Kong has used cognitive dysfunction in psychosis as a connecting theme between the clinical disorder and its underlying brain system dysfunctions. The study of cognitive dysfunction in psychotic disorders has an interesting history over the last few decades. Broadly speaking, two main levels of cognitive involvement in psychosis have been identified, a generic component involving basic cognitive operations, and a more specific component of complex cognitive functions. The generic component is often used to relate to functional outcomes whereas the specific component can involve specific functions that may help to understand the generation of psychotic symptoms, as well as other traits in psychotic disorders. Among specific cognitive functions, our team has taken a special interest in language and related semantic functions as we appreciate that linguistic processes underlie much of the complex social representations that may be involved in the psychopathology of psychosis.

Much of the research studies in Hong Kong have been motivated by clinical questions. Our primary concern has been to improve the outcome of psychotic disorders. We have invested in some strategic directions such as early intervention

10 • *Psychosis and Schizophrenia in Hong Kong*

with particular emphasis on the reduction of DUP through public awareness campaigns. In addition, we have focused on improving symptomatic outcomes through early phase-specific intervention, relapse prevention, and improving cognition via physical exercise. We have also been conducting studies on youth mental health and suicide prevention. These studies will only be mentioned to the extent that they are relevant to the understanding and management of psychotic disorders. Some of our research collaborations have involved studies carried out in China. These will only be considered when they have arisen directly as a joint research project and when the studies are relevant to the themes of the research programme in Hong Kong.

We hope readers will find the overview of research undertaken in Hong Kong and the views presented in this book stimulating. Throughout the book, our emphasis has been on the subjective experience of our patients, and we have therefore discussed our research findings in this area in the first part. In addition, we wish to facilitate a greater understanding of the population diversity in the neurobiological and environmental processes involved in the emergence and course of psychosis. If our findings can inspire curiosity in developing future research paradigms to enhance knowledge of this devastating disorder and to support patients in leading meaningful and fulfilling lives, our research efforts will have served their purpose.

References

1. Geddes JR, Andreasen NC, Goodwin GM, eds. *New Oxford Textbook of Psychiatry*. 3rd ed. Oxford University Press; 2020: 526-527.
2. Harvey PD, Bosia M, Cavallaro R, et al. Cognitive dysfunction in schizophrenia: an expert group paper on the current state of the art. *Schizophr Res Cogn*. 2022;29:100249. Published Mar 22, 2022. doi:10.1016/j.scog.2022.100249
3. Hui CLM. Relapse in Schizophrenia. *Medical Bulletin*. 2011;16(5):8-9.
4. Morgan C, Lappin J, Heslin M, et al. Reappraising the long-term course and outcome of psychotic disorders: the AESOP-10 study [published correction appears in *Psychol Med*. Oct 2014;44(13):2727]. *Psychol Med*. 2014;44(13):2713-2726. doi:10.1017/S0033291714000282
5. Madeira N, Caldeira S, Bajouco M, et al. Social cognition, negative symptoms and psychosocial functioning in schizophrenia. *Int J Clin Neurosci Ment Health*. 2016;3:1.
6. de Winter L, Couwenbergh C, van Weeghel J, et al. Changes in social functioning over the course of psychotic disorders-A meta-analysis. *Schizophr Res*. 2022;239:55-82. doi:10.1016/j.schres.2021.11.010
7. Collins PY, Patel V, Joestl SS, et al. Grand challenges in global mental health. *Nature*. 2011;475(7354):27-30. Published Jul 6, 2011. doi:10.1038/475027a
8. Hegarty JD, Baldessarini RJ, Tohen M, Waternaux C, Oepen G. One hundred years of schizophrenia: a meta-analysis of the outcome literature. *Am J Psychiatry*. 1994;151(10):1409-1416. doi:10.1176/ajp.151.10.1409
9. Bora E, Yalincetin B, Akdede BB, Alptekin K. Duration of untreated psychosis and neurocognition in first-episode psychosis: a meta-analysis. *Schizophr Res*. 2018;193:3-10. doi:10.1016/j.schres.2017.06.021

Introduction • 11

10. Bertolote J, McGorry P. Early intervention and recovery for young people with early psychosis: consensus statement. *Br J Psychiatry Suppl.* 2005;48:s116-s119. doi:10.1192/bjp.187.48.s116

11. Hawton K, Sutton L, Haw C, Sinclair J, Deeks JJ. Schizophrenia and suicide: systematic review of risk factors. *Br J Psychiatry.* 2005;187:9-20. doi:10.1192/bjp.187.1.9

12. Barnes TR, Drake R, Paton C, et al. Evidence-based guidelines for the pharmacological treatment of schizophrenia: updated recommendations from the British Association for Psychopharmacology. *J Psychopharmacol.* 2020;34(1):3-78. doi:10.1177/0269881119889296

13. Rössler W. The stigma of mental disorders: a millennia-long history of social exclusion and prejudices. *EMBO Rep.* 2016;17(9):1250-1253. doi:10.15252/embr.201643041

14. Windell DL, Norman R, Lal S, Malla A. Subjective experiences of illness recovery in individuals treated for first-episode psychosis. *Soc Psychiatry Psychiatr Epidemiol.* 2015;50(7):1069-1077. doi:10.1007/s00127-014-1006-x

15. Andreasen NC, Carpenter WT Jr, Kane JM, Lasser RA, Marder SR, Weinberger DR. Remission in schizophrenia: proposed criteria and rationale for consensus. *Am J Psychiatry.* 2005;162(3):441-449. doi:10.1176/appi.ajp.162.3.441

16. Burkhard C, Cicek S, Barzilay R, Radhakrishnan R, Guloksuz S. Need for ethnic and population diversity in psychosis research. *Schizophr Bull.* 2021;47(4):889-895. doi:10.1093/schbul/sbab048

17. Kirkbride JB. Migration and psychosis: our smoking lung? *World Psychiatry.* 2017;16(2):119-120. doi:10.1002/wps.20406

18. Jongsma HE, Turner C, Kirkbride JB, Jones PB. International incidence of psychotic disorders, 2002-17: a systematic review and meta-analysis. *Lancet Public Health.* 2019;4(5):e229-e244. doi:10.1016/S2468-2667(19)30056-8

19. Lam M, Chen CY, Li Z, et al. Comparative genetic architectures of schizophrenia in East Asian and European populations. *Nat Genet.* 2019;51(12):1670-1678. doi:10.1038/s41588-019-0512-x

20. Yang Y, Wang L, Li L, et al. Genetic association and meta-analysis of a schizophrenia GWAS variant rs10489202 in East Asian populations. *Transl Psychiatry.* 2018;8(1):144. Published Aug 7, 2018. doi:10.1038/s41398-018-0211-x

21. Chang WC, Tang JYM, Hui CLM, et al. Gender differences in patients presenting with first-episode psychosis in Hong Kong: a three-year follow up study. *Aust N Z J.* 2011;45(3):199-205. doi:10.3109/00048674.2010.547841

22. Hui CL-M, Tang JY-M, Leung C-M, et al. A 3-year retrospective cohort study of predictors of relapse in first-episode psychosis in Hong Kong. *Aust N Z J Psychiatry.* 2013;47(8):746-753. doi:10.1177/0004867413487229

23. Hunt GE, Large MM, Cleary M, Lai HMX, Saunders JB. Prevalence of comorbid substance use in schizophrenia spectrum disorders in community and clinical settings, 1990-2017: systematic review and meta-analysis. *Drug Alcohol Depend.* 2018;191:234-258. doi:10.1016/j.drugalcdep.2018.07.011

24. Sartorius N, Jablensky A, Shapiro R. Cross-cultural differences in the short-term prognosis of schizophrenic psychoses. *Schizophrenia Bulletin.* 1978; 4(1), 102-113. doi:10.1093/schbul/4.1.102

25. Ng RMK, Mui J, Cheung HK, Leung, SP. Expressed emotion and relapse of schizophrenia in Hong Kong. *Hong Kong Journal of Psychiatry.* 2001; 11(1), 4-11. https://link.gale.com/apps/doc/A169678953/HRCA?u=anon~608761c2&sid=googleScholar&xid=305ee1f1

26. Tsang HWH, Tam PKC, Chan F, Cheung WM. Stigmatizing attitudes towards individuals with mental illness in Hong Kong: implications for their recovery. *J Community Psychology.* 2003;31:383-396. doi:10.1002/jcop.10055

27. Lee EH, Hui CL, Ching EY, et al. Public stigma in China associated with schizophrenia, depression, attenuated psychosis syndrome, and psychosis-like experiences. *Psychiatr Serv.* 2016;67(7):766-770. doi:10.1176/appi.ps.201500156

28. Chen ES, Chang WC, Hui CL, Chan SK, Lee EH, Chen EY. Self-stigma and affiliate stigma in first-episode psychosis patients and their caregivers. *Soc Psychiatry Psychiatr Epidemiol.* 2016;51(9):1225-1231. doi:10.1007/s00127-016-1221-8

29. Lee SH. Economic development and city-systems in East Asia, 1880-1980. *Asian Perspective.* 1987;11(1):120-151. http://www.jstor.org/stable/42705284

30. McGee TG. Managing the rural-urban transformation in East Asia in the 21st century. *Sustain Sci.* 2008;3:155-167. doi:10.1007/s11625-007-0040-y

31. Liu J, Ma H, He YL, et al. Mental health system in China: history, recent service reform and future challenges. *World Psychiatry.* 2011;10(3):210-216. doi:10.1002/j.2051-5545.2011.tb00059.x

32. Chong SA. Mental healthcare in Singapore. *Int Psychiatry.* 2007;4(4):88-90. Published Oct 1, 2007.

33. Kanata, T. Japanese mental health care in historical context: why did Japan become a country with so many psychiatric care beds? *Social Work.* 2016;52(4):471-489. doi:org/10.15270/52-2-526

34. Roh S, Lee SU, Soh M, et al. Mental health services and R&D in South Korea. *Int J Ment Health Syst.* 2016;10:45. Published Jun 2, 2016. doi:10.1186/s13033-016-0077-3

35. van Os J, Tamminga C. Deconstructing psychosis. *Schizophr Bull.* 2007;33(4):861-862. doi:10.1093/schbul/sbm066

36. Reininghaus U, Böhnke JR, Chavez-Baldini U, et al. Transdiagnostic dimensions of psychosis in the Bipolar-Schizophrenia Network on Intermediate Phenotypes (B-SNIP). *World Psychiatry.* 2019;18(1):67-76. doi:10.1002/wps.20607

37. Kovacs TZ, Hill RW, Watson S, Turkington D. Clusters, lines and webs-so does my patient have psychosis? Reflections on the use of psychiatric conceptual frameworks from a clinical vantage point. *Philos Ethics Humanit Med.* 2022;17(1):6. Published Feb 14, 2022. doi:10.1186/s13010-022-00118-0

38. Morgan AJ, Reavley NJ, Ross A, Too LS, Jorm AF. Interventions to reduce stigma towards people with severe mental illness: systematic review and meta-analysis. *J Psychiatr Res.* 2018;103:120-133. doi:10.1016/j.jpsychires.2018.05.017

39. Singh SP. Early intervention in psychosis. *Br J Psychiatry.* 2010;196(5):343-345. doi:10.1192/bjp.bp.109.075804

40. Ramachandraiah CT, Subramaniam N, Tancer M. The story of antipsychotics: past and present. *Indian J Psychiatry.* 2009;51(4):324-326. doi:10.4103/0019-5545.58304

41. Hamm JA, Leonhardt BL, Ridenour J, et al. Phenomenological and recovery models of the subjective experience of psychosis: discrepancies and implications for treatment. *Psychosis.* 2018;10(4):340-350. doi:10.1080/17522439.2018.1522540

42. Legge SE, Santoro ML, Periyasamy S, Okewole A, Arsalan A, Kowalec K. Genetic architecture of schizophrenia: a review of major advancements. *Psychol Med.* 2021;51(13):2168-2177. doi:10.1017/S0033291720005334

43. Mallet J, Le Strat Y, Dubertret C, Gorwood P. Polygenic risk scores shed light on the relationship between schizophrenia and cognitive functioning: review and meta-analysis. *J Clin Med.* 2020;9(2):341. Published Jan 25, 2020. doi:10.3390/jcm9020341

44. Reay WR, Cairns MJ. Pairwise common variant meta-analyses of schizophrenia with other psychiatric disorders reveals shared and distinct gene and gene-set associations. *Transl Psychiatry.* 2020;10(1):134. Published May 12, 2020. doi:10.1038/s41398-020-0817-7

45. Zamanpoor M. Schizophrenia in a genomic era: a review from the pathogenesis, genetic and environmental etiology to diagnosis and treatment insights. *Psychiatr Genet.* 2020;30(1):1-9. doi:10.1097/YPG.0000000000000245

46. Patel PK, Leathem LD, Currin DL, Karlsgodt KH. Adolescent neurodevelopment and vulnerability to psychosis. *Biol Psychiatry.* 2021;89(2):184-193. doi:10.1016/j.biopsych.2020.06.028

47. Zipursky RB, Reilly TJ, Murray RM. The myth of schizophrenia as a progressive brain disease. *Schizophr Bull.* 2013;39(6):1363-1372. doi:10.1093/schbul/sbs135

48. Kiburi SK, Molebatsi K, Ntlantsana V, Lynskey MT. Cannabis use in adolescence and risk of psychosis: are there factors that moderate this relationship? A systematic review and meta-analysis. *Subst Abus.* 2021;42(4):527-542. doi:10.1080/08897077.2021.1876200

49. Murrie B, Lappin J, Large M, Sara G. Transition of substance-induced, brief, and atypical psychoses to schizophrenia: a systematic review and meta-analysis. *Schizophr Bull.* 2020;46(3):505-516. doi:10.1093/schbul/sbz102

50. Castillejos MC, Martín-Pérez C, Moreno-Küstner B. A systematic review and meta-analysis of the incidence of psychotic disorders: the distribution of rates and the influence of gender, urbanicity, immigration and socio-economic level. *Psychol Med.* 2018;48(13):2101-2115. doi:10.1017/S0033291718000235

51. Henssler J, Brandt L, Müller M, et al. Migration and schizophrenia: meta-analysis and explanatory framework [published correction appears in *Eur Arch Psychiatry Clin Neurosci.* Sep 2020;270(6):787]. *Eur Arch Psychiatry Clin Neurosci.* 2020;270(3):325-335. doi:10.1007/s00406-019-01028-7

52. Croft J, Heron J, Teufel C, et al. Association of trauma type, age of exposure, and frequency in childhood and adolescence with psychotic experiences in early adulthood [published correction appears in *JAMA Psychiatry.* Jan 1, 2019;76(1):102] [published correction appears in *JAMA Psychiatry.* Feb 1, 2020;77(2):218]. *JAMA Psychiatry.* 2019;76(1):79-86. doi:10.1001/jamapsychiatry.2018.3155

53. Nettis MA, Pariante CM, Mondelli V. Early-life adversity, systemic inflammation and comorbid physical and psychiatric illnesses of adult life. *Curr Top Behav Neurosci.* 2020;44:207-225. doi:10.1007/7854_2019_89

54. Taylor SF, Grove TB, Ellingrod VL, Tso IF. The fragile brain: stress vulnerability, negative affect and GABAergic neurocircuits in psychosis. *Schizophr Bull.* 2019;45(6):1170-1183. doi:10.1093/schbul/sbz046

14 • *Psychosis and Schizophrenia in Hong Kong*

55. Braff DL, Freedman R, Schork NJ, Gottesman II. Deconstructing schizophrenia: an overview of the use of endophenotypes in order to understand a complex disorder. *Schizophr Bull.* 2007;33(1):21-32. doi:10.1093/schbul/sbl049

56. Greenwood TA, Shutes-David A, Tsuang DW. Endophenotypes in schizophrenia: digging deeper to identify genetic mechanisms. *J Psychiatr Brain Sci.* 2019;4(2):e190005. doi:10.20900/jpbs.20190005

57. Kircher T, Wöhr M, Nenadic I, et al. Neurobiology of the major psychoses: a translational perspective on brain structure and function-the FOR2107 consortium. *Eur Arch Psychiatry Clin Neurosci.* 2019;269(8):949-962. doi:10.1007/s00406-018-0943-x

58. Vanasse TJ, Fox PT, Fox PM, et al. Brain pathology recapitulates physiology: a network meta-analysis. *Commun Biol.* 2021;4(1):301. Published Mar 8, 2021. doi:10.1038/s42003-021-01832-9

59. Schiwy LC, Forlim CG, Fischer DJ, Kühn S, Becker M, Gallinat J. Aberrant functional connectivity within the salience network is related to cognitive deficits and disorganization in psychosis. *Schizophr Res.* 2022;246:103-111. doi:10.1016/j.schres.2022.06.008

60. Raabe FJ, Slapakova L, Rossner MJ, et al. Oligodendrocytes as a new therapeutic target in schizophrenia: from histopathological findings to neuron-oligodendrocyte interaction. *Cells.* 2019;8(12):1496. Published Nov 23, 2019. doi:10.3390/cells8121496

61. Knight S, McCutcheon R, Dwir D, et al. Hippocampal circuit dysfunction in psychosis [published correction appears in Transl Psychiatry. Sep 12, 2022;12(1):382]. *Transl Psychiatry.* 2022;12(1):344. Published Aug 25, 2022. doi:10.1038/s41398-022-02115-5

62. Kraguljac NV, Carle M, Frölich MA, et al. Mnemonic discrimination deficits in first-episode psychosis and a ketamine model suggest dentate gyrus pathology linked to NMDA receptor hypofunction. *Biol Psychiatry Cogn Neurosci Neuroimaging.* 2021;6(12):1185-1192. doi:10.1016/j.bpsc.2021.09.008

63. Norbom LB, Doan NT, Alnæs D, et al. Probing brain developmental patterns of myelination and associations with psychopathology in youths using gray/white matter contrast. *Biol Psychiatry.* 2019;85(5):389-398. doi:10.1016/j.biopsych.2018.09.027

64. Smucny J, Dienel SJ, Lewis DA, Carter CS. Mechanisms underlying dorsolateral prefrontal cortex contributions to cognitive dysfunction in schizophrenia. *Neuropsychopharmacology.* 2022;47(1):292-308. doi:10.1038/s41386-021-01089-0

65. Krajcovic B, Fajnerova I, Horacek J, et al. Neural and neuronal discoordination in schizophrenia: from ensembles through networks to symptoms. *Acta Physiol (Oxf).* 2019;226(4):e13282. doi:10.1111/apha.13282

66. Exposito-Alonso D, Rico B. Mechanisms underlying circuit dysfunction in neurodevelopmental disorders. *Annu Rev Genet.* 2022;56:391-422. doi:10.1146/annurev-genet-072820-023642

67. Calvo A, Roddy DW, Coughlan H, et al. Reduced hippocampal volume in adolescents with psychotic experiences: a longitudinal population-based study. *PLoS One.* 2020;15(6):e0233670. Published Jun 3, 2020. doi:10.1371/journal.pone.0233670

68. Ho NF, Lee BJH, Tng JXJ, et al. Corticolimbic brain anomalies are associated with cognitive subtypes in psychosis: a longitudinal study. *Eur Psychiatry.* 2020;63(1):e40. Published Apr 27, 2020. doi:10.1192/j.eurpsy.2020.36

69. Stahl SM. Beyond the dopamine hypothesis of schizophrenia to three neural networks of psychosis: dopamine, serotonin, and glutamate. *CNS Spectr.* 2018;23(3):187-191. doi:10.1017/S1092852918001013

70. Howes OD, Shatalina E. Integrating the neurodevelopmental and dopamine hypotheses of schizophrenia and the role of cortical excitation-inhibition balance. *Biol Psychiatry.* 2022;92(6):501-513. doi:10.1016/j.biopsych.2022.06.017

71. Menon V, Palaniyappan L, Supekar K. Integrative brain network and salience models of psychopathology and cognitive dysfunction in schizophrenia [published online ahead of print, Oct 4, 2022]. *Biol Psychiatry.* 2022;S0006-3223(22)01637-7. doi:10.1016/j.biopsych.2022.09.029

72. Valt C, Quarto T, Tavella A, et al. Reduced magnetic mismatch negativity: a shared deficit in psychosis and related risk [published online ahead of print, Nov 2, 2022]. *Psychol Med.* 2022;1-9. doi:10.1017/S003329172200321X

73. Park SH, Kim T, Ha M, et al. Intrinsic cerebellar functional connectivity of social cognition and theory of mind in first-episode psychosis patients. *NPJ Schizophr.* 2021;7(1):59. Published Dec 3, 2021. doi:10.1038/s41537-021-00193-w

74. Picó-Pérez M, Vieira R, Fernández-Rodríguez M, De Barros MAP, Radua J, Morgado P. Multimodal meta-analysis of structural gray matter, neurocognitive and social cognitive fMRI findings in schizophrenia patients. *Psychol Med.* 2022;52(4):614-624. doi:10.1017/S0033291721005523

75. Sheffield JM, Karcher NR, Barch DM. Cognitive deficits in psychotic disorders: a lifespan perspective. *Neuropsychol Rev.* 2018;28(4):509-533. doi:10.1007/s11065-018-9388-2

76. Fusar-Poli P, Bonoldi I, Yung AR, et al. Predicting psychosis: meta-analysis of transition outcomes in individuals at high clinical risk. *Arch Gen Psychiatry.* 2012;69(3):220-229. doi:10.1001/archgenpsychiatry.2011.1472

77. Lam MM, Hung SF, Chen EY. Transition to psychosis: 6-month follow-up of a Chinese high-risk group in Hong Kong. *Aust N Z J Psychiatry.* 2006;40(5):414-420. doi:10.1080/j.1440-1614.2006.01817.x

78. Barnow S, Arens EA, Sieswerda S, Dinu-Biringer R, Spitzer C, Lang S. Borderline personality disorder and psychosis: a review. *Curr Psychiatry Rep.* 2010;12(3):186-195. doi:10.1007/s11920-010-0107-9

79. Dickson H, Hedges EP, Ma SY, et al. Academic achievement and schizophrenia: a systematic meta-analysis. *Psychol Med.* 2020;50(12):1949-1965. doi:10.1017/S0033291720002354

80. Catalan A, Salazar de Pablo G, Aymerich C, et al. Neurocognitive functioning in individuals at clinical high risk for psychosis: a systematic review and meta-analysis [published online ahead of print, Jun 16, 2021]. *JAMA Psychiatry.* 2021;78(8):859-867. doi:10.1001/jamapsychiatry.2021.1290

81. Marshall M, Lewis S, Lockwood A, Drake R, Jones P, Croudace T. Association between duration of untreated psychosis and outcome in cohorts of first-episode patients: a systematic review. *Arch Gen Psychiatry.* 2005;62(9):975-983. doi:10.1001/archpsyc.62.9.975

82. Boonstra N, Klaassen R, Sytema S, et al. Duration of untreated psychosis and negative symptoms – a systematic review and meta-analysis of individual patient data. *Schizophr Res.* 2012;142(1-3):12-19. doi:10.1016/j.schres.2012.08.017

83. Chan SKW, Hui CLM, Chang WC, Lee EHM, Chen EYH. Ten-year follow up of patients with first-episode schizophrenia spectrum disorder from an early intervention service: predictors of clinical remission and functional recovery. *Schizophr Res*. 2019;204:65-71. doi:10.1016/j.schres.2018.08.022

84. Chan SKW, Chan HYV, Devlin J, et al. A systematic review of long-term outcomes of patients with psychosis who received early intervention services. *Int Rev Psychiatry*. 2019;31(5-6):425-440. doi:10.1080/09540261.2019.1643704

85. Chan SKW, Pang HH, Yan KK, et al. Ten-year employment patterns of patients with first-episode schizophrenia-spectrum disorders: comparison of early intervention and standard care services. *Br J Psychiatry*. 2020;217(3):491-497. doi:10.1192/bjp.2019.161

86. Birchwood M, Todd P, Jackson C. Early intervention in psychosis. The critical period hypothesis. *Br J Psychiatry Suppl*. 1998;172(33):53-59.

87. Chan SKW, Chan SWY, Pang HH, et al. Association of an early intervention service for psychosis with suicide rate among patients with first-episode schizophrenia-spectrum disorders. *JAMA Psychiatry*. 2018;75(5):458-464. doi:10.1001/jamapsychiatry.2018.0185

88. Alvarez-Jiménez M, Parker AG, Hetrick SE, McGorry PD, Gleeson JF. Preventing the second episode: a systematic review and meta-analysis of psychosocial and pharmacological trials in first-episode psychosis. *Schizophr Bull*. 2011;37(3):619-630. doi:10.1093/schbul/sbp129

89. Chen EY, Hui CL, Dunn EL, et al. A prospective 3-year longitudinal study of cognitive predictors of relapse in first-episode schizophrenic patients. *Schizophr Res*. 2005;77(1):99-104. doi:10.1016/j.schres.2005.02.020

90. Baldez DP, Biazus TB, Rabelo-da-Ponte FD, et al. The effect of antipsychotics on the cognitive performance of individuals with psychotic disorders: network meta-analyses of randomized controlled trials. *Neurosci Biobehav Rev*. 2021;126:265-275. doi:10.1016/j.neubiorev.2021.03.028

91. Lutgens D, Gariepy G, Malla A. Psychological and psychosocial interventions for negative symptoms in psychosis: systematic review and meta-analysis. *Br J Psychiatry*. 2017;210(5):324-332. doi:10.1192/bjp.bp.116.197103

92. Wykes T, Huddy V, Cellard C, McGurk SR, Czobor P. A meta-analysis of cognitive remediation for schizophrenia: methodology and effect sizes. *Am J Psychiatry*. 2011;168(5):472-485. doi:10.1176/appi.ajp.2010.10060855

93. Lin J, Chan SK, Lee EH, et al. Aerobic exercise and yoga improve neurocognitive function in women with early psychosis. *NPJ Schizophr*. 2015;1(0):15047. Published Dec 2, 2015. doi:10.1038/npjschz.2015.47

94. Jiang Y, Guo Z, Xing G, et al. Effects of high-frequency transcranial magnetic stimulation for cognitive deficit in schizophrenia: a meta-analysis. *Front Psychiatry*. 2019;10:135. Published Mar 29, 2019. doi:10.3389/fpsyt.2019.00135

95. Chan KW, Wong MH, Hui CL, Lee EH, Chang WC, Chen EY. Perceived risk of relapse and role of medication: comparison between patients with psychosis and their caregivers. *Soc Psychiatry Psychiatr Epidemiol*. 2015;50(2):307-315. doi:10.1007/s00127-014-0930-0

PART I

THE IMPACT OF PSYCHOSIS ON THE LIVES OF PATIENTS

1

The Experience of Psychosis as One of the Most Devastating Illnesses

The Subjective Illness Perspective in Psychotic Disorders

Having a continuous and coherent subjective experience in daily life is something that most people take for granted. When we wake up in the morning, we are aware that we are starting another day with a sense of the reality of what went on the previous day. It does not require effort to be in touch with our surroundings and form an internal representation of our environment. Psychosis affects the brain systems that are responsible for allowing us to have a continuous sense of experiencing ourselves and our environment. The disorders most frequently begin in late adolescence and early adulthood. This is an important developmental stage during which identity is formed and consolidated. Restoring the coherence of the sense of self embedded in their surroundings is probably the most important treatment goal. Supporting patients during the initial treatment phase as well as the long-term management of their condition is rarely a straightforward process.

Systematic efforts have been made to gain a better understanding of the subjective experience in psychosis to tailor treatments and broader psychosocial support to the individual needs of patients (1, 2, 3). Apart from the familiar psychopathology of hallucinations and delusions, some patients have difficulties processing familiar words, people, objects, and experiences. Memory deficits, disturbances in language production and comprehension, mistaking identities, and a distorted sense of time have also been reported (1).

Negative symptoms impact motivation and functioning. Loss of concentration, motivation, withdrawal, and 'feeling but not feeling' are symptoms patients have identified. Subjects have also described factors that they believed contributed to the onset of their symptoms, namely the impact of traumatic events, the perceived impact of their social network, as well as recreational and prescribed drug use (4).

How someone who is recovering from a psychotic episode understands the nature of their illness is likely to affect their appraisal of treatment, recovery, and relapse prevention (5, 6). In addition, premorbid personality, sociocultural factors, prior knowledge of mental disorders and the information provided by psychoeducation also impact the subjective illness experience (7, 8, 9, 10, 11).

More recently, research has focused on understanding issues affecting insight and treatment adherence in the hope of tailoring psychoeducation more effectively (12, 13). Since the development of standardised rating instruments measuring insight, insight repairment has been studied and considered as one of the itemised factors. Despite its clinical utility, the item is, in fact, far more complex than other symptoms ascertained by rating scales. In Jaspers' *General Psychopathology*, insight repairment was not represented as a single 'symptom' but accommodated in a broader concept of 'self-knowledge' (14). When examining the impact of psychotic disorders on insight, a more holistic framework should be employed to gain a richer understanding of the issues faced by patients. In addition to a rather narrow definition of insight and its impairment, these approaches also tended to utilise clinician-centred perspectives of psychotic symptoms as an illness rather than taking into account more complex illness narratives. To achieve a more nuanced approach several rating tools were developed in the 1990s to enhance knowledge of patients' awareness of symptoms, attribution of illness, and attitudes towards treatment (15, 16, 17, 18, 19).

Despite advances in the understanding of patients' views about their illness and its treatment, crucial aspects of the therapeutic relationship between patient, carer, and clinician remain under-researched. Sendt et al. (2015) conducted a systematic review of factors influencing adherence to antipsychotic medication based on thirteen observational studies and found that a positive attitude to medication and illness insight were most consistently associated with better adherence (20). Issues affecting treatment adherence will be further explored in Chapter 9 with a particular focus on psychopharmacological interventions. Our review of the experience of carers revealed the emotional challenges, uncertainty, and stigma-related burden associated with looking after a relative with psychosis and highlighted the need to offer high-quality caregiver interventions to support recovery (21).

Other important aspects to consider when formulating individualised treatment plans are patients' hopes for recovery and how this should be achieved as well as the potential impact of relapse and how this should best be managed. Windell et al. (2015) carried out semi-structured interviews with 30 individuals in early recovery following a first episode of psychosis. Participants spoke about their recovery from psychotic symptoms and having to reconcile the meaning of their illness experience, as well as regaining control over their illness, and having to negotiate and accept treatment. They argued for the importance of assisting individuals with the

The Subjective Experience of Psychosis in Hong Kong

In Hong Kong, research has focused on the subjective experience of illness onset, help-seeking, and perceived recovery.

Recovery is thought to be a multidimensional concept. Clinically, recovery is defined as symptomatic improvement and adequate functioning in the community, socially and vocationally. Although clinicians and patients broadly agree that symptom and functional recovery are essential features of being able to lead a meaningful life, it appears that certain health beliefs and aspects of functioning important to patients are mostly neglected. This disregard has the potential to significantly impact our patients' ability to maintain improvements following the initial treatment phase.

Culture and language are important reflections of these complex processes. In Chinese, it is hard to find a term that closely resembles the meaning of the English term 'recovery'. The term 'recovery' in English has the meaning of reclaiming what is lost. There are two senses of the word. One is reclaiming something we once had before the disorder. The other sense is the patient is re-establishing control and functioning as much as he can despite the overall impact of the disorder. These two aspects of recovery are represented by different words in Chinese. The Chinese term for recovery *fuyuan* (復元) is closer to the meaning of rehabilitation, i.e., making progress in adapting and coping with the impact of a disorder. In the Cantonese vocabulary, there is another term for 'getting well', i.e., regaining the premorbid state *houfaan* (好番).

To aid the development of a recovery-centred service model that is based on effective treatment and encompasses a culturally sensitive understanding of the concept of 'recovery' (復元; *fuyuan; to resume, renew, recover, regain, restore, reinstate, and rehabilitate*), several Chinese language mental health recovery measures that were based on the United States Compendium of Outcome Measures were cross-validated in Hong Kong (23, 24, 25). In addition, we developed a self-administered instrument to systematically explore patients' experience of recovery after the first episode of psychosis, the Psychosis Recovery Inventory (PRI, 26). The rating scale was designed to measure the experience of illness, attitudes toward treatment, and the complex issues surrounding recovery and risk of relapse. Prior to the development of the questionnaire, we undertook a series of qualitative interviews with recovering first-episode psychosis patients. Relevant themes were extracted, and 42 items were initially generated using clear and simple language. This was refined and led to the final validated Chinese version comprising 25 core items, with each item having a declarative statement to which a six-point Likert scale is applied that ranges from 1 ('strongly disagree') to 6 ('strongly agree'). Two quantitative items were also included measuring the extent of perceived recovery and perceived risk of relapse. Two follow-up questions address misattributions for abnormal experiences and the perceived nature of non-recovery. The PRI was found to have good test-retest reliability and validity.

It appears that patients vary in their conceptualisation of symptoms and recovery during different stages of their illness (27, 28, 29). Individuals, following their first episode of psychosis, reported feelings of loss and fear of an uncertain future, particularly in relation to the possibility of experiencing a relapse. They were very focused on regaining their previous functional abilities. Compared to chronic patients, early psychosis patients described a very narrow view of recovery, namely one in which they did not require psychiatric support or medication. Psychosis patients were also wary about disclosing their mental illness for fear of discrimination. However, many patients also thought of psychosis as having allowed personal growth and development (27, 28). Those with a chronic illness seemed to be more accepting of the need for medication as well as professional and family support for optimal functioning (29).

The Subjective Perception of Recovery

According to the PRI, on a 0–100 percentage scale, subjective ratings of full recovery (100%) have been found in only around 10% of first-episode psychosis cases, with half of the surveyed participants regarding themselves to have made a good recovery of 75% or more. Only around 20% considered themselves as having made a limited recovery of less than 50% (26, 30). Those who did not perceive themselves to have fully recovered rated the following reasons for their non-recovery: 'cognitive dysfunction', 'social functioning impairment', 'occupational functioning impairment', and 'need to continue with medication' (26). It appears that subjectively perceived recovery is not associated with positive, negative, and depressive symptoms or measurement-based criteria of recovery (31). We observed that patients who reported greater subjective recovery had fewer perseverative errors in the Modified Wisconsin Card Sorting Test, although the variance explained by this correlation was small. These data support the view that patients likely consider a much broader range of factors important to their perceived recovery than symptomatic remission and adequate psychosocial functioning (31).

One such factor appears to be patients' beliefs about ongoing treatment. It seems that patients considered themselves to have recovered only once they no longer required medication (26). Psychopharmacological treatment for psychotic disorders consists of antipsychotic medication in the acute and maintenance phase of the illness and patients are usually advised to continue medication for at least one year following the resolution of all symptoms. Psychoeducation on the nature of psychosis as a potentially chronic condition, its treatment, and relapse prevention are part of a standard package of care and it may therefore be surprising that patients appear to have adopted a different understanding of recovery. Patients might be concerned about having to continue medication despite feeling well, whether this may be due to troublesome side effects such as drowsiness, metabolic effects, extrapyramidal symptoms, or the need for monitoring of side effects as well as regular psychiatric and nursing reviews. In further qualitative interviews, we asked patients, who rated higher on the need to take medication as an indication of not having yet recovered, whether they would still regard taking medication as a problem if the medication had no side effects. Their replies indicated that even if medication had no side effects, patients would still consider that they had not completely recovered, simply because they still had to take medication (26). For patients, complete recovery meant neither having to take medication nor receiving other treatments, even if they were offered as a preventative measure. In other words, the bare fact of having to take medication prevented patients from regarding themselves as fully recovered.

Patients may also feel that they have had to make numerous adjustments to their work environment, daily routines, and social life to cope with side effects of medication such as tiredness. It is well known that a significant proportion of psychosis patients lose employment or drop out of education. This might be experienced as a significant loss of healthy functioning despite having recovered from psychotic symptoms per se. Indeed, we showed in our ten-year follow-up study that patients with a diagnosis of schizophrenia and non-affective psychosis cited loss of working ability as a major concern. Patients also reported reduced self-confidence, particularly in social situations as a result of weight gain (32).

The Subjective Experience of Cognitive Abilities

We also observed that subjective awareness of changes in cognitive ability is vital to patients. Some individuals recognise even subtle cognitive abnormalities during the early course of their illness. Cognitive dysfunction is now considered a core feature of psychotic disorders and is often present in first-episode psychosis (FEP) (33, 34, 35). We will consider cognitive impairments in psychotic disorders more fully in Chapter 14 and will concentrate here on subjective aspects of cognitive dysfunction.

Conventional clinical evaluations do not routinely include detailed cognitive assessments. We observed in our longitudinal studies that when the psychotic episode is successfully treated, psychotic symptoms subside but subtle cognitive impairments often remain. It appears that the recovery trajectory of cognitive functions is substantially different from that of psychotic symptoms. Some cognitive impairments are already present twelve to eighteen months prior to onset, and a further decline is seen at the time when psychotic symptoms emerge (36, 37, 38).

Several cognitive domains gradually improve following the remission of psychotic symptoms, while others remain significantly diminished.

When clinical assessments focus on symptom remission, there is thus often a failure to appreciate the residual cognitive difficulties that patients may be experiencing as psychotic symptoms recede. This can lead to subjective perceptions of not having fully recovered, whereas clinicians believe that their patients have regained their symptom-free state. The discrepancy may affect the therapeutic relationship and patients may lose confidence in their treating clinician. Sometimes, patients may attribute lingering cognitive impairments to side effects of antipsychotic medication and decide to stop treatment without discussing this with their psychiatrist.

Although some studies have examined the subjective experience of cognitive functioning in early psychosis, there has been far less data on how patients perceive their cognitive abilities in real-life situations (39, 40). Given the paucity of data on the subject, Chang et al. (2015) developed the Subjective Cognitive Impairment Scale to facilitate research into associations between measures of subjective and objective cognitive measures. The scale was proven to have adequate psychometric properties (41). What has been shown so far is that subjective cognitive impairment (SCI) does not appear to be strongly correlated with objective cognitive test performance and that depression and anxiety seem to be correlated with SCI (39, 41).

In clinical practice, perceived successful treatment is largely based on objective measures of recovery. Although side effects are regularly monitored, the complex interplay between often subtle residual positive and negative symptoms, mood disturbance, cognitive impairment, medication effects, and psychosocial functioning can be difficult to manage in a low-resource, high-volume outpatient clinic. Failure to address these points has potential consequences for adherence to treatment.

Perception of Relapse Risk

In Hong Kong, early psychosis patients are routinely provided with psychoeducational information on their illness including the potential risk of relapse. Relapse following FEP in the first three years is estimated to be around 50%, and the five-year relapse rate was found to be as high as 82% (42, 43). These figures are shared with patients in such a way that the risk of relapse can be easily comprehended and can open up further conversations on how to reduce the chances of a further psychotic episode. It is therefore somewhat surprising that more than three-quarters of patients who were asked about their own risk of relapse considered it to be 50% or less, just over half regarded their risk of relapse as 30% or less, and 20% did not think they would relapse at all (26). Subjects who perceived their risk of relapse to be less than 30% were found to have significantly fewer cognitive problems, exercised less effort in understanding their illness, perceived less impact of their illness, and reported more control over relapse and recovery. A similar profile was obtained

The Experience of Psychosis as One of the Most Devastating Illnesses • 25

for those who perceived their risk of relapse to be less than 50% (26). The findings might be explained by limited insight but 'optimism bias' may have also played a role.

Optimism bias is a cognitive bias characterised by a belief that one, as compared to others, is less likely to experience a negative event. Four factors are proposed to be involved in this: one's desired end state, one's cognitive mechanisms, the information one has about oneself versus others, and overall mood (44). In our study, patients who considered themselves to be at low risk of relapse also reported fewer cognitive problems and less perceived impact of their illness (26). This may reflect the cognitive mechanism of representative heuristics, whereby patients compare themselves to other patients who are more cognitively and functionally impaired, thereby underestimating their own risk of relapse. The belief of being able to exercise more control is likely to be related to the wishes or goals a patient may have or wants to achieve. The patients in the study had been ill for an average of 19 months and some had not experienced a relapse. It has been shown that the perception of personal control is influenced by prior experience of a negative event. It might well be that chronic patients develop a more realistic view of their prognosis over time (45, 46).

Our data, however, suggests that having had a previous relapse was not found to have an impact on the perception of the chance of future relapse (47). Perhaps even more surprisingly, around 20% of patients did not believe that they would relapse at all. Patients who indicated that there was no possibility of a relapse explained that relapse involved a resurgence of psychotic symptoms. In their view, psychotic symptoms were subjective experiences under their direct control, therefore ruling out further relapses. They had forgotten that during their previous psychotic episode, this had not been the case. This may indicate either there is difficulty in accessing the memory of their psychotic experiences, or that patients deliberately adopt this position in order to cope. This position corresponds to that of a 'sealing over' recovery style (48). One may understand this as a lack of insight or a denial of reality. Those patients who had made less effort to understand their illness could be understood as denying important aspects of it. This, of course, can be a protective mechanism to allow patients to process having been diagnosed with a severe and enduring mental disorder and adjust to having to live with a chronic illness. However, it might also lead to non-adherence and disengagement from services.

Insight and denial of illness are likely to play a significant role in patients' perception of relapse. It might also be that patients have difficulties accessing the memory of their symptoms due to the altered state of mind during the acute psychotic phase of their illness. It has been shown in several studies that memory and attention are dependent on emotional context (49, 50, 51). Velakoulis et al. (2006) reported that patients with first-episode schizophrenia showed left hippocampal volume reduction and those with chronic schizophrenia had reduced bilateral hippocampal volume (52). Furthermore, in another study, patients with chronic schizophrenia had significantly decreased left anterior and posterior hippocampal volumes. These volume reductions were associated with episodic and semantic autobiographical memory deficits (53).

Deficits in meta-memory have also been demonstrated in patients suffering from psychosis. Meta-memory includes the recognition of one's memory competency, adapting one's beliefs about one's memory capacities, as well as employing adequate strategies to recognise and correct false memories (54, 55). Patients with FEP and chronic schizophrenia are overconfident in errors while at the same time being under-confident in responses that are, in fact, correct. The inflation of inaccurate but confidently held memories is thought to be a vulnerability factor for the development of delusions. It may also play a role in patients' beliefs of being able to control their symptoms and accurately predict future relapse (56).

Another important aspect to consider is how patients understand the concepts of risk and probability of an event occurring. It has been shown repeatedly that the general public does not appreciate the risks and benefits of medical interventions in a strictly logical numerical manner. It has also been argued that low numeracy may increase susceptibility to the effects of mood or how information is presented and to biases in judgement and decision-making (57). We have made attempts to capture patients' understanding of numerical concepts and their effect on medical decision-making. However, these efforts have been hampered by a high degree of complexity of how numerical terms can best reflect and be mapped onto patients' experiences of their illness. Advances in the understanding of mathematical cognition have been made in recent years. It might be interesting to revisit this area of research to understand patients' perceptions of risk and risk predictors in more tangible ways (57, 58, 59).

Caregiver's Perspective on Relapse

Another important area of study has been the views of family and caregivers on issues of recovery, relapse, and treatment of psychosis. This is of particular importance in Hong Kong, where more than 50% of people with schizophrenia live with or depend on the care and assistance of their families (60). We interviewed 80 patients and 80 caregivers who had been attending the early psychosis service on perceived relapse and the role of medication (47). Like in our previous findings, the majority of patients thought they had recovered 80% or more (31, 47). Caregivers rated recovery similarly, however only around 60% of patient–caregiver pairs agreed on the extent of recovery. More patients than caregivers thought medication could be stopped within a year. However, more caregivers thought the condition would get worse after discontinuing medication. There were significantly more caregivers than patients who endorsed the positive effects of medication.

Almost half of the patients were considered to be non-adherent to medication. Unsurprisingly, those who took medication regularly were more likely to think that stopping medication could lead to a relapse. Caregivers of patients who had good adherence were also more likely to believe that stopping medication would worsen the condition. However, interestingly, medication adherence was not directly related to the perceived risk of relapse in patients or their caregivers. Patients were also much more optimistic about their chances of relapse with 60% believing that their risk of relapse was 20% or less, compared to around 28% of caregivers. Significantly more caregivers than patients thought stopping medication, not engaging in meaningful activities, and being stressed could lead to a relapse of the illness (47). Caregivers who perceived their relatives to be at higher perceived relapse risk were more likely to have greater knowledge of psychosis and were caring for patients with more positive symptoms.

As we have shown, fewer caregivers underestimated the risk of and potential contributing factors for relapse, and caregivers' perception of the probability of relapse was not associated with a previous history of relapse (47). One might postulate that similar to patients, caregivers may lack knowledge of the nature of psychosis and have a limited understanding of numerical concepts of risk. However, denial and difficulties in accepting the reality of having to care for a family member with a severe enduring mental illness may also play a role. Differing views on the likelihood of relapse and the role of medication may lead to family conflict and high-expressed emotions, a known risk factor for relapse in psychosis. Paying attention to the views and opinions of caregivers and working collaboratively with both patients and their families is likely to improve understanding of the illness, its treatment, and medication adherence.

Reflections: The Subjective Experience of Psychosis and Its Clinical Implications

The impact of psychosis on subjective experience is not only a core manifestation but indeed a defining feature of the disorder and can directly affect treatment and outcome. Phenomenological approaches detailing subjective experiences have a long tradition and have contributed to descriptive psychopathology, which has provided the foundation of modern diagnostic systems and contemporary classifications. The experiential aspect of the disorder, however, has received less than its fair share of attention over the last three or four decades. As progress is being made in the biological understanding of the disorder, subjective experiences risk being viewed merely as epiphenomena and dismissed as irrelevant by-products of objectively measurable core brain abnormalities. This perspective is potentially misleading as it may lead to a premature closure towards subjective experiences as being informative for the understanding of the causes and outcomes of the disorder.

Psychotic disorders profoundly affect one's ability to judge the validity of one's own experiences in such a way that patients are often not aware that their perceptions and beliefs are, in fact, psychotic symptoms. Having to come to terms with the possibility that what one experiences as real over a period of time could be the result of a psychotic disorder is one of the most disorienting aspects of the condition.

When we view psychosis from the perspective of patients, it is crucial to acknowledge personal accounts of lived experience. Subjective illness narratives are not only important in understanding patients' attitudes towards the causes and treatment of their illness, but they may actually also reflect the structure of how the experience of illness has been processed in memory. This may have an important impact on illness attitudes. In this regard, it is an extremely important aspect of the illness that has been relatively under-studied.

When patients emerge from a psychotic episode, they need to make sense of their memories during the time of their illness. Psychotic symptoms will have been experienced alongside other 'real' events during an acute episode. A revision of what has been consolidated in memory will be required as the patient slowly recovers and discovers that what had been experienced as real would retrospectively be reconsidered as the result of an illness. This is likely to be disorienting to patients and they will require professional support to come to terms with the fact that their sense of reality has been clouded by their symptoms.

Given the broad range of subjective experiences in psychosis and research in this area, it might feel rather overwhelming for professionals to consider how best to translate research findings into daily clinical practice. Perhaps the most important aspect to consider is that patients' and carers' understanding and experiences of psychotic illness will likely differ from that of clinicians. It is important to appreciate that some of the clinicians' ideas about patients' perspectives have failed to recognise the fact that patients, like other human beings, do not think in a purely rational manner, and that heuristics and biases are parts of normal human cognition. As has been shown, patients' beliefs on recovery include being able to fully function cognitively, socially, and occupationally as well as not having to take medication. A careful and sensitive inquiry into illness beliefs, subjective understanding of the acute illness phase and recovery, prediction of relapse, as well as assessment of subjective residual symptoms and impairment will likely be beneficial. Considering that a significant proportion of patients will have at least some cognitive difficulties that will likely persist beyond the resolution of positive symptoms, it might be helpful to review psychoeducational material to better suit patients' needs. An assessment of cognitive abilities is also likely to be beneficial. However, resources may limit the availability of extensive cognitive testing. Nonetheless, clinicians should remember that although patients may not show obvious signs of cognitive impairment, they might still experience a subjective sense of cognitive dysfunction and may attribute this to their antipsychotic medication. Another important aspect to consider is the skilful use of language to manage patients' beliefs around their recovery and relapse and to support them in developing a meaningful and constructive illness narrative.

References

1. Marshall M, Lewis S, Lockwood A, Drake R, Jones P, Croudace T. Association between duration of untreated psychosis and outcome in cohorts of first-episode patients: a systematic review. *Arch Gen Psychiatry*. 2005;62(9):975-983. doi:10.1001/archpsyc.62.9.975

2. Wadeson H, Carpenter WT Jr. Subjective experience of schizophrenia. *Schizophr Bull*. 1976;2(2):302-316. doi:10.1093/schbul/2.2.302

3. Cutting J, Dunne F. Subjective experience of schizophrenia. *Schizophr Bull*. 1989;15(2):217-231. doi:10.1093/schbul/15.2.217

4. Butcher I, Berry K, Haddock G. Understanding individuals' subjective experiences of negative symptoms of schizophrenia: a qualitative study. *Br J Clin Psychol*. 2020;59(3):319-334. doi:10.1111/bjc.12248

5. Andresen R, Oades L, Caputi P. The experience of recovery from schizophrenia: towards an empirically validated stage model. *Aust N Z J Psychiatry*. 2003;37(5):586-594. doi:10.1046/j.1440-1614.2003.01234.x

6. Sells DJ, Stayner DA, Davidson L. Recovering the self in schizophrenia: an integrative review of qualitative studies. *Psychiatr Q*. 2004;75(1):87-97. doi:10.1023/b:psaq.0000007563.17236.97

7. Strauss JS. The person with schizophrenia as a person. II: approaches to the subjective and complex. *Br J Psychiatry Suppl*. 1994;(23):103-107.

8. White R, Bebbington P, Pearson J, Johnson S, Ellis D. The social context of insight in schizophrenia. *Soc Psychiatry Psychiatr Epidemiol*. 2000;35(11):500-507. doi:10.1007/s001270050271

9. Davidson L, Strauss JS. Beyond the biopsychosocial model: integrating disorder, health, and recovery. *Psychiatry*. 1995;58(1):44-55. doi:10.1080/00332747.1995.11024710

10. Thompson KN, McGorry PD, Harrigan SM. Recovery style and outcome in first-episode psychosis. *Schizophr Res*. 2003;62(1-2):31-36. doi:10.1016/s0920-9964(02)00428-0

11. Tait L, Birchwood M, Trower P. Predicting engagement with services for psychosis: insight, symptoms and recovery style. *Br J Psychiatry*. 2003;182:123-128. doi:10.1192/bjp.182.2.123

12. McEvoy JP, Apperson LJ, Appelbaum PS, et al. Insight in schizophrenia: its relationship to acute psychopathology. *J Nerv Ment Dis*. 1989;177(1):43-47. doi:10.1097/00005053-198901000-00007

13. David AS. Insight and psychosis. *Br J Psychiatry*. 1990;156:798-808. doi:10.1192/bjp.156.6.798

14. Jaspers K. *General Psychopathology*. 7th ed. Manchester University Press; 1946/1963.

15. Marková IS, Berrios GE. The assessment of insight in clinical psychiatry: a new scale. *Acta Psychiatr Scand.* 1992;86(2):159-164. doi:10.1111/j.1600-0447.1992.tb03245.x

16. Amador XF, Flaum M, Andreasen NC, et al. Awareness of illness in schizophrenia and schizoaffective and mood disorders. *Arch Gen Psychiatry.* 1994;51(10):826-836. doi:10.1001/archpsyc.1994.03950100074007

17. Jaeger J, Bitter I, Czobor P, Volavka J. The measurement of subjective experience in schizophrenia: the Subjective Deficit Syndrome Scale. *Compr Psychiatry.* 1990;31(3):216-226. doi:10.1016/0010-440x(90)90005-d

18. Haddock G, Wood L, Watts R, Dunn G, Morrison AP, Price J. The Subjective Experiences of Psychosis Scale (SEPS): psychometric evaluation of a scale to assess outcome in psychosis. *Schizophr Res.* 2011;133(1-3):244-249. doi:10.1016/j.schres.2011.09.023

19. Hogan TP, Awad AG, Eastwood R. A self-report scale predictive of drug compliance in schizophrenics: reliability and discriminative validity. *Psychol Med.* 1983;13(1):177-183. doi:10.1017/s0033291700050182

20. Sendt KV, Tracy DK, Bhattacharyya S. A systematic review of factors influencing adherence to antipsychotic medication in schizophrenia-spectrum disorders. *Psychiatry Res.* 2015;225(1-2):14-30. doi:10.1016/j.psychres.2014.11.002

21. Mui EYW, Chan SKW, Chan PY, et al. Systematic review (meta-aggregation) of qualitative studies on the experiences of family members caring for individuals with early psychosis. *Int Rev Psychiatry.* 2019;31(5-6):491-509. doi:10.1080/09540261.2019.16 59236

22. Windell DL, Norman R, Lal S, Malla A. Subjective experiences of illness recovery in individuals treated for first-episode psychosis. *Soc Psychiatry Psychiatr Epidemiol.* 2015;50(7):1069-1077. doi:10.1007/s00127-014-1006-x

23. Tse S, Siu BW, Kan A. Can recovery-oriented mental health services be created in Hong Kong? Struggles and strategies. *Adm Policy Ment Health.* 2013;40(3):155-158. doi:10.1007/s10488-011-0391-7

24. Bola J, Chan THC, Chen EH, Ng R. Cross-validating Chinese language mental health recovery measures in Hong Kong. *Research on Social Work Practice.* 2016;26(6):630-640. doi:10.1177/1049731515625326

25. Campbell-Orde T, Chamberlin J, Carpenter J, Leff HS. *Measuring the Promise: A Compendium of Recovery Measures.* Vol II. Human Services Research Institute, Cambridge, MA; 2005.

26. Chen EY, Tam DK, Wong JW, Law CW, Chiu CP. Self-administered instrument to measure the patient's experience of recovery after first-episode psychosis: development and validation of the Psychosis Recovery Inventory. *Aust N Z J Psychiatry.* 2005;39(6):493-499. doi:10.1080/j.1440-1614.2005.01609.x

27. Lam MML, Chan KPM, Law CW, et al. Subjective experience of first episode psychosis in Hong Kong: IPSOS Report. *Early Intervention in Psychiatry.* 2008;2(Suppl. 1):A27-SP09.2.

28. Lam MM, Pearson V, Ng RM, Chiu CP, Law CW, Chen EY. What does recovery from psychosis mean? Perceptions of young first-episode patients. *Int J Soc Psychiatry.* 2011;57(6):580-587. doi:10.1177/0020764010374418

The Experience of Psychosis as One of the Most Devastating Illnesses • 31

29. Ng RM, Pearson V, Lam M, Law CW, Chiu CP, Chen EY. What does recovery from schizophrenia mean? Perceptions of long-term patients. *Int J Soc Psychiatry*. 2008;54(2):118-130. doi:10.1177/0020764007084600

30. Tam D, Chen E, Law C, Chiu C, Wong JGWS. Perceived extent of recovery and risk of relapse following first-episode psychosis. The 20th International Congress on Schizophrenia Research, Savannah, GA, April 2–6, 2005. *Schizophr Bull*. 2005;31(2):552. doi:10.1093/schbul/sbi024

31. Tang JYM, Chiu CPY, Hui CLM, et al. Clinical and cognitive correlates of perceived extent of recovery in Chinese patients with psychosis. The 2nd Biennial Schizophrenia International Research Conference, Florence, Italy, 10–14 April 2010. In *Schizophr Res*. 2010; 117(2-3):516. doi:10.1016/j.schres.2010.02.990

32. Hui CLM, Lo MCL, Chan EHC, et al. Perception towards relapse and its predictors in psychosis patients: A qualitative study. *Early Interv Psychiatry*. 2018;12(5):856-862. doi:10.1111/eip.12378

33. Mohamed S, Paulsen JS, O'Leary D, Arndt S, Andreasen N. Generalized cognitive deficits in schizophrenia: a study of first-episode patients. *Arch Gen Psychiatry*. 1999;56(8):749-754. doi:10.1001/archpsyc.56.8.749

34. Reichenberg A, Harvey PD. Neuropsychological impairments in schizophrenia: integration of performance-based and brain imaging findings [published correction appears *in Psychol Bull*. 2008 May;134(3):382]. *Psychol Bull*. 2007;133(5):833-858. doi:10.1037/0033-2909.133.5.833

35. Aas M, Dazzan P, Mondelli V, Melle I, Murray RM, Pariante CM. A systematic review of cognitive function in first-episode psychosis, including a discussion on childhood trauma, stress, and inflammation. *Front Psychiatry*. 2014;4:182. Published Jan 8, 2014. doi:10.3389/fpsyt.2013.00182

36. Fusar-Poli P, Deste G, Smieskova R, et al. Cognitive functioning in prodromal psychosis: a meta-analysis. *Arch Gen Psychiatry*. 2012;69(6):562-571. doi:10.1001/archgenpsychiatry.2011.1592

37. Bozikas VP, Andreou C. Longitudinal studies of cognition in first episode psychosis: a systematic review of the literature. *Aust N Z J Psychiatry*. 2011;45(2):93-108. doi:10.31 09/00048674.2010.541418

38. Lewandowski KE, Cohen BM, Ongur D. Evolution of neuropsychological dysfunction during the course of schizophrenia and bipolar disorder. *Psychol Med*. 2011;41(2):225-241. doi:10.1017/S0033291710001042

39. Wright AL, Phillips LJ, Bryce S, et al. Subjective experiences of cognitive functioning in early psychosis: a qualitative study. *Psychosis*. 2019;11(1):63-74. doi:10.1080/1752243 9.2019.1571623

40. Wood H, Cupitt C, Lavender T. The experience of cognitive impairment in people with psychosis. *Clin Psychol Psychother*. 2015;22(3):193-207. doi:10.1002/cpp.1878

41. Chang WC, Chan TC, Chiu SS, et al. Self-perceived cognitive functioning and its relationship with objective performance in first-episode schizophrenia: the Subjective Cognitive Impairment Scale. *Compr Psychiatry*. 2015;56:42-50. doi:10.1016/j.comppsych.2014.10.004

42. Alvarez-Jimenez M, Priede A, Hetrick SE, et al. Risk factors for relapse following treatment for first episode psychosis: a systematic review and meta-analysis of longitudinal studies. *Schizophr Res.* 2012;139(1-3):116-128. doi:10.1016/j.schres.2012.05.007

43. Robinson D, Woerner MG, Alvir JM, et al. Predictors of relapse following response from a first episode of schizophrenia or schizoaffective disorder. *Arch Gen Psychiatry.* 1999;56(3):241-247. doi:10.1001/archpsyc.56.3.241

44. Shepperd JA, Carroll P, Grace J, Terry M. Exploring the causes of comparative optimism. *Psychologica Belgica.* 2002;42(1-2):65-98.

45. Helweg-Larsen M, Shepperd JA. Do moderators of the optimistic bias affect personal or target risk estimates? A review of the literature. *Personality and Social Psychology Review.* 2001;5(1):74-95.

46. Weinstein, ND. Unrealistic optimism about future life events. *Journal of Personality and Social Psychology.* 1980;39(5):806-820. doi:10.1037/0022-3514.39.5.806

47. Chan KW, Wong MH, Hui CL, Lee EH, Chang WC, Chen EY. Perceived risk of relapse and role of medication: comparison between patients with psychosis and their caregivers. *Soc Psychiatry Psychiatr Epidemiol.* 2015;50(2):307-315. doi:10.1007/s00127-014-0930-0

48. McGlashan TH, Levy ST. Sealing-over in a therapeutic community. *Psychiatry.* 2019;82(1):1-12. doi:10.1080/00332747.2019.1594437

49. Erk S, Kiefer M, Grothe J, Wunderlich AP, Spitzer M, Walter H. Emotional context modulates subsequent memory effect. *Neuroimage.* 2003;18(2):439-447. doi:10.1016/s1053-8119(02)00015-0

50. Kim JS, Vossel G, Gamer M. Effects of emotional context on memory for details: the role of attention. *PLoS One.* 2013;8(10):e77405. Published Oct 7, 2013. doi:10.1371/journal.pone.0077405

51. Moore MM, Urban-Wojcik EJ, Martin EA. Emotional context effects on memory accuracy for neutral information. *Cogn Emot.* 2021;35(4):774-789. doi:10.1080/02699931.2021.1874880

52. Velakoulis D, Wood SJ, Wong MT, et al. Hippocampal and amygdala volumes according to psychosis stage and diagnosis: a magnetic resonance imaging study of chronic schizophrenia, first-episode psychosis, and ultra-high-risk individuals. *Arch Gen Psychiatry.* 2006;63(2):139-149. doi:10.1001/archpsyc.63.2.139

53. Herold CJ, Lässer MM, Schmid LA, et al. Hippocampal volume reduction and autobiographical memory deficits in chronic schizophrenia. *Psychiatry Res.* 2013;211(3):189-194. doi:10.1016/j.pscychresns.2012.04.002

54. Eisenacher S, Zink M. The Importance of metamemory functioning to the pathogenesis of psychosis. *Front Psychol.* 2017;8:304. Published Mar 6, 2017. doi:10.3389/fpsyg.2017.00304

55. Moritz S, Woodward TS, Chen E. Investigation of metamemory dysfunctions in first-episode schizophrenia. *Schizophr Res.* 2006;81(2-3):247-252. doi:10.1016/j.schres.2005.09.004

56. Reyna VF, Nelson WL, Han PK, Dieckmann NF. How numeracy influences risk comprehension and medical decision making. *Psychol Bull.* 2009;135(6):943-973. doi:10.1037/a0017327

The Experience of Psychosis as One of the Most Devastating Illnesses • 33

57. Paling J. Strategies to help patients understand risks. *BMJ.* 2003;327(7417):745-748. doi:10.1136/bmj.327.7417.745

58. Gigerenzer G. *Calculated Risks: How to Know When Numbers Deceive You.* Simon & Schuster; 2002.

59. Fagerlin A, Zikmund-Fisher BJ, Ubel PA. Helping patients decide: ten steps to better risk communication. *J Natl Cancer Inst.* 2011;103(19):1436-1443. doi:10.1093/jnci/djr318

60. Chen EY, Tang JY, Hui CL, et al. Three-year outcome of phase-specific early intervention for first-episode psychosis: a cohort study in Hong Kong. *Early Interv Psychiatry.* 2011;5(4):315-323. doi:10.1111/j.1751-7893.2011.00279.x

2

The Stigma of Psychosis: How It Affects Illness Outcome

Background

Historical Context

Patients with a severe mental disorder such as psychosis not only have to manage the devastating effects of their illness but are also exposed to stigmatising attitudes and social exclusion. In Ancient Greece, the word 'stigma' referred to a mark that was cut or burnt into the skin of slaves, criminals, or traitors so that these individuals could be easily identified and avoided by 'respectable' citizens (1). The negative connotations associated with the word 'stigma' have endured and occur most frequently in relation to race, culture, gender, and disease. In many cultures, despite being recognised in ancient medical texts, mental symptoms have been viewed as a supernatural phenomenon, either as a spiritual experience, punishment from the gods, or demonic possession (2). Often, as a consequence of this attribution, mental illness was considered a moral failing and patients were thought of as being dangerous. During the Middle Ages in Europe, treatments such as exorcism, prayer, and fasting were common (3). Later, with the beginning of the Enlightenment, mental illness was increasingly viewed as having a physical cause and patients were admitted to so-called 'madhouses'. Interventions included physical restraint with chains and harsh physical treatments, like those in the Middle Ages, although occasionally attention was paid to inmates' physical well-being and diet. More personalised, therapeutic, and comprehensive approaches emerged at the end of the eighteenth century. However, with the expansion of asylums in the nineteenth century, patients were again confined in overcrowded and understaffed institutions (4). The emergence of the eugenics movement in the late nineteenth century culminated in the systematic sterilisation of psychiatric patients and the extermination of mentally ill persons in the Nazi era (5). Following World War II, the deinstitutionalisation movement beginning in the 1960s led to the widespread introduction of community treatment and greater social integration of individuals with severe mental health disorders. However, community psychiatric services remain woefully underfunded worldwide and psychiatric patients are overrepresented in the homeless and prison population (6).

In ancient China, despite mental symptoms being described in early medical texts, association with supernatural phenomena was common. Health was thought to be related to balance in nature. Mental symptoms were considered to be part of an integral systemic imbalance between the five natural elements, as well as yin and yang. Practitioners of traditional Chinese medicine offered herbs and acupuncture (7, 8, 9). A move towards a somatic and psychological understanding and more comprehensive bio-psycho-social models developed over time (10). Western ideas were slowly incorporated into traditional Chinese conceptualisations of mental illness with the establishment of the first Western-style psychiatric hospital at the end of the nineteenth century (8). In oriental culture, which emphasises family bonding, mental illness has carried immense connotations of weakness, moral failure, and shame for the individual and their family. The intense fear of social isolation and shame prevents patients and their relatives from talking about their mental health difficulties to this day (11).

The Different Types of Stigma

Social stigma was first explored by the French sociologist Émile Durkheim in the late nineteenth century (12). However, it was not before the 1960s that a scientific concept of stigma was developed for mental health research (13). In his book *Stigma: Notes on the Management of Spoiled Identity*, Erving Goffman defined stigma as an attribute, behaviour, or reputation that is socially discredited and consequently leads to an individual being rejected by society. He considered it a 'special discrepancy between virtual and actual social identity' (1). Bruce Link was one of the first to describe the vicious cycle experienced by people with mental illness (14). He and his colleagues argued that patients became increasingly socially withdrawn as a consequence of negative reactions due to deviating from accepted societal standards and norms. Social isolation then leads to diminished self-esteem and increases vulnerability to psychosocial stress, thereby compounding mental health difficulties. In their 'modified labelling theory', the stigma associated with a diagnosis of mental illness tangibly affects employment chances, earnings, psychosocial functioning, and life itself (15). In addition to labelling, stigma is characterised by stereotyping, separation, status loss, and discrimination (16).

Stereotyping refers to preconceived attitudes and opinions towards certain groups of people, whether these groups are based on race or illness. Although stereotyping can be advantageous, particularly when quick judgements are necessary in urgent situations, they are too generalised and not an accurate reflection of the individual. Individuals with mental illness are commonly thought to be dangerous, violent, unreliable, unpredictable, and uncontrollable. Other stereotypes include an inability to recover, work or live independently, and patients being themselves responsible for their mental health difficulties and should therefore be ashamed (13, 17). In their *Stigma in Global Context-Mental Health Study*, Pescosolido and colleagues (2013) measured knowledge of and prejudice towards schizophrenia and depression using case vignettes in 16 countries across the world (18). They showed that despite high levels of recognition, neurobiological attribution, and treatment endorsement, core stigmatising attitudes were commonly expressed concerning persons with mental illness marrying into the family, providing childcare, engaging in self-injurious acts, holding positions of authority, and interacting with others. These attitudes were prevalent even in countries and cultures considered to be more accepting of mental illness.

Stigma research has been criticised for focussing on stereotyping and prejudice at an individual level and neglecting the devastating effects of structural discrimination experienced by patients (19). For example, in a survey of schizophrenia patients from 27 countries, almost 50% reported discrimination in their personal relationships and nearly 30% had experienced discrimination while looking for or maintaining employment. Almost two-thirds anticipated negative discrimination when applying for work and more than 50% when looking for a close relationship. More than 70% felt the need to conceal their diagnosis (20). Hatzenbuehler (2016) has convincingly argued that structural stigma negatively affects stigma processes at the individual level, impacts the efficacy of psychological interventions and contributes to health inequalities (21).

Differences in stigmatisation depend on the type of mental disorder. The general population prefers a greater social distance to someone with schizophrenia compared to someone with depression (22). Surprisingly, despite an attribution of biological aetiology and endorsement of treatment, the desire for social distance has increased in the twenty-first century. It has been postulated that this may be associated with high perceived risks of patients who have been increasingly treated in the community over the last 50 years.

Schizophrenia is one of the most stigmatised disorders alongside alcohol dependence, with only drug dependence being perceived more negatively (13).

Personal or self-stigma refers to internalised stigmatisation of persons with mental disorders. A recent meta-analysis of self-stigma of psychosis patients showed that demographic factors such as age, employment, economic status, and rural residence showed small correlations with personal stigma. It was inversely related to medication adherence and well-being, as well as positively associated with insight and positive symptoms. Higher self, perceived, and experienced stigma has also been associated with lower quality of life in psychosis (23).

It has been shown that self-stigma affects help-seeking behaviour very early in the course of psychotic disorders (24). A systematic review of 38 studies by Colizzi et al. (2020) showed that those at risk of psychosis already face stigmatising attitudes. Negative views were held particularly by members of the general public with low educational attainment and no direct experience of at-risk states. Persons at risk of psychosis also report more internalised stigma and perceive more discrimination compared to healthy controls or patients with non-psychotic disorders, and these attitudes are associated with increased distress, shame, and fear. Furthermore, self-stigma increased the likelihood of poor outcomes, including the transition to frank psychosis, suicidality, disengagement from services, and family stigma (25). Delayed help-seeking and disengagement from services are associated with poor outcomes and likely lead to more pronounced and publicly displayed symptoms, emergency presentations, and police involvement. This then further impacts the public perception of psychosis patients being dangerous and untreatable creating a vicious cycle (26). However, it is important to note that the labelling of at-risk states also carries positive effects as it can provide validation and relief (25).

Stigma and the Media

The mass media has had an important role in perpetuating negative stereotypes of mental illness, but also in educating the public on the nature and treatment of mental disorders (27, 28, 29). It has been shown that prejudiced media reporting can have detrimental effects on recovery, lead to an increase in experienced discrimination, and discourage help-seeking in sufferers (30). The general population is more likely to respond with fear, hostility, and intolerance towards the mentally ill when exposed to negative media reporting (31). However, with careful engagement, the media can be a helpful ally to challenge stigma and contribute to more positive reporting on mental ill health (32). Maiorano et al. (2017) showed that anti-stigma interventions for media professionals appear to have some effect in improving reporting style, with contact-based educational programmes being the most promising approach (29).

Interventions to Reduce Stigma

Increasingly, stigma has been recognised as an important public health problem and it has become the focus of national strategies across the world. In 2013, the World Health Organization called for action to reduce stigma (33). Stigma reduction interventions have been implemented in many countries. Three different strategies have been employed to change perceptions of mental illness. Protesting the inaccurate portrayal of mental illness is one such strategy. Although this approach may lead to fewer negative representations in the media, it has been criticised for being reactive, not offering a more positive appraisal of mental illness, and possibly creating negative reactions to being told what to think (34, 35). Education is another strategy and has been most widely researched. Several approaches, including public service announcements, flyers, lectures, films, and other audiovisual materials have been used to educate and reach large audiences. The third strategy is face-to-face contact between members of the general public and persons with mental illness (35). Corrigan and colleagues (1999, 2002) reported that interpersonal contact leads to greater improvements in attitudes than protest and education, as well as participants' willingness to donate money to a mental health advocacy group (36, 37). However, these findings have not been confirmed in systematic reviews and meta-analyses.

Interventions addressing personal stigma or social distance result in small significant improvements for all mental disorders including psychosis. Educational interventions, with or without patient contact, reduced personal stigma and internet-based interventions were as effective as face-to-face delivery (38). Similarly, Morgan et al. (2018) showed small to medium reductions in stigmatising attitudes and desire for social distance for both contact and educational interventions. Small improvements in social distance persist for educational programmes after six months, but following face-to-face contact, attitudes reverted to preintervention levels and improvements did not endure (39). To date, there is little evidence that educational or contact interventions improve perceived or self-stigma. However, cognitive approaches might be a promising avenue to address this neglected area (24, 38).

There have been several comparative studies investigating the attitudes of Western and Chinese cultures towards individuals with mental illness. These studies suggest that Chinese groups were more likely to endorse greater negative stereotypes and attitudes than their Western counterparts (40, 41, 42, 43).

Studies on Stigma in Hong Kong

In Hong Kong, stigma for mental conditions has been investigated to gain a better understanding of its contributory factors and to inform public stigma campaigns in the city.

Attitudes and Knowledge of Mental Illness in Hong Kong

In Hong Kong, the knowledge of and attitudes towards mental illness have been explored not only in the general population but also in secondary schools, undergraduate students, medical students, and healthcare professionals using case vignettes and psychoeducational material. Adolescent boys appeared to have more stereotyping, restrictive, pessimistic, and stigmatising attitudes towards mental illness than girls (44). However, among undergraduate students, young women were more likely to endorse greater social distance towards patients (45). University students had less stigmatising attitudes towards individuals with mental illness when they studied medicine or when they had previous contact with patients. They were more willing to interact with someone who was receiving ongoing psychiatric care compared to those who were labelled as mentally ill and those who had never been hospitalised (45). Students without previous contact with patients would only consider having contact with someone who had fully recovered from their illness.

In a large survey, Tsang et al. (2003) distributed stigma questionnaires to primary and secondary schools, for students' friends and relatives over the age of 16 years to complete (46). Just over 1,000 questionnaires were returned. They showed rather severe stigmatising attitudes in the community, such as beliefs about parents causing the illness, strong opposition to setting up psychiatric community facilities near one's residence, and limited employment opportunities for people with mental illness. Such beliefs likely increase the burden on clients' relatives by denying them support. Like university students, respondents who had had a higher level of previous contact with mentally ill persons had fewer stigmatising attitudes (46). In addition, those with a lower education level held more negative beliefs about those with schizophrenia or an attenuated psychosis syndrome. Having frequent encounters with a person appearing mentally ill in public was also associated with more exclusionary sentiments and negative affect (47).

Moreover, we showed that schizophrenia is one of the most stigmatised mental illnesses in Hong Kong and that public stigma already exists towards individuals who experience prepsychotic states. Persons known to have received treatment for the condition likely face long-term discrimination (47).

Anti-stigma Interventions in Hong Kong

Several anti-stigma interventions have been explored in Hong Kong, among them were comparisons between videos of a person with lived experience sharing their story with educational videos provided by an expert. Among medical students, psychoeducation delivered by either a patient or an expert reduced fear of someone with a mental illness. Knowledge and attitudes improved only in those who saw the patient video (48).

The Early Psychosis Foundation (EPISO) developed a school-based programme called 'The School Tour'. The programme comprised an engaging drama performance based on the theme of mental conditions in a school setting and was delivered to 4520 students. Knowledge of and attitudes towards psychosis significantly improved following the programme illustrating that innovative and engaging activities may help to reduce stigma (49).

Renaming Psychosis and Stigmatising Attitudes

A Chinese term for psychosis was adopted in 2001 as part of a comprehensive and wide-ranging public awareness campaign to facilitate a reduction in public stigma and improve help-seeking. The previously used term for psychosis *zhongxing jingshenbing* (重性精神病), literally 'severe mental disorder', was associated with a negative stereotype. It was replaced by the term *sijueshitiao* (思覺失調), translated as 'dysregulation of thoughts and perception' (50). The new name covered a broader concept of psychosis and it was hoped that it would portray the illness more objectively. In recognition of the fact that stigma is already associated with the very early stages of psychosis, the acceptability of a new Chinese term to describe the condition for people at risk of psychosis was also investigated (26, 51). The term *yunniangqi* (醞釀期) denoting an 'incubation period' was the most widely endorsed term by both health professionals and the general population (51). The Hong Kong experience of changing the terms for psychosis and at-risk states is further explored in Chapter 5.

In 2009, we investigated public stigma in a randomised telephone survey of a representative sample of the adult Hong Kong population (52). Despite using the new term for psychosis, stigmatising attitudes were widespread. Almost 90% thought that most employers would not consider a job application from an individual with psychosis, three-quarters of participants considered a person with psychosis dangerous and unpredictable, and more than 70% agreed that most people would take the opinion of a person with psychosis less seriously. Women and those with higher educational levels and better knowledge of symptoms and treatment of psychosis had more prejudiced views.

A further telephone survey 9 years later revealed female gender, older age, and being a pensioner or homemaker as significant predictors of more stigmatising attitudes (53). Surprisingly, unlike in the previous survey, lower education was associated with higher stigma. This is possibly a reflection of population change, as well as the impact of public awareness on the better educated.

Following the widely reported homicide of a young boy committed by a schizophrenia patient in 2009, we conducted a random telephone survey to explore the effects of media reporting on the knowledge of and stigma towards psychosis, and the use of the terms for schizophrenia and psychosis in Hong Kong (54). 506 participants were asked to answer questions about their knowledge, treatment, and belief of the dangerousness of psychosis as well as their emotional reaction to the tragic news. Significantly more subjects agreed that people with psychosis were a danger to the public. However, no significant differences were observed in overall attitudes. Women and older people reported greater distress related to the news, and participants who reported a high level of distress were more likely to perceive people with psychosis as dangerous.

We repeated our telephone survey in 2014 to gain an understanding of the change in population knowledge about psychosis and public stigma (55). 1018 subjects with similar demographic characteristics to the 2009 cohort completed the survey. Significantly more respondents endorsed medication as a treatment and had a better understanding of psychosis; however, knowledge of symptoms did not change. There was also no significant change in public stigma. In fact, male subjects were found to report higher levels of stigma but also endorsed medication as the treatment of choice for psychosis. Female participants reported similar levels of stigma and knowledge of treatment in 2009 and 2014.

We also questioned randomly selected members of the public regarding their willingness to disclose psychotic symptoms and found that higher stigmatising attitudes, more recent life stressors, and lower life satisfaction were associated with more reluctance to reveal unusual experiences, particularly in women and youth. Worryingly, almost 15% of respondents were unwilling to disclose their difficulties to anyone, and those who were more open to the idea of sharing their experiences said they would prefer to speak to family members (56).

Stigma, Aetiological Attribution, and Social Contact

The finding that a biological account of mental disorders is associated with persistent or even higher levels of stigma has been observed in countries across the world (22). We have also shown that females were more likely to endorse psychosocial aetiologies that may affect their acceptance of medication and biological explanations (49, 50). Persistent high levels of stigma among women might be related to the presumed dangerousness of people with mental illness (57, 58, 59). Despite improvements in knowledge, 40% of the public in Hong Kong thought that psychosis could be treated solely by psychotherapy and 40% still considered anxiety attacks a common symptom of psychosis. Also, over 60% of the population continued to associate *jingshenfenlie* (精神分裂) with psychosis, although significantly fewer respondents endorsed this term following the introduction of *sijueshitiao* (思覺失調). The term has been increasingly used since its introduction in 2001 (60).

Fang et al. (2021) also observed that when relatives, members of the general public, and professionals had more frequent contact with people who have a mental illness, they had better knowledge of mental health conditions, were less prejudiced, and endorsed fewer discriminatory behaviours. Experiential contact seemed to be directly related to less prejudice. Lower levels of prejudice were associated with fewer biased behaviours; however, better knowledge did not appear to directly affect discriminatory behaviour (61).

Internalised and Affiliate Stigma in Hong Kong

In addition to public stigma, several studies have examined the characteristics of self-stigma in the Chinese population of Hong Kong. In order to comprehensively assess internalised stigma, Ho et al. (2015) validated the Chinese version of the Stigma Scale in persons living with mental illness in Hong Kong (62). Of concern has been the realisation that first-episode psychosis (FEP) patients who had a longer duration of untreated psychosis, more symptoms, and more hospitalisations experienced more severe self-stigma over the long term (63). There were also direct associations between internalised stigma and functioning (64). On the other hand, patients who were able to maintain employment were less likely to report internalised stigma (65).

Chen et al. (2016) were also interested in the interplay of self-stigma and affiliated stigma in FEP patients and their caregivers (66). Lee et al. (2005, 2006) had already shown that 40% of patients with schizophrenia, compared with 15% of diabetes patients, experienced stigma from family members, partners, friends, and colleagues (67, 68). More than half of patients who reported anticipated stigma concealed their illness and experienced dysphoria (67). Almost half of psychosis patients encountered stigma related to medication and their hospital admission (68).

'Face concern' represents an important concept in Chinese culture and refers to an individual's occupation with preserving their social image or status and avoiding 'loss of face' (69). Insight, loss of face, and perceived public stigma were positively correlated with self-stigma. Conversely, quality of life was inversely correlated with self-stigma. Greater concern for loss of face and a higher degree of perceived public stigma were independently associated with patients' self-stigma. Face concern partially mediated the relationship between perceived public stigma and self-stigma. Affiliate stigma was positively correlated with higher levels of stress and symptoms of depression and anxiety in caregivers, but it was not associated with perceived public stigma or face concern. In addition, we observed that poor neurocognitive functioning and negative symptoms were associated with higher levels of discriminatory experiences and increased self-stigma (70).

Personal Reflections on Stigma

Stigma, consisting of a negative stereotype of mental illness and its treatment, can kill people. We have come across the tragic case of a young person committing suicide as a consequence of intense stigma towards psychosis in one of our psychological autopsy studies (demographic details have been changed to protect the identity of the case). An adolescent boy had developed typical symptoms of a psychotic condition. His situation had been known by the school, yet a referral to the specialised Early Assessment Service for Young People (EASY) was declined by his parents. He continued to suffer from psychotic symptoms and, three months later, he jumped to his death from a building. The early psychosis service would likely have controlled his psychotic symptoms within weeks. When we interviewed the parents, they expressed that they had no regrets about the fatal outcome. They thought it was probably best that their son had died. On further enquiry, we learned that another member of the extended family had been suffering from psychosis. The relative, despite treatment, continued to experience disabling symptoms and also had significant side effects from medication. The parents anticipated that their son would likely suffer the same fate. The family had not been aware that the treatment of psychotic illnesses had significantly improved over the last two decades, in both pharmacological and psychological aspects. Thus, a negative perception of psychosis and its treatment cost the boy his life.

The root of stigma is probably embedded deep in human nature. Survival in an early evolutionary environment depended upon the ability to function collaboratively in groups. Humans have developed the capacity to recognise group members and to identify outsiders and free riders. Since reciprocal altruism underlies prosocial behaviour, it is important for individuals to be able to recognise conspecifics that could potentially not return their contributions. Stigma towards chronic conditions that result in changes in external appearances such as leprosy is intense. Stigma towards medical conditions such as infectious disease is also intensified by fear of contagion. In mental disorders, the issue of contagiousness is unclear, yet from time to time, the possibility of being rendered mentally ill through contact with people with mental health problems is being raised. For instance, it has been suggested by a prominent legislator in Hong Kong that psychiatrists are themselves at risk of mental disorders because of contagion from prolonged interaction with psychiatric patients. Perhaps more than the risk of contagion, the risks of violence and unpredictable behaviour are prominent in the minds of the public. In densely populated cities such as Hong Kong and many East Asian cities, there are understandable concerns about the mental health of neighbours we encounter in the course of daily life. In housing estates with thousands of residents, it is inevitable that conflicts and disorderly behaviour occur, and a number of people will experience mental health problems in the neighbourhood. Individuals who fared well with a mental health condition would not be visible. It will be those with symptoms who are noticed by the general public. In large housing estates, such as those in which a significant proportion of the population dwells in Asian cities, estate managers can play a significant gatekeeper role. In the course of empowering estate managers in their ability to support individuals with emerging psychotic disorders, we have offered basic training for the recognition of symptoms and provided guidance on how best to respond. To our surprise, we discovered that there are more than 200,000 estate

44 • *Psychosis and Schizophrenia in Hong Kong*

managers in Hong Kong, and they could have a significant role in the early detection of psychosis.

In a major city like Hong Kong, from time to time, there are violent incidents involving patients with psychosis. Several years ago, one such tragedy involved the death of an estate manager. From what can be ascertained, a known psychosis patient had relapsed and developed persecutory ideas towards his estate manager. His wife noted the deterioration and escorted him to an accident and emergency department to seek help. However, upon arrival, the wife was directed to a separate seating area from the cubicle in which the patient was waiting for a clinician. After many hours of waiting, the patient was seen by a clinician and sent home with some cough medicine. The wife had apparently not been interviewed. Several hours later, the patient fatally attacked the estate manager. When the incident was reported in the media, the hospital spokesperson indicated that in the accident and emergency department, the mental state of the patient was 'normal'. This created panic in the population, as the perception was that someone with a mental health condition could be deemed normal at one point in time and then transformed into someone who could act on psychotic experiences and kill another person within a few hours. This, of course, is not the usual time course of psychotic episodes, which develops over days and weeks rather than hours. However, as a result of this, people living in crowded housing estates demanded to be told which of their neighbours suffered from mental health conditions. This is one regrettable incident where tragedy is reinforced by an inaccurate public message and thus intensifies and deepens stigma in the population.

In another incident, a middle-aged man with a history of a psychotic disorder and violence was involved in an apparently random killing of two young women in a busy shopping mall, despite regular outpatient attendance, treatment, and community monitoring. The incident was widely reported and videos were circulated via social media. Cases like this understandably raise fear, particularly as the shopping mall was popular with many local residents. The immediacy of the incident brings home the emotional impact and the sense of danger potentially associated with psychosis patients. The extent to which these associations could be addressed by reminders that this is a rare event is doubtful. The situation is not helped by the incident being described by officials as 'murders' rather than 'incidents'. The tragic nature of the case is reinforced by the fact that apparently, the mental health teams had done all they could within the constraints of the healthcare system. What is regrettable is that the 'system' is one with a chronic manpower shortage, which has perpetuated a minimal standard of clinical care necessitated by high service volumes, short consultation times, and the resulting lack of the kind of clinical sensitivity that would have been required to detect subtle changes in mental states.

The negative stereotype of patients with psychotic illness is fuelled by lack of contact. When the voices of recovered patients are silenced by stigma, the public only has biased access to psychosis patients when they are unwell in public places or are involved in incidents. This creates a distorted prototypical image of a patient with a psychotic disorder as disorganised and unpredictable. Having patients share their experiences in person is the antidote to this silencing effect of stigma. Hong Kong is still early in the process of having the first group of patients willing to brave stigma and share their stories.

We have gained a greater understanding of sociodemographic factors affecting stigmatising attitudes in the general public. With our wide-ranging anti-stigma campaigns using a variety of strategies, and the introduction of a new term for psychosis and the at-risk state, there has been an increase in knowledge of mental illness among the population of Hong Kong. However, similar to findings in the Western world, the endorsement of a biological aetiology has not changed public attitudes, but has, in fact, increased stigma, particularly among men. This might be due to genetic and brain imaging information being unjustifiably associated with an underlying deterministic view on the treatability of psychosis.

Building on our work, ongoing public anti-stigma campaigns will require a multipronged approach and need to target particular populations to address negative preconceptions of psychosis. For example, our team has regularly encouraged secondary school students in our 'Mindshift programme' to join sports activities with recovered psychosis patients. The experience of interacting in non-clinical settings has been overwhelmingly positive. Students have reported positive exchanges with patients, having developed a better understanding of illness trajectory, and feeling less fearful when meeting a person with psychosis.

Alongside public campaigns, patients will also require additional support to manage the effects of pervasive discrimination and self-stigma. Preliminary evidence has pointed towards cognitive-behavioural approaches being beneficial and neurocognitive strategies may also play a role given the negative effects of poor neurocognitive functioning on internalised stigma (25).

References

1. Goffman E. *Stigma: Notes on the Management of Spoiled Identity*. Simon & Schuster; 2009.
2. Porter R. *Madness: A Brief History*. Oxford University Press; 2002.
3. Laffey P. Psychiatric therapy in Georgian Britain. *Psychol Med*. 2003;33(7):1285-1297. doi:10.1017/s0033291703008109
4. Wright D. Getting out of the asylum: understanding the confinement of the insane in the nineteenth century. *Soc Hist Med*. 1997;10(1):137-155. doi:10.1093/shm/10.1.137

46 • Psychosis and Schizophrenia in Hong Kong

5. Strous RD. Psychiatry during the Nazi era: ethical lessons for the modern professional. *Ann Gen Psychiatry.* 2007;6:8. Published Feb 27, 2007. doi:10.1186/1744-859X-6-8

6. Torrey EF, Stieber J, Ezekiel J, et al. *Criminalizing the Seriously Mentally Ill: The Abuse of Jails as Mental Hospitals (Report).* National Alliance for the Mentally Ill & Public Citizen Health Research Group, Washington, DC; 1992.

7. Aung SK, Fay H, Hobbs RF III. Traditional Chinese medicine as a basis for treating psychiatric disorders: a review of theory with illustrative cases. *Med Acupunct.* 2013;25(6):398-406. doi:10.1089/acu.2013.1007

8. Liu J, Ma H, He YL, et al. Mental health system in China: history, recent service reform and future challenges. *World Psychiatry.* 2011;10(3):210-216. doi:10.1002/j.2051-5545.2011.tb00059.x

9. Lam CS, Tsang H, Corrigan P, et al. Chinese lay theory and mental illness stigma: implications for research and practices. *Journal of Rehabilitation.* 2010;76 (1):35-40.

10. Tseng WS. The development of psychiatric concepts in traditional Chinese medicine. *Arch Gen Psychiatry.* 1973;29(4):569-575. doi:10.1001/archpsyc.1973.04200040109018

11. Wynaden D, Chapman R, Orb A, McGowan S, Zeeman Z, Yeak S. Factors that influence Asian communities' access to mental health care. *Int J Ment Health Nurs.* 2005;14(2):88-95. doi:10.1111/j.1440-0979.2005.00364.x

12. Durkheim É. *The Rules of Sociological Method and Selected Texts on Sociology and Its Method.* Edited with an introduction by Lukes S; translated by Halls WD. The Free Press; 1982:34-47.

13. Rössler W. The stigma of mental disorders: a millennia-long history of social exclusion and prejudices. *EMBO Rep.* 2016;17(9):1250-1253. doi:10.15252/embr.201643041

14. Link B. Mental patient status, work, and income: an examination of the effects of a psychiatric label. *Am Sociol Rev.* 1982;47(2):202-215.

15. Link BG, Phelan JC, Sullivan G. Mental and physical health consequences of the stigma associated with mental illnesses. In: Major B, Dovidio JF, Bruce G. Link BG, eds. *The Oxford Handbook of Stigma, Discrimination, and Health.* Oxford University Press; 2018. doi:10.1093/oxfordhb/9780190243470.013.2

16. Link BG, Phelan JC. Conceptualizing Stigma. *Annual Review of Sociology.* 2001;27:363-385.

17. Angermeyer MC, Dietrich S. Public beliefs about and attitudes towards people with mental illness: a review of population studies. *Acta Psychiatr Scand.* 2006;113(3):163-179. doi:10.1111/j.1600-0447.2005.00699.x

18. Pescosolido BA, Medina TR, Martin JK, Long JS. The 'backbone' of stigma: identifying the global core of public prejudice associated with mental illness. *Am J Public Health.* 2013;103(5):853-860. doi:10.2105/AJPH.2012.301147

19. Corrigan PW, Markowitz FE, Watson AC. Structural levels of mental illness stigma and discrimination. *Schizophr Bull.* 2004;30(3):481-491. doi:10.1093/oxfordjournals.schbul.a007096

20. Thornicroft G, Brohan E, Rose D, Sartorius N, Leese M; INDIGO Study Group. Global pattern of experienced and anticipated discrimination against people with schizophrenia: a cross-sectional survey. *Lancet.* 2009;373(9661):408-415. doi:10.1016/S0140-6736(08)61817-6

21. Hatzenbuehler ML. Structural stigma: research evidence and implications for psychological science. *Am Psychol.* 2016;71(8):742-751. doi:10.1037/amp0000068

22. Schomerus G, Schwahn C, Holzinger A, et al. Evolution of public attitudes about mental illness: a systematic review and meta-analysis. *Acta Psychiatr Scand.* 2012;125(6):440-452. doi:10.1111/j.1600-0447.2012.01826.x

23. Degnan A, Berry K, Humphrey C, Bucci S. The relationship between stigma and subjective quality of life in psychosis: a systematic review and meta-analysis. *Clin Psychol Rev.* 2021;85:102003. doi:10.1016/j.cpr.2021.102003

24. Gronholm PC, Thornicroft G, Laurens KR, Evans-Lacko S. Mental health-related stigma and pathways to care for people at risk of psychotic disorders or experiencing first-episode psychosis: a systematic review. *Psychol Med.* 2017;47(11):1867-1879. doi:10.1017/S0033291717000344

25. Colizzi M, Ruggeri M, Lasalvia A. Should we be concerned about stigma and discrimination in people at risk for psychosis? A systematic review. *Psychol Med.* 2020;50(5):705-726. doi:10.1017/S0033291720000148

26. Chen EYH, Lee H, Chan GH, Wong GHY, eds. *Early Psychosis Intervention: A Culturally Adaptive Clinical Guide.* Hong Kong University Press; 2013:75.

27. Wahl O. News media portrayal of mental illness implications for public policy. *Am Behav Sci.* 2003;46(12):1594-1600.

28. Schomerus G, Stolzenburg S, Angermeyer MC. Impact of the Germanwings plane crash on mental illness stigma: results from two population surveys in Germany before and after the incident. *World Psychiatry.* 2015;14(3):362-363. doi:10.1002/wps.20257

29. Maiorano A, Lasalvia A, Sampogna G, Pocai B, Ruggeri M, Henderson C. Reducing stigma in media professionals: is there room for improvement? Results from a systematic review. *Can J Psychiatry.* 2017;62(10):702-715. doi:10.1177/0706743717711172

30. Lyons AC. Examining media representations: benefits for health psychology. *J Health Psychol.* 2000;5(3):349-358. doi:10.1177/135910530000500307

31. Hallam A. Media influences on mental health policy: long-term effects of the Clunis and Silcock cases. *Int Rev Psychiatry.* 2002;14(1):26-33.

32. Clement S, Lassman F, Barley E, et al. Mass media interventions for reducing mental health-related stigma. *Cochrane Database Syst Rev.* 2013; (7):CD009453. Published Jul 23, 2013. doi:10.1002/14651858.CD009453.pub2

33. World Health Organization. *Mental Health Action Plan: 2013-2020.* World Health Organization; 2013.

34. Corrigan PW, Watson AC. Understanding the impact of stigma on people with mental illness. *World Psychiatry.* 2002;1(1):16-20.

35. Corrigan P, Gelb B. Three programs that use mass approaches to challenge the stigma of mental illness. *Psychiatr Serv.* 2006;57(3):393-398. doi:10.1176/appi.ps.57.3.393

36. Corrigan PW, Penn DL. Lessons from social psychology on discrediting psychiatric stigma. *Am Psychol.* 1999;54(9):765-776. doi:10.1037//0003-066x.54.9.765

37. Corrigan PW, Rowan D, Green A, et al. Challenging two mental illness stigmas: personal responsibility and dangerousness. *Schizophr Bull.* 2002;28(2):293-309. doi:10.1093/oxfordjournals.schbul.a006939

38. Griffiths KM, Carron-Arthur B, Parsons A, Reid R. Effectiveness of programs for reducing the stigma associated with mental disorders. A meta-analysis of randomized controlled trials. *World Psychiatry*. 2014;13(2):161-175. doi:10.1002/wps.20129

39. Morgan AJ, Reavley NJ, Ross A, Too LS, Jorm AF. Interventions to reduce stigma towards people with severe mental illness: systematic review and meta-analysis. *J Psychiatr Res*. 2018;103:120-133. doi:10.1016/j.jpsychires.2018.05.017

40. Knifton L, Gervais M, Newbigging K, et al. Community conversation: addressing mental health stigma with ethnic minority communities. *Soc Psychiatry Psychiatr Epidemiol*. 2010;45(4):497-504. doi:10.1007/s00127-009-0095-4

41. Shokoohi-Yekta M, Retish PM. Attitudes of Chinese and American male students towards mental illness. *Int J Soc Psychiatry*. 1991;37(3):192-200. doi:10.1177/002076409103700306

42. Yang LH, Wonpat-Borja AJ, Opler MG, Corcoran CM. Potential stigma associated with inclusion of the psychosis risk syndrome in the DSM-V: an empirical question. *Schizophr Res*. 2010;120(1-3):42-48. doi:10.1016/j.schres.2010.03.012

43. Yang LH, Purdie-Vaughns V, Kotabe H, et al. Culture, threat, and mental illness stigma: identifying culture-specific threat among Chinese-American groups. *Soc Sci Med*. 2013;88:56-67. doi:10.1016/j.socscimed.2013.03.036

44. Ng P, Chan KF. Sex differences in opinion towards mental illness of secondary school students in Hong Kong. *Int J Soc Psychiatry*. 2000;46(2):79-88. doi:10.1177/002076400004600201

45. Chung KF, Chen EY, Liu CS. University students' attitudes towards mental patients and psychiatric treatment. *Int J Soc Psychiatry*. 2001;47(2):63-72. doi:10.1177/002076400104700206

46. Tsang HWH, Tam PKC, Chan F, Cheung WM. Stigmatizing attitudes towards individuals with mental illness in Hong Kong: implications for their recovery. *J Community Psychology*. 2003;31:383-396. doi:10.1002/jcop.10055

47. Lee EH, Hui CL, Ching EY, et al. Public stigma in China associated with schizophrenia, depression, attenuated psychosis syndrome, and psychosis-like experiences. *Psychiatr Serv*. 2016;67(7):766-770. doi:10.1176/appi.ps.201500156

48. Tsoi OYY, Chan SKW, Chui AHC, et al. Effect of brief social contact video compared with expert information video in changing knowledge and attitude towards psychosis patients among medical students. *Early Interv Psychiatry*. 2021;15(2):278-285. doi:10.1111/eip.12938

49. Hui CLM, Leung WWT, Wong AKH, et al. Destigmatizing psychosis: investigating the effectiveness of a school-based programme in Hong Kong secondary school students. *Early Interv Psychiatry*. 2019;13(4):882-887. doi:10.1111/eip.12692

50. Chiu CP, Lam MM, Chan SK, et al. Naming psychosis: the Hong Kong experience. *Early Interv Psychiatry*. 2010;4(4):270-274. doi:10.1111/j.1751-7893.2010.00203.x

51. Lee EHM, Ching EYN, Hui CLM, et al. Chinese label for people at risk for psychosis. *Early Interv Psychiatry*. 2017;11(3):224-228. doi:10.1111/eip.12232

52. Chan SK, Tam WW, Lee KW, et al. A population study of public stigma about psychosis and its contributing factors among Chinese population in Hong Kong. *Int J Soc Psychiatry*. 2016;62(3):205-213. doi:10.1177/0020764015621941

53. Lo LLH, Suen YN, Chan SKW, et al. Sociodemographic correlates of public stigma about mental illness: a population study on Hong Kong's Chinese population. *BMC Psychiatry*. 2021;21(1):274. Published May 29, 2021. doi:10.1186/s12888-021-03301-3

54. Chan SKW, Li OWT, Hui CLM, Chang WC, Lee EHM, Chen EYH. The effect of media reporting of a homicide committed by a patient with schizophrenia on the public stigma and knowledge of psychosis among the general population of Hong Kong. *Soc Psychiatry Psychiatr Epidemiol*. 2019;54(1):43-50. doi:10.1007/s00127-018-1610-2

55. Chan SK, Lee KW, Hui CL, Chang WC, Lee EH, Chen EY. Gender effect on public stigma changes towards psychosis in the Hong Kong Chinese population: a comparison between population surveys of 2009 and 2014. *Soc Psychiatry Psychiatr Epidemiol*. 2017;52(3):259-267. doi:10.1007/s00127-016-1317-1

56. Suen YN, Chan KWS, Siu LTT, et al. Relationship between stressful life events, stigma and life satisfaction with the willingness of disclosure of psychotic illness: a community study in Hong Kong. *Early Interv Psychiatry*. 2021;15(3):686-696. doi:10.1111/eip.13008

57. Holzinger A, Floris F, Schomerus G, Carta MG, Angermeyer MC. Gender differences in public beliefs and attitudes about mental disorder in western countries: a systematic review of population studies. *Epidemiol Psychiatr Sci*. 2012;21(1):73-85. doi:10.1017/s2045796011000552

58. Hinkelman L, Haag D. Biological sex, adherence to traditional gender roles, and attitudes toward persons with mental illness: an exploratory investigation. *J Ment Health Couns*. 2003;25:259-270.

59. Phelan JE, Basow SA. College students' attitudes toward mental illness: an examination of the stigma process. *J Appl Soc Psychol*. 2007;37:2877-2902.

60. Chan SKW, Ching EYN, Lam KSC, et al. Newspaper coverage of mental illness in Hong Kong between 2002 and 2012: impact of introduction of a new Chinese name of psychosis. *Early Interv Psychiatry*. 2017;11(4):342-345. doi:10.1111/eip.12298

61. Fang Q, Zhang TM, Wong YLI, et al. The mediating role of knowledge on the contact and stigma of mental illness in Hong Kong. *Int J Soc Psychiatry*. 2021;67(7):935-945. doi:10.1177/0020764020975792

62. Ho AH, Potash JS, Fong TC, et al. Psychometric properties of a Chinese version of the Stigma Scale: examining the complex experience of stigma and its relationship with self-esteem and depression among people living with mental illness in Hong Kong. *Compr Psychiatry*. 2015;56:198-205. doi:10.1016/j.comppsych.2014.09.016

63. Ho RWH, Chang WC, Kwong VWY, et al. Prediction of self-stigma in early psychosis: 3-Year follow-up of the randomized-controlled trial on extended early intervention. *Schizophr Res*. 2018;195:463-468. doi:10.1016/j.schres.2017.09.004

64. Sum MY, Chan SKW, Tse S, et al. Elucidating the relationship between internalized stigma, cognitive insight, illness severity, and functioning in patients with schizophrenia using a path analysis approach. *J Ment Health*. 2022;31(1):29-38. doi:10.1080/09638237.2020.1836553

65. Sum MY, Chan SKW, Tse S, Bola JR, Chen EYH. Internalized stigma as an independent predictor of employment status in patients with schizophrenia. *Psychiatr Rehabil J*. 2021;44(3):299-302. doi:10.1037/prj0000451

66. Chen ES, Chang WC, Hui CL, Chan SK, Lee EH, Chen EY. Self-stigma and affiliate stigma in first-episode psychosis patients and their caregivers. *Soc Psychiatry Psychiatr Epidemiol.* 2016;51(9):1225-1231. doi:10.1007/s00127-016-1221-8

67. Lee S, Lee MT, Chiu MY, Kleinman A. Experience of social stigma by people with schizophrenia in Hong Kong. *Br J Psychiatry.* 2005;186:153-157. doi:10.1192/bjp.186.2.153

68. Lee S, Chiu MY, Tsang A, Chui H, Kleinman A. Stigmatizing experience and structural discrimination associated with the treatment of schizophrenia in Hong Kong. *Soc Sci Med.* 2006;62(7):1685-1696. doi:10.1016/j.socscimed.2005.08.016

69. Ho DY. On the concept of face. *Am J Soc.* 1976;81:867-884.

70. Chan SKW, Kao SYS, Leung SL, et al. Relationship between neurocognitive function and clinical symptoms with self-stigma in patients with schizophrenia-spectrum disorders. *J Ment Health.* 2019;28(6):583-588. doi:10.1080/09638237.2017.1340599

3

Quality of Life and Functional Outcomes in Psychotic Disorders as Ultimate Intervention Targets

Health-related quality of life (QoL) encompasses physical, psychological, and social determinants that are influenced by an individual's experiences, expectations, beliefs, and perceptions (1). In contrast, QoL covers a much broader range of concerns and is defined by the World Health Organization as 'an individual's perception of their position in life in the context of the culture and value systems in which they live and in relation to their goals, expectations, standards and concerns' (2). In addition to health, other aspects such as relationships, educational attainment, work and social status, wealth, freedom and autonomy, spiritual and religious beliefs, a sense of security and safety, the environment, social belonging, and recreation affect the well-being of the individual (3). A uniform definition of QoL has been lacking and efforts have focused on delineating the sub-domains of ecology, economics, politics, and culture in order to allow for more accurate and meaningful assessment (3, 4).

In this chapter, we will focus on subjective health-related QoL and psychosocial functioning pertaining to first-episode psychosis (FEP).

Background: Short- and Long-Term Functional Outcomes and Quality of Life in Psychosis

It has been shown that short-term functional outcomes improve after treatment of the first episode, but longer-term outcomes remain relatively poor for a substantial proportion of patients. Poorer outcomes appear to be associated with early age of onset, poor premorbid adjustment, poor cognitive functioning, and negative symptoms during the prodromal and post-onset phases. In contrast, poor QoL is related to residual psychopathology, long delays in treatment, and poor premorbid adjustment (5).

Research in this area has been hampered by a lack of operational definitions, the choice of specific instruments to measure outcomes, and the use of large enough samples to generate meaningful results (5). Despite the lack of consensus definitions, attempts have been made to conceptualise outcomes as multidimensional constructs. For example, subjective quality of life (SQoL) is generally defined as an individual's perceived satisfaction with various life domains encompassing physical health, mental well-being, and social functioning (6, 7).

The overall QoL in FEP has been shown to be impaired, and there are complex interactions between QoL domains in relation to psychological well-being, symptoms, outlook, and physical health (8). There appears to be little correlation between patients' appraisal of their QoL and clinician assessment regarding their health status, whereas there is more agreement on functional outcomes such as occupational status, social relations, economic circumstances, and activities of daily living (8). However, measuring SQoL offers an opportunity to understand patients' illness experiences, their appraisal of self during different illness stages, as well as sociocultural beliefs, priorities, and values regarding their health. SQoL is not only impaired in FEP but also has been shown to predict symptomatic remission, relapse and functional outcomes (9, 10). Data has further suggested the potential clinical utility of integrating SQoL assessment with feedback in routine psychiatric care for schizophrenia patients to enhance patient-clinician communication and service satisfaction (11).

The severity of symptoms and duration of untreated psychosis have been identified as predictors of overall QoL, and depression has consistently been found to be a robust predictor of SQoL in first-episode populations (12, 13, 14, 15). Other important clinical variables such as premorbid adjustment and functioning have not been found to be consistently associated with SQoL (8, 13, 16, 17). The majority of studies have been conducted at initial presentation, likely showing higher impaired SQoL, and possibly skewing or obscuring potential factors related to SQoL. It is also possible that predictors of SQoL vary during the course of illness (18). For example, Gardsjord et al. (2016) followed up 186 FEP patients after their initial presentation and found that SQoL had significantly improved (13). More contact with family and a better financial situation at baseline had a positive and longstanding effect on SQoL. Higher depressive symptoms and fewer daily activities had a negative independent impact; however, these effects diminished over time. Conversely, a decrease in depressive symptoms and increased daily activities were associated with higher SQoL over time (13).

Only a handful of studies have examined the relationship between treatment-related factors and SQoL. Patients with chronic schizophrenia who reported anti-psychotic-induced extrapyramidal side effects experienced lower SQoL (19, 20, 21). Anxiety symptoms, including social anxiety, experienced by chronic schizophrenia patients are also associated with lower SQoL (22, 23, 24, 25). However, little evidence exists regarding the effects of co-occurring mental health difficulties in FEP.

The Outcome of Psychosis in Hong Kong

Functional Outcomes and Their Measurement

In Hong Kong, several studies have been undertaken to gain a better understanding of the interplay between clinical characteristics, cognitive functioning, treatment variables, remission, and psychosocial functioning in patients experiencing a first episode of psychosis.

Measurement of functional outcomes is often challenging. We reported on an improved measure to capture psychosocial outcomes in a more objective and comprehensive manner, the Life Functioning Assessment Inventory (L-FAI), which assesses four life domains including work, social relationships, leisure, and homemaking (26). The scale focuses on assessing the actual performance of individuals across different life domains rather than their capacities. The scale was found to have good reliability and validity and correlated well with some commonly used measures such as the Social and Occupational Functioning Assessment Scale and Role Functioning Scale.

Demographic Variables, Symptom Dimensions, and Functional Outcomes

From a follow-up study conducted over 13 years, Chang et al. (2019) established that most of our adult FEP patient cohort exhibited minimal or mild and stable negative symptoms. Only around 10% of psychosis patients experienced severe negative symptoms with a worsening course. Unsurprisingly, those who were most symptomatic had the worst long-term outcomes (27). In addition, general psychopathology and insight were shown to impact functioning and to have a mediating effect between cognitive ability and functional outcome (28).

The amotivational dimension of negative symptoms, as well as neurocognition and general self-efficacy, also directly affect global functioning during the early stages of psychosis with amotivation and anhedonia appearing to have a most critical impact on psychosocial outcome (29, 30, 31). In addition, amotivation appears to mediate a significant indirect effect of neurocognition and general self-efficacy on functioning (32). Impairments in effort-based decision-making, particularly the ability or willingness of FEP patients to proactively pursue effortful and highly rewarding goals, may underlie clinically observed amotivation (33, 34). This finding might be explained by the observation that patients were less likely to consider the benefits of a reward (34). Diminished cognitive flexibility may also play a role in amotivation (35). Chang et al. (2018) showed that lower levels of amotivation and better functioning at study intake independently predicted functional remission after three years of extended treatment in an early intervention (EI) service (36). An interesting finding has been that FEP individuals are more likely to be risk-averse compared to healthy controls (37). Whether this also contributes to the clinical picture of amotivation and affects functional outcomes remains to be seen.

In relation to demographic variables, functional outcomes at four months were correlated to the highest-ever occupational level rather than the levels immediately prior to contact with EI services (38). Also, cognitive functioning at initial contact was not predictive of outcome. However, following clinical stabilisation measures on visual memory and sustained attention were correlated to outcomes at four months follow-up (38). Another study reported that factors predictive of psychosocial functioning differed over time. At baseline, the severity of acute psychotic symptoms was the most determinant of the level of functioning. At six months, those with better insight at baseline actually had poorer functioning. At one year, only the basic demographics of gender and educational attainment predicted functioning levels. Female patients generally achieved better functional outcomes at all time points (39, 40, 41). After three years of EI, female gender remained a significant predictor of functional remission. In addition, lower levels of positive symptoms at intake, fewer premorbid schizoid-schizotypal traits, and better baseline functioning independently predicted functional remission (42). However, women in persistent socioeconomic difficulty, who represent up to half of all female FEP patients attending our EI programmes, had more severe depressive and negative symptoms, poorer cognitive ability, and worse social and occupational functioning at illness onset and warrant additional assistance and attention (43).

Chang et al. (2014) examined the vocational outcome of 93 FEP patients and its clinical and cognitive predictors over the course of three years (44). Approximately half of the patients were engaged in full-time work at the initial presentation and at three years. Of the 43 subjects who were not working at intake, just over half remained unemployed over three years. The sample's median length of full-time employment over the three-year follow-up period was eight months (mean = 13.6, SD = 14.6, range 0–36). Premorbid adjustment, baseline occupational status, and Wisconsin Card Sorting Test (WCST) performance were found to predict vocational outcomes. Analysis of a sub-group of patients who were unemployed at intake showed that subjects who remained unemployed over three years had poorer WCST performance and more severe positive symptoms at baseline than those having attained employment during follow-up (45). In addition to lower educational attainment and more severe negative symptoms after one year of treatment, more months of unemployment during the first three years of illness were also predictive of negative symptoms at ten-year follow-up (46).

Subjective Quality of Life Outcomes and Issues of Capacity

One of the challenges of using SQoL as an outcome measure in psychosis is that for some patients the difficulty in appraising and communicating their circumstances may affect SQoL ratings. To support the measurement of SQoL in patients with FEP or schizophrenia an inventory was developed to measure the capacity of patients to report on their QoL (47). It has been recognised that it is not uncommon for patients, particularly during the chronic stages of their illnesses, to lack the ability to accurately describe or assess their QoL. Cognitive impairment, communication difficulties, co-occurring mental health difficulties, symptom distress, and the burden of having to complete a SQoL assessment have also been cited as reasons for difficulties in appraising SQoL. The Capacity to report subjective Quality of Life (CapQOL) screening tool was designed with the aim of identifying people who are unable to complete SQoL measures. It is an interview questionnaire designed for use in people with a wide range of mental health and intellectual difficulties, that focuses on the cognitive ability of respondents to appraise and make judgements on their SQoL and their ability to complete a SQoL questionnaire. The measure consists of 12 questions based on five key areas, namely acquiescence (is the respondent likely to agree to any question asked), consistency in evaluations (is the individual answering questions consistently), understanding of the format of responses such as a 5-point scale, understanding of and values attached to each domain, and awareness of own situation and comparison with own standard or desirable ideal.

In addition to scores in each of the five key areas, a final global score is included at the end of the CapQOL. Utilising a 5-point scale, the global score records a score given by raters based on their general impression of the respondent's ability to complete the CapQOL, informed by their performance in the five key areas (47).

The CapQOL was administered to 442 young people with FEP at the point of entry into the Early Assessment Service for Young People (EASY) and its satisfactory psychometric properties were confirmed (47). 89% of participants obtained a global score of 4 or 5, indicating that the majority of participants had the ability to complete SQoL measures (47).

Remission, Subjective Quality of Life, and Psychosocial Functioning

Another focus of inquiry has centred on the relationship between remission status, SQoL, and functional outcome in FEP. The type of antipsychotic medication has been shown to influence the SQoL and psychosocial functioning of FEP patients (48). Also, it appears that those who experience impairments in one domain such as sexual dysfunction also have difficulties in other functional areas (49). In addition, it was established that higher levels of depression were associated with lower SQoL during the first five years of illness (49, 50, 51, 52, 53, 54). Patients who experienced significant psychosocial stressors and who had more pronounced positive symptoms, as well as marked extrapyramidal side effects and negative attitudes towards medication were more likely to suffer from depressive symptoms (54). Social anxiety also predicted lower SQoL scores, as did more severe positive symptoms, more pronounced negative attitudes towards medication, akathisia, and poorer functioning (49, 50, 52). We showed that psychosocial functioning may have an intermediary role in linking amotivation, neurocognitive impairment, and positive symptoms to SQoL in FEP patients (52). It also appears that younger age of onset and shorter EI intervention are correlated with a poor SQoL trajectory (50). A coping style characterised by difficulties discriminating threatening information may moreover affect SQoL (51). Another factor implicated in SQoL is whether a service is perceived to be recovery-oriented by patients (55).

Subjective Quality of Life and Duration of Untreated Psychosis

The length of untreated psychosis negatively impacts the general health of young people (56, 57). Those with a duration of untreated psychosis (DUP) greater than 12 months have lower general health scores on the 36-item short-form health survey (SF-36) compared to those with a shorter DUP, and low SQoL scores were correlated with negative symptoms. This is on a background of already significantly reduced SQoL experienced by psychosis sufferers when compared to healthy controls (56, 57, 58).

Reflections: The Importance of Context

There are several difficulties associated with measuring functional outcomes. The expected role functioning of an individual is not only affected by cognitive, emotional, and physical abilities but also influenced by sociocultural expectations, subjective values, and life stage. Whether a person is able to function to their fullest abilities thus is context-dependent. With the development of the Life Functioning Assessment Inventory (L-FAI), we have included a much broader set of domains paying particular attention to context to improve the reliability of functional assessments. Subsequent studies showed that less severe illness and better baseline functioning predict better psychosocial outcomes over the course of a patient's illness. The outcomes of EI are discussed in more detail in Chapter 8.

The SQoL of individuals with psychosis is perceived to be significantly lower compared to the general population and is not only determined by the psychotic illness per se but also affected by the presence of depressive and anxiety symptoms, side effects of medication, cognitive ability, functioning, motivation, coping style, and stigma.

The measurement of SQoL can be challenging due to its subjective nature. Patients' views on what is important to living 'a good life' likely change during the course of illness due to habituation and adaptation to living with a chronic disorder. SQoL is also a highly individual concept, even more so than functional outcome, and not necessarily reflective of a person's life circumstances.

Motivation and an adaptive coping style have emerged as potential therapeutic targets. Life coaching adapted to the needs of FEP patients has been introduced at the Jockey Club Early Psychosis Project (JCEP) programmes. In a group setting, patients are encouraged to identify a goal and are supported to achieve their objectives using a reward-based strategy.

Supporting patients to improve their SQoL and psychosocial functioning remains a complex and challenging endeavour. Individualised treatment with a focus on appropriate psychopharmacological treatment, addressing co-occurring mental health conditions, and co-producing treatment plans taking individual values and goals into account will likely go a long way to improving SQoL. In addition to offering psychopharmacological treatment, the provision of motivational approaches, cognitive remediation, and tailored exercise programmes, as well as addressing stigma may positively impact clinical and functional remission or recovery. This individualised and holistic approach appears promising in helping patients to adapt to living with a chronic illness, develop meaningful relationships and find purpose in life.

References

1. Testa MA, Simonson DC. Assessment of quality-of-life outcomes. *N Engl J Med.* 1996;334(13):835-840. doi:10.1056/NEJM199603283341306
2. World Health Organization. *WHOQOL: Measuring Quality of Life.* World Health Organization. Mar 1, 2012. Accessed May 5, 2023. https://www.who.int/toolkits/whoqol
3. Teoli D, Bhardwaj A. Quality of Life. Updated Mar 26, 2022. In: *StatPearls* [Internet]. Treasure Island (FL): StatPearls Publishing; Jan- 2023. Accessed May 5, 2023. https://www.ncbi.nlm.nih.gov/books/NBK536962/#
4. Magee, L, Scerri A, James P. Measuring social sustainability: a community-centred approach. *Applied Research Quality Life.* 2012; 7:239-261. doi:10.1007/s11482-012-9166-x
5. Malla A, Payne J. First-episode psychosis: psychopathology, quality of life, and functional outcome. *Schizophr Bull.* 2005;31(3):650-671. doi:10.1093/schbul/sbi031
6. Lehman AF. Measures of quality of life among persons with severe and persistent mental disorders. *Soc Psychiatry Psychiatr Epidemiol.* 1996;31(2):78-88. doi:10.1007/BF00801903

7. Development of the World Health Organization WHOQOL-BREF quality of life assessment. The WHOQOL Group. *Psychol Med.* 1998;28(3):551-558. doi:10.1017/s0033291798006667

8. Renwick L, Drennan J, Sheridan A, et al. Subjective and objective quality of life at first presentation with psychosis. *Early Interv Psychiatry.* 2017;11(5):401-410. doi:10.1111/eip.12255

9. Lambert M, Naber D, Eich FX, Schacht M, Linden M, Schimmelmann BG. Remission of severely impaired subjective wellbeing in 727 patients with schizophrenia treated with amisulpride. *Acta Psychiatr Scand.* 2007;115(2):106-113. doi:10.1111/j.1600-0447.2006.00862.x

10. Boyer L, Millier A, Perthame E, Aballea S, Auquier P, Toumi M. Quality of life is predictive of relapse in schizophrenia. *BMC Psychiatry.* 2013;13:15. Published Jan 9, 2013. doi:10.1186/1471-244X-13-15

11. Boyer L, Lançon C, Baumstarck K, Parola N, Berbis J, Auquier P. Evaluating the impact of a quality of life assessment with feedback to clinicians in patients with schizophrenia: randomised controlled trial. *Br J Psychiatry.* 2013;202:447-453. doi:10.1192/bjp.bp.112.123463

12. Watson P, Zhang JP, Rizvi A, Tamaiev J, Birnbaum ML, Kane J. A meta-analysis of factors associated with quality of life in first episode psychosis. *Schizophr Res.* 2018;202:26-36. doi:10.1016/j.schres.2018.07.013

13. Gardsjord ES, Romm KL, Friis S, et al. Subjective quality of life in first-episode psychosis: a ten-year follow-up study. *Schizophr Res.* 2016;172(1-3):23-28. doi:10.1016/j.schres.2016.02.034

14. Malla AK, Norman RM, McLean TS, et al. Determinants of quality of life in first-episode psychosis. *Acta Psychiatr Scand.* 2004;109(1):46-54. doi:10.1046/j.0001-690x.2003.00221.x

15. Renwick L, Jackson D, Foley S, et al. Depression and quality of life in first-episode psychosis. *Compr Psychiatry.* 2012;53(5):451-455. doi:10.1016/j.comppsych.2011.07.003

16. MacBeth A, Gumley A, Schwannauer M, Fisher R. Self-reported quality of life in a Scottish first-episode psychosis cohort: associations with symptomatology and premorbid adjustment. *Early Interv Psychiatry.* 2015;9(1):53-60. doi:10.1111/eip.12087

17. Cotton SM, Gleeson JF, Alvarez-Jimenez M, McGorry PD. Quality of life in patients who have remitted from their first episode of psychosis. *Schizophr Res.* 2010;121(1-3):259-265. doi:10.1016/j.schres.2010.05.027

18. Bow-Thomas CC, Velligan DI, Miller AL, Olsen J. Predicting quality of life from symptomatology in schizophrenia at exacerbation and stabilization. *Psychiatry Res.* 1999;86(2):131-142. doi:10.1016/s0165-1781(99)00023-2

19. Awad AG, Voruganti LN, Heslegrave RJ. A conceptual model of quality of life in schizophrenia: description and preliminary clinical validation. *Qual Life Res.* 1997;6(1):21-26. doi:10.1023/a:1026409326690

20. Browne S, Garavan J, Gervin M, Roe M, Larkin C, O'Callaghan E. Quality of life in schizophrenia: insight and subjective response to neuroleptics. *J Nerv Ment Dis.* 1998;186(2):74-78. doi:10.1097/00005053-199802000-00002

21. Hofer A, Kemmler G, Eder U, Edlinger M, Hummer M, Fleischhacker WW. Quality of life in schizophrenia: the impact of psychopathology, attitude toward medication, and side effects. *J Clin Psychiatry*. 2004;65(7):932-939.
22. Huppert JD, Smith TE. Longitudinal analysis of subjective quality of life in schizophrenia: anxiety as the best symptom predictor. *J Nerv Ment Dis*. 2001;189(10):669-675. doi:10.1097/00005053-200110000-00003
23. Braga RJ, Mendlowicz MV, Marrocos RP, Figueira IL. Anxiety disorders in outpatients with schizophrenia: prevalence and impact on the subjective quality of life. *J Psychiatr Res*. 2005;39(4):409-414. doi:10.1016/j.jpsychires.2004.09.003
24. Pallanti S, Quercioli L, Hollander E. Social anxiety in outpatients with schizophrenia: a relevant cause of disability. *Am J Psychiatry*. 2004;161(1):53-58. doi:10.1176/appi.ajp.161.1.53
25. Kumazaki H, Kobayashi H, Niimura H, et al. Lower subjective quality of life and the development of social anxiety symptoms after the discharge of elderly patients with remitted schizophrenia: a 5-year longitudinal study. *Compr Psychiatry*. 2012;53(7):946-951. doi:10.1016/j.comppsych.2012.03.002
26. Hui CL, Li YK, Leung KF, et al. Reliability and validity of the life functioning assessment inventory (L-FAI) for patients with psychosis. *Soc Psychiatry Psychiatr Epidemiol*. 2013;48(10):1687-1695. doi:10.1007/s00127-013-0679-x
27. Chang WC, Ho RWH, Tang JYM, et al. Early-stage negative symptom trajectories and relationships with 13-year outcomes in first-episode nonaffective psychosis. *Schizophr Bull*. 2019;45(3):610-619. doi:10.1093/schbul/sby115
28. Lee EHM, Hui CLM, Chan KPK, et al. The role of symptoms and insight in mediating cognition and functioning in first episode psychosis. *Schizophr Res*. 2019;206:251-256. doi:10.1016/j.schres.2018.11.009
29. Chang WC, Wong CSM, Or PCF, et al. Inter-relationships among psychopathology, premorbid adjustment, cognition and psychosocial functioning in first-episode psychosis: a network analysis approach. *Psychol Med*. 2020;50(12):2019-2027. doi:10.1017/S0033291719002113
30. Chang WC, Hui CL, Chan SK, Lee EH, Chen EY. Impact of avolition and cognitive impairment on functional outcome in first-episode schizophrenia-spectrum disorder: a prospective one-year follow-up study. *Schizophr Res*. 2016;170(2-3):318-321. doi:10.1016/j.schres.2016.01.004
31. Hu HX, Lau WYS, Ma EPY, et al. the important role of motivation and pleasure deficits on social functioning in patients with schizophrenia: a network analysis. *Schizophr Bull*. 2022;48(4):860-870. doi:10.1093/schbul/sbac017
32. Chang WC, Kwong VW, Hui CL, Chan SK, Lee EH, Chen EY. Relationship of amotivation to neurocognition, self-efficacy and functioning in first-episode psychosis: a structural equation modeling approach. *Psychol Med*. 2017;47(4):755-765. doi:10.1017/S0033291716003044
33. Chang WC, Chu AOK, Treadway MT, et al. Effort-based decision-making impairment in patients with clinically-stabilized first-episode psychosis and its relationship with amotivation and psychosocial functioning. *Eur Neuropsychopharmacol*. 2019;29(5):629-642. doi:10.1016/j.euroneuro.2019.03.006

34. Chang WC, Westbrook A, Strauss GP, et al. Abnormal cognitive effort allocation and its association with amotivation in first-episode psychosis. *Psychol Med*. 2020;50(15):2599-2609. doi:10.1017/S0033291719002769

35. Chang WC, Liu JTT, Hui CLM, et al. Executive dysfunctions differentially predict amotivation in first-episode schizophrenia-spectrum disorder: a prospective 1-year follow-up study. *Eur Arch Psychiatry Clin Neurosci*. 2019;269(8):887-896. doi:10.1007/s00406-018-0918-y

36. Chang WC, Kwong VWY, Or Chi Fai P, et al. Motivational impairment predicts functional remission in first-episode psychosis: 3-Year follow-up of the randomized controlled trial on extended early intervention. *Aust N Z J Psychiatry*. 2018;52(12):1194-1201. doi:10.1177/0004867418758918

37. Msk L, Wc C, Csy C, et al. Altered risky decision making in patients with early non-affective psychosis. *Eur Arch Psychiatry Clin Neurosci*. 2021;271(4):723-731. doi:10.1007/s00406-019-00994-2

38. Chen EYH, Dunn ELW, Chen RYL, et al. Predictors of short-term functional outcome following first episode psychosis. The 10th Biennial Winter Workshop on Schizophrenia; Feb 5–11, 2000; Davos, Switzerland. In *Schizophr Res*. 2000;41(1):297, abstract B.331. doi:10.1016/S0920-9964(00)91056-9

39. Chong CS, Siu MW, Kwan CH, et al. Predictors of functioning in people suffering from first-episode psychosis 1 year into entering early intervention service in Hong Kong. *Early Interv Psychiatry*. 2018;12(5):828-838. doi:10.1111/eip.12374

40. Chang WC, Tang JY, Hui CL, et al. Gender differences in patients presenting with first-episode psychosis in Hong Kong: a three-year follow up study. *Aust N Z J Psychiatry*. 2011;45(3):199-205. doi:10.3109/00048674.2010.547841

41. Hui CL, Leung CM, Chang WC, Chan SK, Lee EH, Chen EY. Examining gender difference in adult-onset psychosis in Hong Kong. *Early Interv Psychiatry*. 2016;10(4):324-333. doi:10.1111/eip.12167

42. Chang WC, Kwong VW, Chan GH, et al. Prediction of functional remission in first-episode psychosis: 12-month follow-up of the randomized-controlled trial on extended early intervention in Hong Kong. *Schizophr Res*. 2016;173(1-2):79-83. doi:10.1016/j.schres.2016.03.016

43. Hui CLM, Ko WT, Chang WC, Lee EHM, Chan SKW, Chen EYH. Clinical and functional correlates of financially deprived women with first-episode psychosis. *Early Interv Psychiatry*. 2019;13(3):639-645. doi:10.1111/eip.12551

44. Chang WC, Man Tang JY, Ming Hui CL, Wa Chan SK, Ming Lee EH, Hai Chen EY. Clinical and cognitive predictors of vocational outcome in first-episode schizophrenia: a prospective 3-year follow-up study. *Psychiatry Res*. 2014;220(3):834-839. doi:10.1016/j.psychres.2014.09.012

45. Chen EY, Tam DK, Dunn EL, et al. Neurocognitive and clinical predictors for vocational outcome following first episode schizophrenia: a 3-year prospective study. The 20th International Congress on Schizophrenia Research; Apr 2–6, 2005; Savannah, GA. In *Schizophr Bull*. 2005;31(2):320. doi:10.1093/schbul/sbi024

46. Chan SKW, Chan HYV, Pang HH, et al. Ten-year trajectory and outcomes of negative symptoms of patients with first-episode schizophrenia spectrum disorders. *Schizophr Res*. 2020;220:85-91. doi:10.1016/j.schres.2020.03.061

47. Wong JG, Cheung EP, Chen EY, et al. An instrument to assess mental patients' capacity to appraise and report subjective quality of life. *Qual Life Res.* 2005;14(3):687-694. doi:10.1007/s11136-004-1215-y

48. Lee EH, Hui CL, Lin JJ, et al. Quality of life and functioning in first-episode psychosis Chinese patients with different antipsychotic medications. *Early Interv Psychiatry.* 2016;10(6):535-539. doi:10.1111/eip.12246

49. Hui CL, Lee EH, Chang WC, et al. Sexual dysfunction in Chinese patients with first-episode psychosis: prevalence, clinical correlates and functioning. *Schizophr Res.* 2013;148(1-3):181-182. doi:10.1016/j.schres.2013.06.004

50. Kwong VW, Chang WC, Chan GH, et al. Clinical and treatment-related determinants of subjective quality of life in patients with first-episode psychosis. *Psychiatry Res.* 2017;249:39-45. doi:10.1016/j.psychres.2016.12.038

51. Kam CTK, Chang WC, Kwong VWY, et al. Patterns and predictors of trajectories for subjective quality of life in patients with early psychosis: three-year follow-up of the randomized controlled trial on extended early intervention. *Aust N Z J Psychiatry.* 2021;55(10):983-992. doi:10.1177/00048674211009603

52. Wong A, Chiu CY, Chen YH. Discriminative facility as a predictor of psychological health amongst patients with schizophrenia. The 9th International Congress on Schizophrenia Research; Mar 29–Apr 2, 2003; Colorado Springs, CO. In *Schizophr Res.* 2003;60(1)(Suppl.):331. doi:10.1016/S0920-9964(03)80309-2

53. Wong SCY, Chang WC, Hui CLM, et al. Relationship of subjective quality of life with symptomatology, neurocognition and psychosocial functioning in first-episode psychosis: a structural equation modelling approach. *Eur Arch Psychiatry Clin Neurosci.* 2021;271(8):1561-1569. doi:10.1007/s00406-021-01309-0

54. Chang WC, Cheung R, Hui CL, et al. Rate and risk factors of depressive symptoms in Chinese patients presenting with first-episode non-affective psychosis in Hong Kong. *Schizophr Res.* 2015;168(1-2):99-105. doi:10.1016/j.schres.2015.07.040

55. Sum MY, Chan SKW, Tse S, et al. Relationship between subjective quality of life and perceptions of recovery orientation of treatment service in patients with schizophrenia and major depressive disorder. *Asian J Psychiatr.* 2021;57:102578. doi:10.1016/j.ajp.2021.102578

56. Law CW, Chen EY, Cheung EF, et al. Impact of untreated psychosis on quality of life in patients with first-episode schizophrenia. *Qual Life Res.* 2005;14(8):1803-1811. doi:10.1007/s11136-005-3236-6

57. Law C, Chen EY, Cheung EF, Chan RC, Lam CL, Lo MS. Study of quality of life in first-episode psychotic patients in the period of untreated psychosis. The 9th International Congress on Schizophrenia Research; Mar 29–Apr 2, 2003; Colorado Springs, CO. In *Schizophr Res.* 2003;60(Suppl. 1):338. doi:10.1016/S0920-9964(03)80330-4

58. Lam CLK, Lauder IJ, Lam TP, Gandek B. Population based norming of the Chinese (HK) version of the SF-36 health survey. *HK Pract.* 1999;21:460-470.

PART II

EARLY INTERVENTION FOR PSYCHOSIS

4

Early Intervention in Psychosis: A Paradigm Shift

Background: Services for Psychotic Disorders in Hong Kong before Early Intervention

In Hong Kong, in the late 1990s, there had been increasing recognition that patients with psychotic disorders were not well served by traditional psychiatric services. With an estimated lifetime prevalence of approximately 2.5%, this represented an increasingly pressing public health concern (1). The majority of psychiatric care for a population of 7.34 million is provided by the government-subsidised public healthcare system. Hong Kong has a high population density, and people typically live with family members due to the high cost of living and stronger family ties compared to Western cultures. Over 90% of the population is Han Chinese, and Cantonese is the primary language (2). Patients with suspected psychosis required a referral from their general practitioner before being seen in public outpatient services. Waiting times for assessment and treatment were often several months. A smaller proportion of acutely ill patients were treated in the private sector. However, psychiatric emergency care and inpatient treatment are predominantly provided by government hospitals.

In the 1990s, individuals with psychotic symptoms often came into contact with services at a time of crisis involving significant risks of self-injury and violence. Late presentations were not unusual and frequently resulted in attendance at accident and emergency departments (AEDs) with subsequent hospitalisation. Upon discharge, patients received ongoing psychiatric reviews in crowded outpatient clinics. Clinic consultation times averaged only five to six minutes, follow-up appointments were infrequent and community therapeutic interventions were limited (3). The duration of untreated psychosis in Hong Kong was long, with a median of 150 days

(4). It was thought that this was due to a lack of symptom awareness in the wider population, mental health stigma, and scarcity of services (5, 6).

Global Background and Historical Context of Early Intervention for Psychosis

Worldwide, a re-focusing on early intervention (EI) as a means to improve outcomes of patients with psychotic disorders started with pioneering programmes such as the Early Psychosis Prevention and Intervention Centre (EPPIC) programme in Melbourne and an early identification and treatment programme in Norway (7, 8). Evidence at the time suggested that EI produced better treatment response and reduced long-term morbidity (9, 10). Also, it had been shown that a long duration of untreated psychosis (DUP) was associated with a longer time to recovery (11). These early research findings led to the implementation of EI services around the world, including in North America, Europe, and Southeast Asia (12, 13, 14, 15, 16).

However, the roots of EI in the treatment of mental illness were laid in the nineteenth century (17). At the time, a number of psychiatrists, such as William Charles Ellis, pointed out that patients admitted to asylums were receiving treatment too late in the course of their illness (18). This view was based on the observation that mental illnesses were generally considered progressive and incurable (17). With the emergence of systematic descriptive psychopathology during the nineteenth century the view that 'insanity' was caused by a disease of the brain became generally accepted. Aetiological hypotheses, including genetic factors, brain abnormalities, and psychological vulnerabilities, were proposed as causative components of the disorder. Ellis further divided 'insanity' into 'incipient' and 'chronic insanity' and expected improvement or cure only for incipient cases, while holding that chronic illness was associated with irrevocable damage (19).

Despite differentiating stages of severe mental illness and advocating for early treatment, interventions in the nineteenth century were often only delivered once disorders had progressed. We thought that this was due to the reluctance of relatives, carers, and the authorities to send patients to asylums (17). In the UK, for example, admission to asylums was regulated by the Lunacy Act. A patient considered to have a serious mental illness had to be certified as 'insane' by a doctor and also required a compulsory reception order from a local magistrate (20).

In the early twentieth century, the notion of EI appeared to have been sidelined, possibly due to the fact that physical and psychological treatments had shown limited effectiveness in treating psychotic disorders. Disagreements regarding aetiology and treatment – i.e., purely biological, psychodynamic, or psychosocial frameworks – were also likely to have played a role in impeding the development of effective models of care.

The discovery of first-generation antipsychotics in the 1950s hastened the deinstitutionalisation of patients (21). However, it was not before the 1980s that the Northwick Park team first reported a correlation between delayed treatment and impaired outcomes in patients with first-episode schizophrenia (22).

We argued that early treatment for schizophrenia may have been neglected because it had been viewed as a disorder with a predetermined poor prognosis during the early and mid-twentieth century (23). In addition to psychopharmacological treatments, we considered paying close attention to balancing antipsychotic therapeutic effects and side effects, and focusing on the assessment and management of co-occurring conditions such as depression, anxiety as well as suicide and serious self-harm. Psychosocial interventions to reduce negative symptoms and improve social skills and occupational functioning are essential treatments (24).

Early Intervention for Psychosis in Hong Kong

The EASY Programme: Its Principles, Aims, and Service Specifications

In order to reduce the duration of untreated psychosis (DUP) and to improve outcomes for patients with psychosis, the Early Assessment Service for Young People (EASY) was launched in Hong Kong in 2001, embedding it within established public psychiatric services, with links to local community networks and non-governmental organisations (NGOs). Alongside providing a specialist clinical service to optimise access and treatment for first-episode psychosis, it aimed to offer a phase-specific intervention to reduce stigma and raise public awareness.

Singapore has also implemented an EI programme in 2001. Both cities developed services based on the shared principles of facilitating easy access, offering individually tailored phase-specific interventions and addressing stigma through public education campaigns. Singapore decided to operate a single service across the city, while Hong Kong favoured smaller localised teams due to the administrative structure of the health service.

The EASY programme was developed to accept patients aged 15 to 25 who would be supported by a specialist team consisting of psychiatrists, nurse case managers, social workers, and a clinical psychologist over a two-year period. Four catchment areas were established with four separate teams each covering a population of around 1.5 million (24, 25).

To allow easy access to the service, an open hotline was offered, which was unprecedented in mental health services. Staff from the EASY service provided telephone-based engagement for potential patients or informants. These intake assessments were carried out by key workers who received training to identify potential cases of first-episode psychosis who would benefit from the EASY programme. Contact was made from a range of sources such as through a hotline,

68 • *Psychosis and Schizophrenia in Hong Kong*

e-mail, walk-ins, NGOs, and school social workers, and within the healthcare system through triage from outpatient departments, non-EASY psychiatrists, consultation-liaison teams, inpatient departments, and AEDs. Eligible patients were provided with a comprehensive psychiatric assessment within days of the initial contact and were offered flexible appointments to facilitate engagement. Whenever possible, assessments were carried out in non-stigmatising settings such as on the premises of an NGO or general hospital to reduce barriers to accessing care (26).

Treatment was based on the principle of offering assertive and phase-specific interventions for patients diagnosed with a psychotic disorder (27). Each patient was assigned a case manager or key worker who provided phase-specific psychosocial care. This included engaging the patient and carers, undertaking a comprehensive assessment of symptoms, psychosocial needs and functioning, offering regular follow-up, and liaising with carers and other relevant professionals. This approach ensured that patients were offered continuity, which facilitated rapport building, a more thorough understanding of patients' histories, and individual needs, as well as better risk management.

A case management protocol was developed based on the International Clinical Practice Guidelines for Early Psychosis, the Psychological Intervention Programme in Early Psychosis (PIPE) (28). PIPE has three modules, (i) enhancing psychological adjustment to early psychosis; (ii) intervention for secondary morbidity; and (iii) cognitive-behavioural therapy (CBT) for drug-resistant psychotic symptoms. The intervention addresses psychological issues at different stages of illness to enhance psychosocial functioning and is delivered in the form of psychoeducation for patients and families, and individual and family psychological support. The programme aims to support patients in developing an understanding of their illness, dealing with the uncertainty about the course of the disorder, the subjective experience of cognitive dysfunction and subtle symptoms, functional recovery, and handling the need for maintenance medication and the risk of relapse. In addition, carers have access to an interactive internet-based carer self-help psychoeducation programme, iPEP. It provides comprehensive written and video-based resources covering subjects such as knowledge about psychosis and carer skills, and provides links to locally available carer support. A forum allows carers to directly communicate with healthcare practitioners to enhance self-management skills (29).

EASY case management is offered during the first two years of treatment. In the third year, patients are stepped down to psychiatric follow-up before being transferred to general psychiatric services. All staff have been trained in the interventions of the PIPE protocol. Regular centralised training sessions are offered to clinicians and annual training days involving all staff are provided. Local and international skill updates are arranged regularly.

In addition, patients are offered community programmes by collaborating NGOs and vocational training centres to facilitate psychosocial rehabilitation. Each EASY team collaborates with a network of local NGOs to co-design engagement programmes for young people recovering from psychosis. These programmes aim at normalisation, social integration, and improvement in functioning. The EASY service hosts an annual workshop where NGOs collaborating with all four regional EASY teams gather to share their ideas and experiences.

Our Public Awareness Campaign

The EASY programme also established a working group of clinicians and media experts to raise public awareness by organising public education programmes. The strategy was a two-pronged approach involving (1) large-scale dissemination of simple information about psychotic symptoms, and the need for assessment, with information on the EASY hotline; and (2) in-depth information for young people aimed at reducing stigma and facilitating detection of psychosis among peer networks. Information about psychotic symptoms was distributed in leaflets, on posters, in exhibitions, in public talks, during school visits and roadshows, via radio and TV interviews, during press releases, in advertisements, as well as on social media and websites. To reduce stigma, the team also sought to rename the Chinese translation of 'psychosis' and introduced the term *sijueshitiao* (思覺失調). A charity, the Early Psychosis Foundation (EPISO), was created in 2007 to enable more agile public awareness and anti-stigma campaigns and the training of frontline staff in public services and NGOs.

During the education campaign, it was emphasised that *sijueshitiao* (思覺失調) referred to a symptom cluster or syndrome of an early abnormal mental state and that it was not a diagnosis. In particular, the term was not just another name for 'schizophrenia'. This approach has helped to increase wider public acceptance of the condition and awareness of its signs and symptoms (24, 30).

Early Outcomes of the EASY Programme

In the first decade of the programme, there was a significant reduction in the DUP from a median of 150 to 105 days (30, 31). More patients in their first episode were managed as outpatients. More positive symptoms were noted at four months of treatment compared to controls, possibly suggesting more cautious use of antipsychotic medication in the EASY population. Negative symptoms were significantly lower in the EASY group after one year of treatment.

A large-scale three-year follow-up case-control study was carried out to compare clinical and functional outcomes between 700 patients in the EASY programme and 700 case controls who had received standard care just before its launch (32).

Subjects were matched for age, sex, diagnosis, and highest premorbid functional levels. They had comparable illness severity in positive and negative symptoms at presentation. Subjects in the EI group had significantly fewer days of hospitalisation, less severe positive and negative symptoms, fewer suicides, fewer dropouts, and a higher likelihood of achieving a period of recovery compared to the control group after three years. Both groups were similar in their rates of relapse and DUP (32). We later revisited whether the two-year duration of the EASY service was optimal using a randomised controlled trial (RCT) comparing two years to three years of case management and observed that the three-year programme offered additional advantages in functional outcomes (33).

On average, EASY receives 3000 hotline enquiries and carries out around 1000 assessments each year. Sources of referrals are predominantly from inpatient and outpatient settings, as well as relatives of patients (26%, 25%, and 23%, respectively). Self-referrals account for 8% of contacts. Each team has an active caseload of around 360 patients, and average caseloads for key workers have been between 1:80 and 1:100 (34). Despite high caseloads, the EASY programme was shown to be more cost-effective than standard care by reducing hospital admissions, AED attendance, and the use of community psychiatric services (35).

The Jockey Club Early Psychosis Project

In recognition of the fact that around half of all psychotic disorders begin over the age of 25 years, a five-year early psychosis pilot project for adult patients called the Jockey Club Early Psychosis Project (JCEP) was introduced in 2009 (34, 36, 37). The programme would also allow us to gain a better understanding of the impacts of EI on later-onset psychotic disorders (38). Like in the EASY programme, close collaboration with NGOs was fostered to deliver a phase-specific case management intervention for 1000 first-episode patients aged 26 to 55 years. Psychosocial interventions included elements of life coaching, cognitive-behavioural therapy for psychosis (CBTp), and case management tailored to patients' illness stage and needs. An RCT to compare functional outcomes and cost-effectiveness of two- versus four-year case management was an integral part of the project. Following its early positive outcomes, the EASY programme was extended in 2011 to cover the entire adult age range, i.e., over 25 years of age, for a period of three years after the first episode (30, 33).

Psychosis Studies: An Innovative Postgraduate Programme

To offer more formal training and education on psychotic disorders, we started offering a postgraduate programme in Psychosis Studies in 2011. The course covers epidemiology, aetiology, and symptomatology of psychosis, as well as specific skills considered to be crucial in early interventions, such as psychopharmacology and psychosocial interventions. The emphasis on hands-on research experience equips students with a critical mindset for evidence-based information. The programme has attracted students from diverse backgrounds and professions (35).

Reflections: Meeting the Local Needs of Psychosis Patients

Early intervention for psychosis has evolved from a recognition of the fact that delayed presentation and treatment may have an impact on outcome. The development of early intervention services has been guided by data on the DUP as well as evidence-based evaluation of treatment outcomes. The essential ingredients of EI have been distilled into three principles (1) early detection and reduction of DUP; (2) the provision of phase-specific treatment in the early years of a psychotic disorder in the so-called critical period; and (3) preventative intervention in the clinical high-risk state (39).

With these objectives in mind, EI services developed their own strategies and priorities to meet the needs of their local population. The components required to achieve the implementation of the global goals should be driven by local data (40).

In Hong Kong, the delay in presentation has been shown to be related to family knowledge of psychosis. In order to reduce the DUP, it will therefore be important to increase the knowledge of psychotic symptoms in families in which psychosis cases could emerge. Since it is impossible to predict which families will be affected by psychosis, a more general psychoeducational strategy for the entire population is necessary. This strategy is supported by gatekeeper training, particularly for young people entering the age of increased risk of psychosis onset. Efforts to reduce the DUP in Hong Kong have been successful in reducing the very long DUP in some patients, especially among the adult-onset population. EI appears to have a more limited effect on the DUP of young people, which was already shorter than the DUP for adults. Since specialised EI targets young people in the initial stage of illness, there is a dissociation between DUP reduction and phase-specific intervention, in that young people received phase-specific intervention but the DUP has not significantly changed. The outcome benefits we saw in the early stages of the EASY service therefore could be attributed to phase-specific intervention rather than DUP reduction.

How do we know that we are not merely engaging individuals with milder symptoms in a population? Three pieces of evidence are relevant: our case-control studies showed that patients from the EASY programme have had the same highest functional levels as control patients. They also have had the same rates of relapse. In addition, a recent epidemiological study of young people confirms that over 85% of young people with psychotic disorders in the community have engaged with the EASY service. The short-term benefits of a specialised EI team were a clear-cut reduction in hospitalisations and improved functional outcomes. Longer-term sustained benefits have also been observed and will be discussed in Chapter 8.

In Hong Kong, we have therefore witnessed the initial success of EI for psychosis with improved outcomes over a sustained period of time without increasing costs. It is also of interest that increasing the length of treatment from two to three years is associated with further functional gains, suggesting that further improvements in functioning can be attained through a longer period of intervention. However, we have also seen that the additional benefits of the third year of treatment appear to be less sustained over time. This may suggest a diminishing return of clinical benefit, with later inputs having a more transient effect on outcome than earlier intervention.

One notable development for the Hong Kong EI programme was the extension of services to cover adult-onset psychosis patients. Age-related differences in the outcome of psychosis are well known in that younger age of onset is associated with poorer outcomes. As a result, we postulated that the scope for improvement in the adult-onset population may be more limited. We observed in our sample that additional case management improved outcomes only for those patients who initially experienced a long treatment delay. In contrast, additional benefits for adult-onset cases with a short DUP were less obvious.

The development of public services for EI in psychosis in Hong Kong has focused on phase-specific intervention for first-episode psychosis patients. Reducing DUP through alleviating stigma and psychoeducation has mainly been undertaken by the charity sector and volunteer organisations. Preventative intervention for high-risk states has been explored in community settings and will be further discussed in Chapter 7.

References

1. Chang WC, Wong CSM, Chen EYH, et al. Lifetime prevalence and correlates of schizophrenia-spectrum, affective, and other non-affective psychotic disorders in the Chinese adult population. *Schizophr Bull.* 2017;43(6):1280-1290. doi:10.1093/schbul/sbx056

2. Population By-census Office. *Domestic Households by Household Size and Type of Quarters, 2016.* Census and Statistics Department. 2016. Accessed Feb 28, 2023. https://www.bycensus2016.gov.hk/en/index.html

3. Hui C, Wong G, Lam C, Chow P, Chen E. Patient-clinician communication and needs identification for outpatients with schizophrenia in Hong Kong: role of the 2-COM instrument. *Hong Kong Journal of Psychiatry.* 2008;18:92-100.

4. Chen EY, Dunn EL, Miao MY, et al. The impact of family experience on the duration of untreated psychosis (DUP) in Hong Kong. *Soc Psychiatry Psychiatr Epidemiol.* 2005;40(5):350-356. doi:10.1007/s00127-005-0908-z

5. Chung KF, Chen EY, Lam LC, Chen RY, Chan CK. How are psychotic symptoms perceived? A comparison between patients, relatives and the general public. *Aust N Z J Psychiatry.* 1997;31(5):756-761. doi:10.3109/00048679709062691

6. Chung KF, Wong MC. Experience of stigma among Chinese mental health patients in Hong Kong. *Psychiatric Bull.* 2004;28:451-454.
7. Larsen TK, McGlashan TH, Moe LC. First-episode schizophrenia: I. Early course parameters. *Schizophr Bull.* 1996;22(2):241-256. doi:10.1093/schbul/22.2.241
8. McGorry PD, Edwards J, Mihalopoulos C, Harrigan SM, Jackson HJ. EPPIC: an evolving system of early detection and optimal management. *Schizophr Bull.* 1996;22(2):305-326. doi:10.1093/schbul/22.2.305
9. Lieberman J, Jody D, Geisler S, et al. Time course and biologic correlates of treatment response in first-episode schizophrenia. *Arch Gen Psychiatry.* 1993;50(5):369-376. doi:10.1001/archpsyc.1993.01820170047006
10. Wyatt RJ. Neuroleptics and the natural course of schizophrenia. *Schizophr Bull.* 1991;17(2):325-351. doi:10.1093/schbul/17.2.325
11. Loebel AD, Lieberman JA, Alvir JM, Mayerhoff DI, Geisler SH, Szymanski SR. Duration of psychosis and outcome in first-episode schizophrenia. *Am J Psychiatry.* 1992;149(9):1183-1188. doi:10.1176/ajp.149.9.1183
12. Malla A, Norman R, McLean T, Scholten D, Townsend L. A Canadian programme for early intervention in non-affective psychotic disorders. *Aust N Z J Psychiatry.* 2003;37(4):407-413. doi:10.1046/j.1440-1614.2003.01194.x
13. Craig TK, Garety P, Power P, et al. The Lambeth Early Onset (LEO) Team: randomised controlled trial of the effectiveness of specialised care for early psychosis. *BMJ.* 2004;329(7474):1067. doi:10.1136/bmj.38246.594873.7C
14. Chong SA, Mythily S, Verma S. Reducing the duration of untreated psychosis and changing help-seeking behaviour in Singapore. *Soc Psychiatry Psychiatr Epidemiol.* 2005;40(8):619-621. doi:10.1007/s00127-005-0948-4
15. Chen EYH. Developing an early intervention service in Hong Kong. In: Ehmann T, MacEwan GW, Honer WG, eds. *Best Care in Early Psychosis Intervention: Global Perspectives.* Taylor & Francis; 2004:125-130.
16. Petersen L, Jeppesen P, Thorup A, et al. A randomised multicentre trial of integrated versus standard treatment for patients with a first episode of psychotic illness [published correction appears in *BMJ.* Nov 5, 2005;331(7524):1065]. *BMJ.* 2005;331(7517):602. doi:10.1136/bmj.38565.415000.E01
17. Chau HS, Chong WS, Wong JGWS, et al. Early intervention for incipient insanity: early notions from the 19th century English literature. *Early Interv Psychiatry.* 2018;12(4):708-714. doi:10.1111/eip.12355
18. Winslow F. *On Obscure Diseases of the Brain, and Disorders of the Mind: Their Incipient Symptoms, Pathology, Diagnosis, Treatment, And Prophylaxis.* Blanchard & Lea; 1860.
19. Ellis WC. *A Treatise on the Nature, Symptoms, Causes, and Treatment of Insanity with Practical Observations on Lunatic Asylums, and a Description of the Pauper Lunatic Asylum for the County of Middlesex, at Hanwell, with a Detailed Account of Its Management.* Samuel Holdsworth, Amen Corner, Paternoster Row; 1838.
20. Killaspy H. From the asylum to community care: learning from experience. *Br Med Bull.* 2006;79-80:245-258. doi:10.1093/bmb/ldl017
21. Carpenter WT Jr, Davis JM. Another view of the history of antipsychotic drug discovery and development. *Mol Psychiatry.* 2012;17(12):1168-1173. doi:10.1038/mp.2012.121

74 • *Psychosis and Schizophrenia in Hong Kong*

22. Johnstone EC, Crow TJ, Johnson AL, MacMillan JF. The Northwick Park Study of first episodes of schizophrenia. I. Presentation of the illness and problems relating to admission. *Br J Psychiatry*. 1986;148:115-120. doi:10.1192/bjp.148.2.115

23. Chen EY. Early intervention in schizophrenia patients – rationale for its implementation and practice. *Hong Kong Med J*. 1999;5(1):57-62.

24. Wong GHY, Hui CLM, Chiu CPY, et al. Early detection and intervention of psychosis in Hong Kong – experience of a population-based intervention programme. The EASY Programme. *Clinical Neuropsychiatry: Journal of Treatment Evaluation*. 2008;5(6):286-289.

25. Tang JY, Wong GH, Hui CL, et al. Early intervention for psychosis in Hong Kong – the EASY programme. *Early Interv Psychiatry*. 2010;4(3):214-219. doi:10.1111/j.1751-7893.2010.00193.x

26. Chen EY, Wong GH, Lam MM, Chiu CP, Hui CL. Real-world implementation of early intervention in psychosis: resources, funding models and evidence-based practice. *World Psychiatry*. 2008;7(3):163-164. doi:10.1002/j.2051-5545.2008.tb00188.x

27. International Early Psychosis Association Writing Group. International clinical practice guidelines for early psychosis. *Br J Psychiatry Suppl*. 2005;48:s120-s124. doi:10.1192/bjp.187.48.s120

28. Wong C, Chong HC, eds. *Psychological Intervention Programmes for People with Early Psychosis (PIPE) Manual*. Early Assessment Service for Young People with Psychosis, Hong Kong; 2002.

29. Chan SK, Tse S, Sit HL, et al. Web-based psychoeducation program for caregivers of first-episode of psychosis: an experience of Chinese population in Hong Kong. *Front Psychol*. 2016;7:2006. Published Dec 26, 2016. doi:10.3389/fpsyg.2016.02006

30. Chang WC. Rationale and the local development of early intervention for psychosis. *Medical Bull*. 2011;16(5):4-5.

31. Chen EYH. Early intervention for psychosis in Hong Kong: initial experience of the EASY programme. *World Psychiatry*. 2003;2(Suppl 1):46.

32. Chen EY, Tang JY, Hui CL, et al. Three-year outcome of phase-specific early intervention for first-episode psychosis: a cohort study in Hong Kong. *Early Interv Psychiatry*. 2011;5(4):315-323. doi:10.1111/j.1751-7893.2011.00279.x

33. Chang WC, Kwong VW, Chan GH, et al. Prediction of functional remission in first-episode psychosis: 12-month follow-up of the randomized-controlled trial on extended early intervention in Hong Kong. *Schizophr Res*. 2016;173(1-2):79-83. doi:10.1016/j.schres.2016.03.016

34. Wong GH, Hui CL, Tang JY, et al. Early intervention for psychotic disorders: real-life implementation in Hong Kong. *Asian J Psychiatr*. 2012;5(1):68-72. doi:10.1016/j.ajp.2012.01.001

35. Wong KK, Chan SK, Lam MM, et al. Cost-effectiveness of an early assessment service for young people with early psychosis in Hong Kong. *Aust N Z J Psychiatry*. 2011;45(8):673-680. doi:10.3109/00048674.2011.586329

36. Häfner H, Maurer K, Löffler W, Riecher-Rössler A. The influence of age and sex on the onset and early course of schizophrenia. *Br J Psychiatry*. 1993;162:80-86. doi:10.1192/bjp.162.1.80

37. The Government of Hong Kong Special Administrative Region (HKSAR). *The 2010-2011 Policy Address: Sharing Prosperity for a Caring Society*; 2010.
38. Suen YN, Wong SMY, Hui CLM, et al. Late-onset psychosis and very-late-onset-schizophrenia-like-psychosis: an updated systematic review. *Int Rev Psychiatry*. 2019;31(5-6):523-542. doi:10.1080/09540261.2019.1670624
39. Chen EYH. Early intervention for psychosis: current issues and emerging perspectives. *Int Rev Psychiatry*. 2019;31(5-6):411-412. doi:10.1080/09540261.2019.1667597
40. Asian Network of Early Psychosis Writing Group. Early psychosis declaration for Asia by the Asian Network of Early Psychosis. *East Asian Arch Psychiatry*. 2012;22(3):90-93.

5

The Naming of Psychosis: Concepts Matter in Community Education

Background: Renaming Schizophrenia in East Asia

With the territory-wide introduction of the Early Assessment Service for Young People (EASY) in Hong Kong in 2001 and recognition of the importance of breaking down barriers to care, questions arose about how best to describe the nature of psychotic disorders in a culturally sensitive way in order to facilitate communication between professionals, service users, and the lay public.

As we described in Chapter 2 on stigma, patients with a schizophrenia diagnosis are particularly vulnerable to all forms of negative attitudes resulting in discrimination in social and occupational relationships, affecting livelihoods and well-being. Although the consequences of stigma have been studied and increasingly recognised, until recently the usefulness of the prevalent concept of schizophrenia has not been questioned outside of Asia, despite increasing evidence that it has hampered research efforts and recovery-oriented practice (1).

The term schizophrenia literally translates from Greek as 'split mind', and was first coined by Eugen Bleuler. He based his conceptualisation of the disorder on Kraepelin's dementia praecox, a mental disorder resulting in severe cognitive and behavioural decline (2). However, Bleuler extended its scope to include less severe 'terminal' psychotic states and non-affective psychoses and stressed that it 'is not a disease in the strict sense, but appears to be a group of diseases' (3). With the introduction of operationalised psychiatric classifications, Bleuler's subtleties in understanding this group of disorders were unfortunately lost.

At the turn of the twenty-first century, there was increasing recognition in several Asian countries that the term and concept of schizophrenia were no longer useful to provide effective and non-stigmatising treatment and care.

The Chinese and East Asian term for schizophrenia *jingshenfenliezheng* (精神分裂症), literally 'mental split mind disorder', was and remains explicitly associated with negative connotations of an irreversibly 'broken brain' (4). The term for psychosis (嚴重精神病, *yanzhong jingshenbing*) translated into 'serious mental illness' giving little indication regarding the nature of the disorder. Like other historical Chinese terms used for mental illness such as *dian* (癲), *xian* (癇), *kuang* (狂) and *feng* (瘋), *jingshenfenliezheng* (精神分裂症) became affiliated with notions of abnormality and carried significant stigma and shame (5, 6, 7). Similarly in Japanese, the term *seishin bunretsu byo* (精神分裂病) translates to 'mind split disease' and sufferers were heavily stigmatised by the label (4, 8, 9). The term denoted a lifelong, hereditary, and untreatable mental disorder characterised by severe mental deterioration, lack of volition, and personal and social dysfunction (9). It had been introduced by the Japanese Society of Psychiatry and Neurology (JSPN) in 1937 and was a literal translation of the Western term 'schizophrenia'. Japanese mental health care had been heavily influenced by German psychiatry from the Meiji Restoration to the end of World War II (10).

In Korea, a similar term *jeongshin-bunyeol-byung* (精神分裂病), 'mind splitting disorder', was used to describe schizophrenia and the term suffered a similar fate to *jingshenfenliezheng* (精神分裂症) and *seishin bunretsu byo* (精神分裂病) (11). Although, there is also significant stigma attached to the term 'schizophrenia' in the West, its Greek origin together with a limited understanding of medical terminology in the general population has meant that associated negative stereotypes might have been less explicit and pervasive than in Asian countries.

In Japan, the National Federation of Families with Mentally Ill in Japan (NFFMIJ) made a formal request to the JSPN in 1993 to change the old term in the hope of lessening the stigma associated with a diagnosis of *seishin bunretsu byo* (精神分裂病) (9). The JSPN decided to replace the old name with *togo shitcho sho* (統合失調症), meaning 'integration disorder'. Alongside the change in name, the society insisted on modernising the concept of schizophrenia by emphasising a stress-vulnerability model and moving away from Kraepelin's conceptualisation of dementia praecox (9, 12). *Togo shitcho sho* (統合失調症) was defined as a clinically significant syndrome that is amenable to treatment and can lead to meaningful and lasting recovery with appropriate psychopharmacological and psychosocial interventions. Following wide consultation with the NFFMIJ, the general public and members of the JSPN the new term was approved in 2002 (4). Similarly in Korea, the old term was replaced by *johyun-byung* (調絃病) or 'attunement disorder', to dispel the stigma associated with *jeongshin-bunyeol-byung* (精神分裂病). The new name was introduced by the Korean Neuropsychiatric Association in 2012 and attunement, akin to tuning a musical instrument, was used as a metaphor for tuning the strings of the mind, implying that neural circuitry is inadequately modulated in the disorder (13).

Naming Psychosis in Hong Kong

In Hong Kong, we took a different approach. Rather than renaming 'schizophrenia', we aimed for a new term for 'psychosis' to emphasise its potentially reversible nature.

Why did we target psychosis rather than schizophrenia for public communication? Our approach was based (1) on accumulating evidence showing that psychotic experiences are prevalent in the general population; and (2) it remains difficult to establish distinct diagnostic boundaries across different psychotic disorders (14, 15, 16, 17).

Another dilemma of targeting 'schizophrenia' in public and clinical communication is that patients are more likely to present with a heterogeneous clinical picture and often do not meet the narrowly defined criteria for schizophrenia (18). Diagnostic instability is common during the early stages of psychosis. It has been established that up to 50% of those diagnosed with acute and transient psychotic disorder eventually meet the criteria for schizophrenia (19, 20, 21). Furthermore, a diagnosis of schizophrenia has become associated with a lifelong chronic condition and disabling course that is difficult to treat. The idea is reminiscent of Kraepelin's concept of dementia praecox. These negative attributes have made clinicians reluctant to diagnose schizophrenia early in the course of the disorder (22). Another argument supporting the use of a spectrum approach is the potentially confusing effect of a change in diagnosis for patients and carers that may jeopardise therapeutic relationships and trust and create hopelessness. It may also negatively affect the developmental trajectory and sense of self of young people, particularly when the course of their psychotic illness changes, for example when symptoms of bipolar disorder emerge, resulting in the reappraisal of the diagnosis (e.g., from schizophrenia to bipolar disorder) (5).

The search for a meaningful and impactful term to describe the psychosis continuum started in 2000. A working group considered over 50 suggestions over a period of nine months (23). The term *sijueshitiao* (思覺失調) was unanimously selected to communicate 'psychotic disorders'. *Si* (思) means thought, *jue* (覺) perception, and *shitiao* (失調) means dysregulation. *Sijue* (思覺) denotes positive symptoms of psychosis with an emphasis on delusions and hallucinations. The term *shitiao* (失調) is commonly used to describe disturbance or imbalance in medical conditions. It implies a reversible imbalance and was considered less stigmatising than terms that have a connotation of irreversible 'brokenness'. The team very deliberately decided to limit their nomenclatural description to positive symptoms, i.e., those of thought and perception, to be able to concisely and precisely communicate the most prominent features of early psychosis and for the symptoms to be easily recognisable by professionals and lay people alike. In addition, its longer four-syllable phonetic structure might have the advantage of being less likely misused as a derogatory term or swear word (5).

Sijueshitiao (思覺失調) was introduced to the wider public as part of a wide-ranging media campaign to improve knowledge and reduce the stigma of psychosis. The new term was accompanied by a brief description of the main features of psychosis with an emphasis on hallucinations and delusions. Alongside this, the public was encouraged to make contact with the EASY hotline should they encounter these symptoms.

Regular meetings were arranged with media professionals. Through these meetings, the Public Affairs Department of the Hospital Authority actively monitored the use of *sijueshitiao* (思覺失調) in the media. It provided immediate feedback and clarification on its use to ensure accurate and less stigmatising reporting, and to minimise inaccurate use of the term. These efforts appeared to bear fruit – the new term became part of the day-to-day vocabulary in Hong Kong. We reported entering *sijueshitiao* (思覺失調) in internet search engines and being directed to the EASY homepage and pages on early psychosis resources. The term also yielded entries referring to psychosis symptoms and the Wikipedia entry for psychosis. We also found that the lay public developed a more differentiated view of psychotic disorders in public discussions and internet groups, viewing schizophrenia as one of several diagnoses of the psychosis spectrum (5). For example, a person with lived experience of psychosis published an autobiographical account of his psychotic illness as *Wode Sijueshitiao* (我的思覺失調, *My Psychosis*) (24). Such personal accounts would have been unlikely or even unthinkable while the term 'serious mental illness' was still widely used (5).

We explored whether the adoption of the new term *sijueshitiao* (思覺失調) for psychosis led to less negative attitudes compared to the traditional name for schizophrenia among secondary school students. Surprisingly, psychiatric labelling did not have a statistically significant main effect on attitude measures. However, students with religious beliefs were more accepting of an individual with a diagnostic label than those without a label (25). To gain a more thorough understanding of wider public perceptions of *sijueshitiao* (思覺失調), we investigated the coverage of the terms *jingshenfenlie* (精神分裂), denoting schizophrenia, and *sijueshitiao* (思覺失調) over ten years in local Hong Kong newspapers (26). We identified 1217 newspaper articles in the three most commonly read papers in Hong Kong. 752 (61.8%) used *jingshenfenlie* (精神分裂) and 465 (38.2%) used *sijueshitiao* (思覺失調). Over the course of ten years, the new term *sijueshitiao* (思覺失調) was increasingly used and *jingshenfenlie* appeared less frequently in newspapers. Over time, *jingshenfenlie* (精神分裂) became less often associated with positive and neutral themes as compared with negative themes. Articles containing the old term also showed a significant increase in the use of stereotypical phrases associated with danger.

The Naming of Clinical High-Risk States in Hong Kong

Given the successful introduction of the term *sijueshitiao* (思覺失調), its wide acceptance and fewer stigmatising views among the general population, we set out to develop a Chinese term to describe a diagnostic label for people at risk of psychosis that may positively impact how the condition is perceived by the general population (27). Four local psychiatrists generated five terms to describe the condition. The search for a culturally acceptable term generated intense discussions among mental health professionals and culminated in the proposal of the following terms: *yunniangqi* (醞釀期) denoting 'incubation period'; *qianquqi* (前驅期) as 'premorbid period'; *zaoxianqi* (早顯期) 'early-manifestation period'; *fengxianqi* (風險期) 'risky period'; and *gaoweiqi* (高危期) also denoting 'high-risk period'. Almost half of the respondents, mental health professionals and members of the general public alike, favoured the Chinese label *yunniangqi* (醞釀期; 'incubation period'). This neutral, non-judgemental label was thought to best reflect the uncertainty and potential reversibility of the condition and it was hoped that it could facilitate help-seeking among individuals and their families. The term itself, however, was non-specific regarding potential symptoms and may need to be used in conjunction with the term psychosis *sijueshitiao* (思覺失調). This would result in the long and complex term *sijueshitiao yunniangqi* (思覺失調醞釀期), which may be less effective in public communications. At the same time, international and local research data has suggested that this clinical high-risk state may not be specific to psychosis, and may be related to the evolution of other disorders as well. A more neutral term *sijueguomin* (思覺過敏) ('sensitivity in thought and perception') is now being used instead.

Reflections: The Evolution of Psychiatric Terminology

It has been encouraging that the term *sijueshitiao* (思覺失調) has not become associated with the same stigmatising attitudes as *jingshenfenlie* (精神分裂). However, it is important to bear in mind that *sijueshitiao* (思覺失調) refers to a nosologically different concept of psychosis rather than schizophrenia. It seems that a broader psychosis spectrum has fewer negative connotations and is considered by the lay public to have a less severe course. Conversely, stigmatising attitudes associated with *jingshenfenlie* (精神分裂) may have actually increased over time and may reflect a view that the term has become associated with the most severe cases.

We investigated the historical evolution of existing terms used to describe 'insanity' and traced the origins of the Cantonese term for 'insanity', *chisin* (痴線), in Hong Kong from 1939 to 2014 by sampling newspaper and magazine articles as well as popular movies from the 1950s and 1960s (28). We also searched available information in newspapers published in Hong Kong, Macau, Taiwan, and Mainland China, and examined several other local historical sources. *Chisin* (痴線), literally meaning 'wires become stuck together', originally denoted 'short-circuiting' and came into more widespread use as the telephone became more commonly used in the 1960s. In 1939, the term was only used in a technical sense to denote short-circuiting. However, as the Strowger telephone exchange system started to support an increasing number of landlines in the 1960s, errors in telephone connections became a common experience for the public. The term *chisin* (痴線) became associated with telephone line misconnection and was commonly used in jokes associated with this experience. The incongruity in dialogues soon was transported to denote notions of 'insanity'. *Chisin* (痴線) then acquired a new meaning in everyday use. Over the decades, it has picked up the connotation of 'insanity' and is used in everyday language as a term for 'craziness'. Perhaps ironically, the idea of brain network abnormalities has since then become a widely endorsed hypothesis in schizophrenia research. The term *chisin* (痴線), in its original literal meaning, would have been a rather apt metaphor to describe the neurobiology of the condition. However, the term has already been so strongly associated with 'craziness' that its literal meaning is hardly perceptible nowadays.

The term *sijueshitiao* (思覺失調) was developed to aid communication in Hong Kong, and in recent years similar efforts to rename schizophrenia and psychosis have been made in Taiwan. *Sijuezhangai* (思覺障礙) ('thought and perceptual impairment') and *sijuegongnengzhangai* (思覺功能障礙) ('thought-perceptual functional impairment') are now commonly used to describe psychotic disorders (5). The effects of introducing the new term *togo shitcho sho* (統合失調症) have been investigated in Japan. The label had been adopted quickly by the majority of psychiatric practices (4). Psychiatrists felt more confident in informing patients of their diagnosis and this facilitated communication and psychoeducational initiatives (10). Evidence also suggests that the new concept of psychosis changed the perception in the general population. Alongside greater optimism for prognosis and treatment, people who were familiar with *togo shitcho sho* (統合失調症) were less likely to support social distancing from patients with the disorder (10).

Yamaguchi et al. (2017) published a systematic review of studies examining the relationship between renaming schizophrenia and related disorders, and stigma-related outcomes (29). Overall, they could show that a name change may be associated with improvements in adults' attitudes towards people with a psychotic disorder and in disclosing of diagnosis.

These encouraging results in Asia have led to prominent researchers in the West calling for a reconceptualisation and renaming of schizophrenia in the hope of reducing stigma and to facilitate communication between clinicians, patients and their families, and the wider public (1, 10, 22, 30, 31). Nonetheless, it is important to recognise that semantic changes and new nosological concepts may only have a limited impact over a period of time unless accompanied by the modernisation of

82 • *Psychosis and Schizophrenia in Hong Kong*

psychiatric care, exploration of new scientific paradigms, changes in legislation, and education of professionals and the public (22, 31).

References

1. Guloksuz S, van Os J. The slow death of the concept of schizophrenia and the painful birth of the psychosis spectrum. *Psychol Med.* 2018;48(2):229-244. doi:10.1017/S0033291717001775
2. Kraepelin E. *Psychiatrie. Ein Lehrbuch für Studierende und Ärzte.* 6 Auflage. Barth; 1899.
3. Bleuler E. *Lehrbuch der Psychiatrie.* Springer Verlag; 1920.
4. Sato M. Renaming schizophrenia: a Japanese perspective. *World Psychiatry.* 2006;5(1):53-55.
5. Chiu CP, Lam MM, Chan SK, et al. Naming psychosis: the Hong Kong experience. *Early Interv Psychiatry.* 2010;4(4):270-274. doi:10.1111/j.1751-7893.2010.00203.x
6. Chen HF. articulating 'Chinese madness': a review of the modern historiography of madness in pre-modern China. The 1st Annual Meeting, Asian Society for the History of Medicine: Symposium on the History of Medicine in Asia: Past Achievements, Current Research and Future Directions; November 4–8, 2003; Taipei, Taiwan. National Chengchi University. http://nccur.lib.nccu.edu.tw/handle/140.119/13429. Accessed January 22 2023.
7. Wynaden D, Chapman R, Orb A, McGowan S, Zeeman Z, Yeak S. Factors that influence Asian communities' access to mental health care. *Int J Ment Health Nurs.* 2005;14(2):88-95. doi:10.1111/j.1440-0979.2005.00364.x
8. Kim Y, Berrios GE. Impact of the term schizophrenia on the culture of ideograph: the Japanese experience. *Schizophr Bull.* 2001;27(2):181-185. doi:10.1093/oxfordjournals.schbul.a006864
9. Sartorius N, Chiu H, Heok KE, et al. Name change for schizophrenia. *Schizophr Bull.* 2014;40(2):255-258. doi:10.1093/schbul/sbt231
10. Shinfuku N. A history of mental health care in Japan: international perspectives. *Taiwan J Psychiatry.* 2019;33:179-91. doi:10.4103/TPSY.TPSY_43_19
11. Kim SW, Jang JE, Kim JM, et al. Comparison of stigma according to the term used for schizophrenia: split-mind disorder vs. attunement disorder. *J Korean Neuropsychiatr Assoc.* 2012;51:210-217.
12. Maruta T, Iimori M. Schizo-nomenclature: a new condition? *Psychiatry Clin Neurosci.* 2008;62(6):741-743. doi:10.1111/j.1440-1819.2008.01872.x
13. Lee YS, Kwon JS. Renaming of schizophrenia. *J Korean Neuropsychiatr Assoc.* 2011;50:16-19.
14. Kendell R, Jablensky A. Distinguishing between the validity and utility of psychiatric diagnoses. *Am J Psychiatry.* 2003;160(1):4-12. doi:10.1176/appi.ajp.160.1.4
15. Marneros A, Pillmann F, Haring A, Balzuweit S, Blöink R. Is the psychopathology of acute and transient psychotic disorder different from schizophrenic and schizoaffective disorders? *Eur Psychiatry.* 2005;20(4):315-320. doi:10.1016/j.eurpsy.2005.02.001

16. Yung AR, Buckby JA, Cotton SM, et al. Psychotic-like experiences in nonpsychotic help-seekers: associations with distress, depression, and disability. *Schizophr Bull.* 2006;32(2):352-359. doi:10.1093/schbul/sbj018

17. Poulton R, Caspi A, Moffitt TE, Cannon M, Murray R, Harrington H. Children's self-reported psychotic symptoms and adult schizophreniform disorder: a 15-year longitudinal study. *Arch Gen Psychiatry.* 2000;57(11):1053-1058. doi:10.1001/archpsyc.57.11.1053

18. Schwartz JE, Fennig S, Tanenberg-Karant M, et al. Congruence of diagnoses 2 years after a first-admission diagnosis of psychosis. *Arch Gen Psychiatry.* 2000;57(6):593-600. doi:10.1001/archpsyc.57.6.593

19. Castagnini A, Bertelsen A, Berrios GE. Incidence and diagnostic stability of ICD-10 acute and transient psychotic disorders. *Compr Psychiatry.* 2008;49(3):255-261. doi:10.1016/j.comppsych.2007.10.004

20. Haahr U, Friis S, Larsen TK, et al. First-episode psychosis: diagnostic stability over one and two years. *Psychopathology.* 2008;41(5):322-329. doi:10.1159/000146070

21. Whitty P, Clarke M, McTigue O, et al. Diagnostic stability four years after a first episode of psychosis. *Psychiatr Serv.* 2005;56(9):1084-1088. doi:10.1176/appi.ps.56.9.1084

22. Guloksuz S, van Os J. Renaming schizophrenia: 5 × 5. *Epidemiol Psychiatr Sci.* 2019;28(3):254-257. doi:10.1017/S2045796018000586

23. Chen EY. Developing an early intervention service in Hong Kong. In: Ehmann T, MacEwan W, Honer WG, eds. *Best Care in Early Psychosis Intervention: Global Perspectives.* Taylor & Francis; 2004:125-30.

24. Wong ML. *My Psychosis.* Ming Man Publications; 2002.

25. Chung KF, Chan JH. Can a less pejorative Chinese translation for schizophrenia reduce stigma? A study of adolescents' attitudes toward people with schizophrenia. *Psychiatry Clin Neurosci.* 2004;58(5):507-515. doi:10.1111/j.1440-1819.2004.01293.x

26. Chan SKW, Ching EYN, Lam KSC, et al. Newspaper coverage of mental illness in Hong Kong between 2002 and 2012: impact of introduction of a new Chinese name of psychosis. *Early Interv Psychiatry.* 2017;11(4):342-345. doi:10.1111/eip.12298

27. Lee EHM, Ching EYN, Hui CLM, et al. Chinese label for people at risk for psychosis. *Early Interv Psychiatry.* 2017;11(3):224-228. doi:10.1111/eip.12232

28. Ng JY, Chen EY. Transformation of a metaphor: semantic shift in a Cantonese term 'Chi Sin' denoting insanity. *East Asian Arch Psychiatry.* 2015;25(1):16-20.

29. Yamaguchi S, Mizuno M, Ojio Y, et al. Associations between renaming schizophrenia and stigma-related outcomes: a systematic review. *Psychiatry Clin Neurosci.* 2017;71(6):347-362. doi:10.1111/pcn.12510

30. George B, Klijn A. A modern name for schizophrenia (PSS) would diminish self-stigma. *Psychol Med.* 2013;43(7):1555-1557. doi:10.1017/S0033291713000895

31. Lasalvia A, Penta E, Sartorius N, Henderson S. Should the label "schizophrenia" be abandoned? *Schizophr Res.* 2015;162(1-3):276-284. doi:10.1016/j.schres.2015.01.031

6

Delays in Help-Seeking: Duration of Untreated Psychosis and Its Determinants

Background

The Concept of the Duration of Untreated Psychosis

It has been known since at least the 1980s that prolonged untreated psychosis is associated with a poorer prognosis (1). Standardised measures of the duration of untreated psychosis (DUP) were introduced in the mid-1990s to study the relationship between the delay in effective treatment and longer-term outcomes in relation to positive and negative symptoms, as well as cognitive, social, and global functioning.

DUP is defined as the time from the clear manifestation of the first psychotic symptom to the initiation of adequate antipsychotic treatment. It needs to be distinguished from the duration of untreated illness, which is related to the emergence of the first symptom of a psychotic illness, which may not be a psychotic symptom itself. Early non-specific symptoms and signs include subtle changes in cognition, affect, drive, stress tolerance, sleep, speech, perception, and motor actions, which are believed to be early expressions of the underlying physiological disturbances for the later development of psychosis (2). Although the definition of DUP seems relatively straightforward, there is an overlap between the very early stages of psychosis and prodromal states such as at-risk mental states (ARMS). This has made it challenging to systematically assess the data on DUP across the world and is likely to have contributed to often inconsistent results as to whether the DUP impacts prognosis and whether early intervention can effectively shorten the DUP and thereby influence outcomes.

The Measurement of the Duration of Untreated Psychosis

DUP can be measured by structured clinical interviews such as the Interview for the Retrospective Assessment of the Onset of Schizophrenia (IRAOS) or the Nottingham Onset Schedule (NOS) (3, 4). To achieve an accurate estimation of DUP, it is important to involve family members or other key informants, particularly to elicit early behavioural disturbances such as disorganised speech, catatonia, and social withdrawal. Both interview schedules have reasonably high reliability and validity. However, both are retrospective assessments by nature and therefore recall bias has been cited as a concern, especially when psychotic symptoms have been present for a very long time prior to help-seeking.

In addition to uncertainties in clearly defining the onset of DUP, the assessment of DUP is complicated by the fact that patients and relatives may provide conflicting information on symptom duration. Other than the already mentioned recall bias, patients' lack of insight and the emergence of symptoms at different time points are likely to contribute to differing estimates.

The Duration of Untreated Psychosis and Its Significance

Several systematic reviews and meta-analyses have demonstrated that DUP has a modest association with a wide range of adverse outcomes including poorer response to treatment, more severe negative and positive symptoms as well as poorer psychosocial and cognitive functioning. An early systematic review by Marshall et al. (2005) demonstrated significant correlations between DUP and symptomatic and psychosocial outcomes at baseline, and at six- and twelve-month follow-up (5). Patients with a long DUP were significantly more likely to have worse outcomes in overall functioning, positive symptoms, and quality of life, and were more likely to not have achieved remission at all follow-up time points. Despite highly consistent associations between DUP and outcome, DUP only accounted for around 13% of the variance at six months, thus showing a modest association. However, a long DUP appeared to be implicated in one-third to one-quarter of patients not achieving remission (5). A long DUP seemed to exert negative effects on outcomes even after years of treatment, including overall global outcome, more severe positive and negative symptoms, a lesser likelihood of remission, and poor social functioning. However, evidence suggests that long DUP may not be associated with employment, quality of life, or hospital treatment (6). Conversely, a shorter DUP has been associated with a greater response to antipsychotic treatment and less severe negative symptoms at intermediate and longer-term follow-ups (7, 8).

The Duration of Untreated Psychosis and Outcomes in Psychotic Disorders

It has been postulated that early intervention reduces the long-term harm caused by a long DUP (9). In 1998, Sheitman and Lieberman suggested a three-stage model of pathophysiological processes underlying disease pathogenesis and progression in psychosis, namely an inability to regulate presynaptic dopamine release in the limbic striatum leading to endogenous neurochemical sensitisation, which eventually results in structural neuronal changes. This last stage is thought to be a consequence of prolonged sensitisation and to be associated with treatment resistance in schizophrenia (10). Other hypotheses have proposed that diminished neuronal connectivity and stress-related hormones affect neuronal architecture and functioning (11, 12).

Studies examining the effects of DUP on structural and functional brain functioning have provided conflicting results. Several studies have supported an association between DUP and morphological changes in the brain, such as a smaller caudate nucleus, reduction in grey matter volume in the left temporal plane and grey matter density in the left fusiform gyrus as well as grey matter loss in the inferior orbital regions and parietal areas (13, 14, 15, 16, 17). The impact of DUP on neurocognitive functioning has been more controversial with most studies not demonstrating a significant association (13). A meta-analysis on neurocognitive impairment and DUP based on 27 studies with over 3000 patients experiencing first-episode psychosis did not show a significant association between impaired cognitive ability and DUP except in the domain of planning and problem-solving (18).

This lack of effect might be explained by the fact that studies varied greatly in quality, but also that neurocognitive impairment and changes in brain morphology are likely to arise during early development with ongoing structural and functional alterations occurring prior to the onset of psychosis or the prodromal phase (13).

Several international studies have found DUPs ranging from a median of 27.3 to 350 days (5). This wide range in DUP has likely been caused by differing study protocols and varying access to psychiatric services across the world. Early intervention (EI) services have been established in the United States, Canada, Australia, the UK, and several European, Asian, and South American countries in the hope of reducing DUP and ameliorating long-term negative outcomes. Two influential studies from Denmark and Canada showed that patients with first-episode psychosis, who have a relatively short DUP of three months or less and who received extended specialist early treatment of up to five years, tended to have better outcomes as compared to participants receiving specialist care for only two years. Albert et al. (2017) reported significant improvements in disorganised and negative symptom domains, and Malla et al. (2018) showed significantly longer remission for positive, negative, and total symptoms compared to regular care (19, 20). However, neither study showed that patients with a DUP of more than 12 weeks benefitted from an extended EI service (19, 20).

Although there appears to be increasing evidence that EI is effective in improving outcomes for patients who present early it has been far less clear whether specialist early care can reduce the DUP. A recent meta-analysis by Oliver et al. (2018) did not show that EI produced a consistent reduction in DUP, but small sample sizes in individual studies, lack of prospective studies, and substantial heterogeneity were likely to have affected their results (21). These findings might be disheartening, nevertheless, improvements in study design and standardisation of definitions may yield better quality data to draw more definitive conclusions about the effects of EI. It has also been suggested that it might be difficult to demonstrate a significant reduction in DUP as increasing numbers of hitherto untreated patients may come forward, particularly in the early phases of a newly established EI service thereby skewing the results towards showing no effect.

Studies on the Duration of Untreated Psychosis in Hong Kong

The Duration of Untreated Psychosis before Early Intervention Programmes

In Hong Kong, DUP was first investigated in patients presenting to mental health services with first-episode psychosis between 1997 and 2000, prior to the launch of the Early Assessment Service for Young People, our EI project for young people. At the time, DUP was found to be a median of 150 days, with a mean of 1.7 years (22). DUP was not predictive of acute symptom profile, the extent of symptom reduction, or the amount of residual symptoms after treatment of the acute episode. Previous family experience of psychiatric illness, i.e., the presence of another family member who had been receiving psychiatric treatment, and an acute mode of onset were significant predictors of a shorter DUP. Having completed secondary education and living alone also had modest effects on DUP, shortening and lengthening it, respectively. However, neither was significant in the binary logistic regression model. Demographic characteristics, symptom profile, and premorbid adjustment were not associated with DUP (23). Interestingly, Chang et al. (2011) did show gender differences affecting DUP in their cohort of 700 first-episode psychosis (FEP) patients aged 15–25 years: young males had a significantly longer median DUP compared to their female counterparts (24).

The Impact of Early Intervention Initiatives on the Duration of Untreated Psychosis in Hong Kong

In 2009, we separately investigated DUP for youth aged 25 and under, as well as adult patients. While there had been no significant change in DUP for youth, DUP for adults was substantially reduced. Originally in 2000, youth had a lower DUP median of 100 days, which shortened to 90 days. DUP for adults over the age of 25 years was longer at 180 days, and it also reduced significantly to 93 days, particularly in those with gradual onset and without a family history (20, 25, 26). Young people had poorer subjective quality of life during the duration of their untreated psychosis and depressive symptoms appeared to be most specifically associated with this outcome (27, 28).

The Duration of Untreated Psychosis and Help-Seeking

To understand factors affecting the DUP more systematically, we broke down DUP into waiting time and help-seeking duration. Waiting time was defined as the time between the occurrence of the first psychotic symptoms and the first help-seeking behaviour. The help-seeking duration was the period from the first help-seeking behaviour until the receipt of effective psychiatric treatment. We examined which processes affected the initiation of help-seeking behaviour of adult Hong Kong patients (29). Initial help-seeking was delayed by an average of around two months and effective treatment was provided within around one month of making contact with services. We also found that family members initiated contact with services nearly half of the time and that only a small minority of clients had approached priests or traditional healers. Unsurprisingly, a gradual mode of onset was associated with a greater delay in help-seeking and longer DUP (29, 30). Premorbid schizoid and schizotypal traits as well as a migrant background also predicted longer help-seeking duration. In addition, stigma and limited knowledge of available services were likely to prolong the initiation of contact (29).

The Impact of the Duration of Untreated Psychosis on Psychosis Outcome in Hong Kong

When considering the impact of the DUP on outcome, a fifth of patients who never experienced a relapse had a DUP of less than 30 days. They were also more likely to be diagnosed with a non-schizophrenia-spectrum disorder, to have less severe negative symptoms, and to be performing better in logical memory, immediate recall, and verbal fluency tests (31). In the medium term, a shorter DUP predicted symptomatic remission (32).

On the other hand, a DUP of more than three months was significantly correlated with male sex, younger age of onset, a schizophrenia-spectrum diagnosis, an insidious development of psychosis, fewer baseline positive symptoms, and poorer insight (30, 33). In addition, a prolonged DUP was significantly predictive of outcomes in relation to positive symptoms, recovery, and sustained full-time employment (33). A prolonged DUP was even shown to affect medium-term outcomes in that patients were more likely to suffer more severe negative symptoms and memory deficits in the domains of visual and verbal memory. Patients with a long DUP also reported higher levels of self-stigma (34, 35, 36).

Although there have been numerous studies examining the short- and medium-term effects of prolonged DUP, there is little data on the enduring impact of untreated psychosis on recovery. In 2014, a prospective cohort of 153 patients with FEP was followed up after 14 years. The patients were categorised into short (≤ 30 days), medium (31–180 days) and long (> 180 days) DUP groups. Long-term outcome was ascertained in 73% of the sample. Nearly half of the patients fulfilled the criteria for symptomatic remission. The short DUP group experienced a significantly higher remission rate over the course of their illness. The odds of long-term symptomatic remission were significantly reduced by 89% in the medium and 85% in the long DUP groups compared to the short DUP group. Further analysis showed that DUP had a specific impact on negative symptom remission (37).

Public Awareness Strategies

To help develop an effective awareness campaign, a survey on attitudes towards mental illness, understanding of its causes, and help-seeking behaviour among patients, their relatives, and the general public was undertaken in Hong Kong (38). The majority of the lay public did not consider psychotic symptoms features of mental illness and, consequently, did not think that medical intervention was required. Of those surveyed, women, individuals with higher education, and previous acquaintance with patients were significantly more likely to have better knowledge of psychotic symptoms, their causes and treatment. In the patient and relatives groups, symptom awareness and an understanding of the need for psychiatric assessment were significantly higher compared to the general population. However, only 18% and 25% of patients and their relatives considered drug treatment to be important. Contrary to previous studies, beliefs in supernatural causes and the need to consult traditional healers were not widespread in any of the groups surveyed (39).

Reflections: Can the Duration of Untreated Psychosis Be Shortened Further?

Despite immense public awareness efforts over long periods of time, the median DUP in Hong Kong has remained at around 90 days for both adolescent and adult-onset psychosis. Notably, until recently, the focus of public awareness programmes in Hong Kong had been to communicate the nature of psychotic symptoms and the need for assessment. However, there is now increasing recognition among professionals that targeting symptoms of ARMS may be effective in shortening the DUP. Several other programmes, such as in Melbourne, have delivered psychoeducational initiatives addressing ARMS, and have managed to reduce DUP to around 30 days. It is possible that promoting knowledge of prodromal symptoms may contribute to further shortening the DUP for FEP patients. These patients, experiencing upstream ARMS, are already engaged with EI services. Even if the intervention did not succeed in preventing the onset of psychosis, it should still facilitate much earlier detection when conversion to psychosis takes place. However, given limited resources in public mental health services, access to EI may become the rate-limiting step in reducing the DUP unless the capacity of these services is increased.

The debate around shortening the DUP to effect better long-term outcomes has been complicated by the fact that it has not been possible to clearly define a meaningful cut-off threshold for DUP at which outcomes are qualitatively different. The DUP had been assumed to have a linear relationship with symptomatic and functional outcomes and studies tended to use arbitrary cut-offs. Only a few more recent studies have questioned this assumption and shed some light on how one might define a short DUP. For example, we showed a clear correlation between a DUP of 30 days or less and higher remission rates (32). Drake et al. (2020) demonstrated that treatment delay exerted significant harm during the early stages of psychosis and then tended to level off as the DUP increased, thus showing a curvilinear relationship between DUP and symptom severity (40). The argument for focusing on shortening treatment delays has strong face validity and services may have to decide whether to focus on reducing DUP further for those whose DUP is already relatively short or to focus on those with relatively long DUPs (40).

Examining the effect of DUP on longer-term outcomes has also been hampered by the fact that studies have had to rely on costly longitudinal cohorts due to the ethical concerns about using an randomised controlled trial design. This has meant that correlations between DUP and clinical outcomes could be studied but causal relationships have been difficult to establish.

Meta-analyses have not provided convincing evidence that DUP can be reduced by EI programmes, probably owing to cultural differences and varying service designs. Interestingly, Robinson et al. (2017) showed that in the Recovery After an Initial Schizophrenia Episode (RAISE) programme patients with a shorter

DUP had greater symptomatic and functional improvements (41). They postulated that outcomes were affected by a complex interplay between time to effective treatment and the components of the offered interventions. However, the Jockey Club Early Psychosis (JCEP) project in Hong Kong actually showed opposite effects in that those with a longer DUP responded more favourably to EI. It was noted that cut-offs for DUP markedly differed between the two studies at 74 and 13 weeks, respectively. Caseloads for case managers in Hong Kong were also much higher. In addition, the average age of participants was higher and there was a preponderance of female patients in the Hong Kong study. These findings might be explained by the fact that there is a ceiling effect for those patients who receive an intervention at an early stage of their illness. Due to their higher level of functioning, relatively little is gained by offering EI as practised in Hong Kong. It is known that later-onset psychosis is more prevalent among women and generally carries a better overall prognosis. These patients may benefit significantly more from treatment, even at a much longer DUP (26). Although this finding has not been replicated in other countries, it may remind clinicians that DUP is only one factor affecting longer-term outcomes and that prognosis can still be favourable for at least some patients who have experienced a long DUP.

It remains to be seen whether the DUP can be reduced further by focusing on ARMS, i.e., an even earlier phase of a psychotic illness. Lack of awareness among family members and insidious onset of psychosis are predictive of prolonged DUP. A combination of public awareness campaigns and offering city-wide effective EI can positively impact DUP.

References

1. Crow TJ, MacMillan JF, Johnson AL, Johnstone EC. A randomised controlled trial of prophylactic neuroleptic treatment. *Br J Psychiatry*. 1986;148:120-127. doi:10.1192/bjp.148.2.120
2. Wong GHY. Early symptomatology of schizophrenia. *Medical Bulletin*. 2011;16(5):14-15.
3. Häfner H, Löffler W, Maurer K, Riecher-Rössler Anita, Stein A. *IRAOS – Interview for the Retrospective Assessment of the Onset and Course of Schizophrenia and Other Psychoses*. Hogrefe Publishing GmbH; 2003.
4. Singh SP, Cooper JE, Fisher HL, et al. Determining the chronology and components of psychosis onset: The Nottingham Onset Schedule (NOS). *Schizophr Res*. 2005;80(1):117-130. doi:10.1016/j.schres.2005.04.018
5. Marshall M, Lewis S, Lockwood A, Drake R, Jones P, Croudace T. Association between duration of untreated psychosis and outcome in cohorts of first-episode patients: a systematic review. *Arch Gen Psychiatry*. 2005;62(9):975-983. doi:10.1001/archpsyc.62.9.975

6. Penttilä M, Jääskeläinen E, Hirvonen N, Isohanni M, Miettunen J. Duration of untreated psychosis as predictor of long-term outcome in schizophrenia: systematic review and meta-analysis. *Br J Psychiatry.* 2014;205(2):88-94. doi:10.1192/bjp.bp.113.127753

7. Boonstra N, Klaassen R, Sytema S, et al. Duration of untreated psychosis and negative symptoms – a systematic review and meta-analysis of individual patient data. *Schizophr Res.* 2012;142(1-3):12-19. doi:10.1016/j.schres.2012.08.017

8. Perkins DO, Gu H, Boteva K, Lieberman JA. Relationship between duration of untreated psychosis and outcome in first-episode schizophrenia: a critical review and meta-analysis. *Am J Psychiatry.* 2005;162(10):1785-1804. doi:10.1176/appi.ajp.162.10.1785

9. Drake RJ, Haley CJ, Akhtar S, Lewis SW. Causes and consequences of duration of untreated psychosis in schizophrenia. *Br J Psychiatry.* 2000;177:511-515. doi:10.1192/bjp.177.6.511

10. Sheitman BB, Lieberman JA. The natural history and pathophysiology of treatment resistant schizophrenia. *J Psychiatr Res.* 1998;32(3-4):143-150. doi:10.1016/s0022-3956(97)00052-6

11. Goldberg TE, Burdick KE, McCormack J, et al. Lack of an inverse relationship between duration of untreated psychosis and cognitive function in first episode schizophrenia. *Schizophr Res.* 2009;107(2-3):262-266. doi:10.1016/j.schres.2008.11.003

12. Wood SJ, Pantelis C, Yung AR, Velakoulis D, McGorry PD. Brain changes during the onset of schizophrenia: implications for neurodevelopmental theories. *Med J Aust.* 2009;190(S4):S10-S13. doi:10.5694/j.1326-5377.2009.tb02367.x

13. Rund BR. Does active psychosis cause neurobiological pathology? A critical review of the neurotoxicity hypothesis. *Psychol Med.* 2014;44(8):1577-1590. doi:10.1017/S0033291713002341

14. Crespo-Facorro B, Roiz-Santiáñez R, Pelayo-Terán JM, et al. Caudate nucleus volume and its clinical and cognitive correlations in first episode schizophrenia. *Schizophr Res.* 2007;91(1-3):87-96. doi:10.1016/j.schres.2006.12.015

15. Takahashi T, Suzuki M, Tanino R, et al. Volume reduction of the left planum temporale gray matter associated with long duration of untreated psychosis in schizophrenia: a preliminary report. *Psychiatry Res.* 2007;154(3):209-219. doi:10.1016/j.pscychresns.2006.10.001

16. Bangalore SS, Goradia DD, Nutche J, Diwadkar VA, Prasad KM, Keshavan MS. Untreated illness duration correlates with gray matter loss in first-episode psychoses. *Neuroreport.* 2009;20(7):729-734. doi:10.1097/WNR.0b013e32832ae501

17. Malla AK, Mittal C, Lee M, Scholten DJ, Assis L, Norman RM. Computed tomography of the brain morphology of patients with first-episode schizophrenic psychosis. *J Psychiatry Neurosci.* 2002;27(5):350-358.

18. Bora E, Yalincetin B, Akdede BB, Alptekin K. Duration of untreated psychosis and neurocognition in first-episode psychosis: a meta-analysis. *Schizophr Res.* 2018;193:3-10. doi:10.1016/j.schres.2017.06.021

19. Albert N, Melau M, Jensen H, Hastrup LH, Hjorthøj C, Nordentoft M. The effect of duration of untreated psychosis and treatment delay on the outcomes of prolonged early intervention in psychotic disorders. *NPJ Schizophr.* 2017;3(1):34. Published Sep 26, 2017. doi:10.1038/s41537-017-0034-4

20. Malla A, Shah J, Dama M et al. Delay in initial treatment may limit the benefit of even extended early intervention service: results from a RCT. *Early Interv Psychiatry*. 2018;12(suppl 1):23. doi:10.1111/eip.12722

21. Oliver D, Davies C, Crossland G, et al. Can we reduce the duration of untreated psychosis? A systematic review and meta-analysis of controlled interventional studies. *Schizophr Bull*. 2018;44(6):1362-1372. doi:10.1093/schbul/sbx166

22. Chen EYH, Dunn ELW, Chen RYL, et al. Duration of untreated psychosis and symptomatic outcome among first-episode schizophrenic patients in Hong Kong. The 7th International Congress on Schizophrenia Research; Apr 17–21, 1999; Santa Fe, NM. In *Schizophr Res*. 1999;36(1-3):15. doi:10.1016/S0920-9964(99)90023-3

23. Chen EY, Dunn EL, Miao MY, et al. The impact of family experience on the duration of untreated psychosis (DUP) in Hong Kong. *Soc Psychiatry Psychiatr Epidemiol*. 2005;40(5):350-356. doi:10.1007/s00127-005-0908-z

24. Chang WC, Tang JY, Hui CL, et al. Gender differences in patients presenting with first-episode psychosis in Hong Kong: a three-year follow up study. *Aust N Z J Psychiatry*. 2011;45(3):199-205. doi:10.3109/00048674.2010.547841

25. Chan SKW, Chau EHS, Hui CLM, Chang WC, Lee EHM, Chen EYH. Long term effect of early intervention service on duration of untreated psychosis in youth and adult population in Hong Kong. *Early Interv Psychiatry*. 2018;12(3):331-338. doi:10.1111/eip.12313

26. Hui CL, Li AW, Leung CM, et al. Comparing illness presentation, treatment and functioning between patients with adolescent- and adult-onset psychosis. *Psychiatry Res*. 2014;220(3):797-802. doi:10.1016/j.psychres.2014.08.046

27. Law CW, Chen EY, Cheung EF, et al. Impact of untreated psychosis on quality of life in patients with first-episode schizophrenia. *Qual Life Res*. 2005;14(8):1803-1811. doi:10.1007/s11136-005-3236-6

28. Law C, Chen EY, Cheung EF, Chan RC, Lam CL, Lo MS. Study of quality of life in first-episode psychotic patients in the period of untreated psychosis. The 9th International Congress on Schizophrenia Research; Mar 29–Apr 2, 2003; Colorado Springs, CO. In *Schizophr Res*. 2003;60(suppl. 1):338. doi:10.1016/S0920-9964(03)80330-4

29. Hui CL, Tang JY, Wong GH, et al. Predictors of help-seeking duration in adult-onset psychosis in Hong Kong. *Soc Psychiatry Psychiatr Epidemiol*. 2013;48(11):1819-1828. doi:10.1007/s00127-013-0688-9

30. Hui CL, Lau WW, Leung CM, et al. Clinical and social correlates of duration of untreated psychosis among adult-onset psychosis in Hong Kong Chinese: the JCEP study. *Early Interv Psychiatry*. 2015;9(2):118-125. doi:10.1111/eip.12094

31. Hui CL, Honer WG, Lee EH, et al. Predicting first-episode psychosis patients who will never relapse over 10 years. *Psychol Med*. 2019;49(13):2206-2214. doi:10.1017/S0033291718003070

32. Chang WC, Tang JY, Hui CL, et al. Prediction of remission and recovery in young people presenting with first-episode psychosis in Hong Kong: a 3-year follow-up study. *Aust N Z J Psychiatry*. 2012;46(2):100-108. doi:10.1177/0004867411428015

33. Chang WC, Tang JY, Hui CL, et al. Duration of untreated psychosis: relationship with baseline characteristics and three-year outcome in first-episode psychosis. *Psychiatry Res*. 2012;198(3):360-365. doi:10.1016/j.psychres.2011.09.006

94 • *Psychosis and Schizophrenia in Hong Kong*

34. Chang WC, Hui CL, Tang JY, et al. Impacts of duration of untreated psychosis on cognition and negative symptoms in first-episode schizophrenia: a 3-year prospective follow-up study. *Psychol Med.* 2013;43(9):1883-1893. doi:10.1017/S0033291712002838
35. Chen EYH, Hui CLM, Dunn ELW, et al. Long duration of untreated psychosis is associated with poorer neurocognitive and negative symptoms recovery after first episode schizophrenia. The 13th Biennial Winter Workshop on Schizophrenia Research; Feb 4–10, 2006; Davos, Switzerland. *Schizophr Res.* 2006;81(suppl.):231, abstract no. 495. doi:10.1016/j.schres.2006.01.006
36. Ho RWH, Chang WC, Kwong VWY, et al. Prediction of self-stigma in early psychosis: 3-year follow-up of the randomized-controlled trial on extended early intervention. *Schizophr Res.* 2018;195:463-468. doi:10.1016/j.schres.2017.09.004
37. Tang JY, Chang WC, Hui CL, et al. Prospective relationship between duration of untreated psychosis and 13-year clinical outcome: a first-episode psychosis study. *Schizophr Res.* 2014;153(1-3):1-8. doi:10.1016/j.schres.2014.01.022
38. Chung KF, Chen EY, Lam LC, Chen RY, Chan CK. How are psychotic symptoms perceived? A comparison between patients, relatives and the general public. *Aust N Z J Psychiatry.* 1997;31(5):756-761. doi:10.3109/00048679709062691
39. Kua EH, Chew PH, Ko SM. Spirit possession and healing among Chinese psychiatric patients. *Acta Psychiatr Scand.* 1993;88(6):447-450. doi:10.1111/j.1600-0447.1993.tb03489.x
40. Drake RJ, Husain N, Marshall M, et al. Effect of delaying treatment of first-episode psychosis on symptoms and social outcomes: a longitudinal analysis and modelling study. *Lancet Psychiatry.* 2020;7(7):602-610. doi:10.1016/S2215-0366(20)30147-4
41. Robinson DG. Randomized comparison of comprehensive versus usual community care for first-episode psychosis: The Raise-ETP Study. *J American Academy of Child and Adolescent Psychiatry.* 2017;56(10):S340. doi:10.1016/j.jaac.2017.07.719

7

Prevention Starts from Risk States: Risk States and Psychotic-Like Experiences

Background: Psychotic-Like Experiences

Psychotic-like experiences (PLEs) are frequently encountered phenomena but, unlike psychotic symptoms proper, they are often difficult to delineate. It has been suggested that sub-clinical psychotic symptoms exist on a continuum with psychotic symptoms that occur in serious mental illness and are therefore an important area of study, as they may be relevant for the early detection and treatment of psychosis. PLEs are commonly experienced by the general population in the absence of psychiatric illness (1). Early studies indicated that adolescents who report PLEs have a five- to sixteen-fold increased risk of developing clinical psychosis (2, 3, 4) and 8% of adults with PLEs were shown to have a psychosis diagnosis at two-year follow-up (5).

Research into the prevalence and phenomenology of PLEs has been hampered by the fact that studies have adopted a wide variety of definitions and methods to capture PLEs. A median prevalence rate of 5% was suggested by van Os et al. (2009) in their meta-analysis, but lifetime prevalence has varied greatly from study to study. In a UK nationwide phone survey, a rate of 75% was reported, a rate of 28.4% was found in the US National Comorbidity Survey, and 17.5% in the Netherlands Mental Health Survey and Incidence Study (NEMESIS) study (6, 7, 8). In New Zealand, youth described delusional and hallucinatory experiences at rates of 20.1% and 13.2%, respectively (3).

It has been pointed out that given the similar prevalence and incidence rates, PLEs were likely to be transitory phenomena for many people but that PLEs may persist in those with a vulnerability for psychotic disorders. Those with persistent symptoms may be prone to developing psychotic symptoms, leading to the subsequent development of clinical symptoms and impairment (9). The 'psychosis proneness-persistence-impairment model' of van Os et al. (2000) postulates that ongoing environmental stress was the cause for biological and psychological sensitisation, thus giving rise to persistent psychotic symptoms. Studies investigating persistence have shown rates ranging from 8–30% in adults and 16–40% in adolescents. However, there is little data on the development of functional impairment further downstream (5, 10, 11, 12, 13).

Studies of Psychotic-Like Experiences in Hong Kong

We undertook a systematic review of definitions of PLEs and assessment tools to elicit the phenomenon in the hope of further guiding ongoing research in this important area (14). We included a wide range of terms referring to a spectrum of experiences resembling features and characteristics of positive psychotic symptoms regardless of whether they preceded clinically significant psychotic symptoms. It was shown that affective response to auditory hallucinations was likely a key difference between benign conditions and future psychotic disorders. Stress, distress, preoccupation, conviction, feelings of persecution, and loss of control associated with delusion-like ideation were also predictive of clinical psychopathology. Bizarre experiences, perceptual abnormalities, and persecutory ideas were strongly correlated with depression, distress, and poor functioning. One study utilised a meta-cognitive approach and reported a significant association between negative beliefs and PLEs. Given the varied definitions and assessments of PLEs, we proposed the development of a consensus definition of PLEs to enable a better understanding of this phenomenon and its association with psychosis. Further phenomenological studies are needed to contribute to a better definition of PLEs and will allow for the development of more comprehensive, valid, and reliable assessment tools, in the hope that it will lead to more reliable detection and effective intervention of very early psychotic states (14).

Background: Clinical High-Risk Studies

The term at-risk mental state (ARMS) was first introduced by McGorry and colleagues in the early 2000s, arguing that a clearly defined sub-threshold syndrome is a risk factor for the development of psychotic illness (15, 16). This prepsychotic or prodromal period encompasses non-specific symptoms such as low mood, anxiety, and sub-threshold psychotic symptoms (17, 18, 19). It has been argued that the boundary between ARMS and actual psychosis is often poorly demarcated (20). Nonetheless, its identification allows for preventative interventions to be developed. The prodromal period is associated with significant impairments in psychosocial functioning and is often prolonged, lasting up to five years (15, 16, 21, 22, 23, 24, 25, 26).

In Germany, Gerd Huber (1983) introduced the term 'basic symptoms' to describe subtle, subjectively experienced symptoms before the onset of a frank psychotic disorder. They involve disturbances in affect, stress tolerance, thinking, perception, attention, motivation, and speech (27, 28). The symptomatology was termed 'basic' due to the fact that these early subjective symptoms were considered to be the expression of underlying neurobiological processes present in psychotic disorders and thought to occur prior to the development of overt symptoms.

The concepts of 'basic symptoms' and ARMS have been complemented by the more clearly defined ultra-high-risk state (UHR) as an attempt to better predict conversion to psychosis and minimise false positives (29). The risk factors used to define UHR include attenuated psychotic symptoms, intermittent psychotic symptoms, and genetic risk together with a decline in functioning. It has been shown that over a 12-month period, more than half of those with UHR had unfavourable trajectories with either unchanged, recurrence or relapse of their symptoms, or progression to psychosis (30).

Several assessment tools have been developed to aid the detection of prodromal symptoms. The Comprehensive Assessment of 'At-Risk Mental State' (CAARMS) prospectively measures sub-threshold psychotic symptoms and covers seven domains of psychopathology, namely positive, negative, cognitive, and emotional symptoms as well as behavioural, motor, and physical changes (31). CAARMS has also included several of the 'basic symptoms'. It has shown good reliability and predictive validity, and has become one of the most widely used assessment tools. Several early studies using the instrument have shown conversion rates, i.e., the progression of ARMS to actual psychosis, of 30% to 58% (32). Interestingly, more recent studies have demonstrated lower conversion rates in the range of 10%–15% over a one to two-year period (30). Klosterkoetter et al. (1997) developed the Bonn Scale for the Assessment of Basic Symptoms (33). They showed that certain 'basic symptoms', among them, thought interference and thought block, pressure of thought, visual distortions, and the disturbed reception of language, were highly predictive of psychosis. Another commonly used instrument to evaluate clinical high-risk states is the Structured Interview for Psychosis Risk Syndromes (SIPS) (34). The diagnostic scale contains a measure of severity covering positive, negative, disorganisation, and general psychopathology symptoms and has shown excellent cross-culturally validated psychometric properties (35).

Given the relatively low conversion rates, a clinical staging model was proposed as a framework to allow for more differentiated treatment approaches offering a better risk–benefit balance for ARMS and UHR individuals (36). Recent attempts in predictive modelling have made use of advanced statistical or machine learning approaches to predict the clinical evolution of UHR at the individual level (37).

Clinical High-Risk Studies in Hong Kong

Conversion Rates in Clinical High-Risk States

In Hong Kong, Lam et al. (2006) investigated conversion rates in clinical high-risk (CHR) individuals using a naturalistic prospective study design (38). They recruited 62 CHR patients referred to the Early Assessment Service for Young People. The mean age at first assessment was 16.2 years, 58.1% of the sample was male, and most of the subjects were born in Hong Kong and were students. Only 14.5% reported substance use, with ketamine being the most commonly used substance, followed by ecstasy, cannabis, amphetamine-like substances, solvents, and opiates. A family history of psychosis was present in 29% of the patients. Most subjects had attenuated symptoms. Brief limited intermittent psychotic symptoms were less common and even fewer patients were found to have a vulnerability to psychosis. Symptom onset and time to study intake varied between 11 days and 6.6 years, with a median of 463 days. The most commonly 'first noticed experiences' were irritability, avolition, subjective cognitive experiences, and disorganised behaviour. Irritability and subjective cognitive impairment were the most commonly reported 'first noticed disturbance' in those subjects who developed psychosis within six months. The six-month transition rate was 29%, with most of the conversion to psychosis taking place within the first three months of study intake. Those who became psychotic significantly differed from those who did not in their baseline scores on the Positive and Negative Syndrome Scale (PANSS), CAARMS, and Global Assessment of Functioning, but not in their demographic profile. Subjective cognitive decline was reported by all patients who converted to psychosis. Eleven of the 18 psychosis patients were diagnosed with schizophreniform psychosis, two cases had schizoaffective disorder, a further two cases developed affective psychosis, and three patients had a psychotic disorder not otherwise specified.

Lam et al. (2008) followed their CHR sample for two further years and found a transition rate of 45% after 24 months (39). Interestingly, despite not fulfilling the criteria for psychotic disorders, high-risk subjects already had moderate levels of functional decline and psychopathology at study intake, including the full range of negative symptoms usually seen in established psychosis (39, 40). Like in established psychosis, functional impairment in ARMS appeared to be closely associated with motivational deficits and to a lesser extent with reduced processing speed (41). In addition, social amotivation was predictive of functioning at 12-month follow-up (42).

Clinical High-Risk and Comorbidity

Chan et al. (2022) also established significant gender differences in those at risk of developing psychosis. Males with ARMS were more withdrawn and had poorer social functioning when compared to their female counterparts (43). Up to half of individuals at risk of psychosis experienced other psychiatric symptoms, most frequently anxiety and depressive disorders. It appears that females more often had co-occurring disorders and that those with comorbid conditions had more severe depressive symptoms, expressed more suicidal ideation, had a lower global cognitive ability, had more limited social networks, and had lower subjective quality of life (44).

The Evolving Nature of Clinical High Risk

Research into prodromal symptoms is challenging, mainly due to difficulties in measuring mild symptoms (45). As a consequence, differentiating between at-risk mental states and actual early psychotic symptoms has posed significant challenges. One way of overcoming some of these issues is to employ qualitative methodologies to closely study the unfolding of symptoms and changes in psychosocial functioning in small patient samples over time. We utilised a clinical staging model developed by McGorry et al. (2006) to explore the evolving nature of prodromal symptoms in a case series of ten patients over the course of 12 months (46, 47).

Two patients with no change in symptoms initially presented with mood or anxiety symptoms. Their presentation remained stable throughout the study period, and functioning was noted to improve slightly by month six. Insight into changes and family support were both strong. The combination of these factors, along with cognitive-behavioural case management, was thought to account for their functional improvement.

Three other patients improved markedly and gradually over 12 months. They had initially presented with distress arising from perceptual disturbances or delusion-like symptoms. Comorbid anxiety and depressive symptoms were common, as was the experience of a recent stressful life event. The patients had good insight in general and good social support from their families.

Four patients who developed a fluctuating course first presented with delusion-like symptoms and perceptual disturbances. In addition, they reported low mood, anxiety, and social withdrawal. Insight and family support were more limited compared to other patient groups, and several patients had reported stressful life events. Some of the symptoms diminished during the follow-up period but were substituted by other symptoms.

One patient transitioned to psychosis within the first month, accompanied by a rapid decline in functioning. This patient had a family history of mental illness and had experienced delusion-like symptoms and anxiety in the previous two years. A decline in functioning and the emergence of more persistent auditory hallucinations and persecutory delusions were observed.

The Study of Psychotic-Like Experiences and Clinical High-Risk States: Bridging the Gaps

Although PLEs and at-risk mental states are considered to be risk indicators for the development of a psychotic illness, the two concepts and the study of their phenomena have emerged from different research traditions. Psychotic-like phenomena were first recognised in the nineteenth century and have not uncommonly been regarded as spiritual or supernatural experiences in many different cultures (48). They are commonly observed in large-scale epidemiological studies. Wüsten et al. (2019) reported that psychotic experiences significantly differed between high and low/middle-income countries in their frequency and associated distress, pointing towards higher endorsement of these symptoms in low/middle-income countries, while being connected with less distress and potentially being less clinically relevant compared to the Western world (49). This indicates that culture may play a role in PLEs and a more culturally sensitive approach may be informative (49). The advantages of studying PLEs in the general population are that these studies likely capture individuals who are in the very early phase of a psychotic disorder and who may never come to the attention of services (50). Due to the size of population samples, self-report measures are used to ascertain the presence of psychotic experiences. However, self-rating instruments risk overestimating the occurrence of psychotic experiences because they usually capture a more diverse range of responses (50).

In contrast, the study of CHR states emerged from an attempt to define the nature of prepsychotic prodromal states in the hope of detecting conversion to frank psychosis early and offering timely preventative intervention. Research in this area has predominantly relied on high-risk samples, such as high genetic risks, or presentation at early intervention (EI) screening to delineate at-risk mental states and understand risk factors associated with the progression to psychosis.

In order to bridge the gap between large-scale epidemiological studies on psychotic experiences and cohort studies typically recruited within a more specialised early intervention context, Chan et al. (2021) analysed data from the Hong Kong Mental Morbidity Survey (HKMMS) and followed up 152 subjects who had reported PLEs (51, 52). At two-year follow-up, the weighted 12-month prevalence of PLEs was 2.7%, being highest among women aged 36–45 years. The PLE-positive group had a higher proportion of women with a lower mean age, a significantly higher divorce and unemployment rate, significantly poorer mental health, and a higher proportion of individuals with a family history of mental disorders. Illicit drug dependence rates were very low in the PLE-positive and PLE-negative groups.

The majority of PLE-positive individuals (n=120, 78.9%) endorsed only one item on the Psychosis Screening Questionnaire (PSQ). A smaller proportion endorsed more than one item (n=32, 21.1%). Three latent classes of PLEs were identified: hallucination, paranoia, and mixed. Most of the subjects in the mixed and paranoia latent classes reported a single PLE, while a considerable number of subjects in the hallucination class reported multiple PLEs. Multiple PLEs and hallucination latent class were associated with higher levels of common mental health symptoms. At two-year follow-up, 15.2% of respondents had persistent PLEs. No significant difference was found in the distribution of persistent PLEs across groups and those with multiple psychotic-like experiences were more likely to present with poorer mental health at two-year follow-up.

Reflections and the Way Forward

The study of psychotic-like symptoms in the community and the identification of CHR states have been areas of active research internationally. Originally motivated by the search for prodromal states preceding the onset of psychotic disorders, research has led to the identification of sub-clinical conditions that have their own significance. Earlier family studies have led to the recognition of schizotypal disorders, a mild expression of schizophrenia-related family traits. Schizotypal disorder, nevertheless, has a low and slightly increased risk of conversion to frank psychosis.

Efforts to identify prodromal states have led to the development of the concepts of CHR or ARMS, with accompanying standardised interview schedules. CHR groups have conversion rates to psychosis of around 10% to 20% within one to two years of initial presentation. A significant proportion develops non-psychotic disorders such as anxiety and depression.

Identifying those at high risk of developing a mental illness, whether this may be psychosis or a non-psychotic disorder, is an opportunity to intervene early and minimise adverse functional outcomes. These interventions may involve psychosocial treatments such as cognitive-behavioural therapy, emotional regulation, or stress management. Successful treatment of CHR states likely reduces healthcare-related costs in the longer term. However, since services are usually organised in such a way that funding streams are specific to particular psychiatric conditions or highly specialised services, it is difficult to offer treatment to everyone without completely overwhelming EI teams.

This constraint has limited the development of at-risk-mental-state work in Hong Kong. One way of overcoming this dilemma is to further improve our ability to identify those who go on to develop psychosis, whether this is through the discovery of specific biomarkers, such as genetic or imaging markers, or stronger psychopathological or cognitive predictors. With the recent development of youth mental health screening platforms, we may now have an opportunity to engage and study the community CHR population in Hong Kong (53, 54).

Observations from epidemiological studies report a relatively high rate of psychotic-like symptoms in the general population. Our findings on the prevalence of PLEs and their association with mental health difficulties are similar to those in other high-income countries (55, 56). Past adversity and current psychosocial stress may be predisposing and precipitating factors for the development of PLEs. Given the low transition rates, psychotic-like experiences, even multiple PLEs and hallucinations, more likely represent an indicator of general mental distress rather than constitute a risk factor for psychosis per se. Clinical differentiation between those who have transient PLEs and others who go on to develop a psychotic illness is important, but not always straightforward. This will need to involve a broader evaluation of potential risk factors for psychosis. In addition to the frequency and severity of PLEs, a positive family history of psychosis, emotional responses – such as distress, preoccupation, and the degree of conviction – and cognitive reserves to manage and control unusual experiences likely play a role in the emergence of clinically significant psychotic symptoms.

It is important to recognise that the identification of psychopathology at an early stage is challenging. A checklist approach with a detailed elaboration of the complex dimensions of symptoms may capture only a portion of the information embedded in unusual experiences. To enable the unmasking of underlying characteristics of symptoms, it will be necessary to carefully examine each symptom within its context. For example, the notion of bizarreness might be a manifestation of a more distinct pattern of cognitive-semantic dysfunction that may have a more specific association with the risk of psychosis.

Mild transitory psychotic experiences are not uncommon in early to mid-adolescence and are often associated with distress, depression, anxiety, or conduct symptoms. These unusual experiences often improve with broad psychosocial interventions and treatment of co-occurring mental health difficulties (57). However, a small minority will go on to develop a psychotic illness in late adolescence or early adulthood, and it is, therefore, important to recognise and monitor individuals most at risk. Undoubtedly, further research to delineate specific psychopathological and other risk factors is needed to more reliably predict the emergence of a psychotic illness and aid early intervention.

References

1. Kelleher I, Cannon M. Psychotic-like experiences in the general population: characterizing a high-risk group for psychosis. *Psychol Med.* 2011;41(1):1-6. doi:10.1017/S0033291710001005

2. Yung AR, Nelson B, Baker K, Buckby JA, Baksheev G, Cosgrave EM. Psychotic-like experiences in a community sample of adolescents: implications for the continuum model of psychosis and prediction of schizophrenia. *Aust N Z J Psychiatry*. 2009;43(2):118-128. doi:10.1080/00048670802607188

3. Poulton R, Caspi A, Moffitt TE, Cannon M, Murray R, Harrington H. Children's self-reported psychotic symptoms and adult schizophreniform disorder: a 15-year longitudinal study. *Arch Gen Psychiatry*. 2000;57(11):1053-1058. doi:10.1001/archpsyc.57.11.1053

4. Welham J, Scott J, Williams G, et al. Emotional and behavioural antecedents of young adults who screen positive for non-affective psychosis: a 21-year birth cohort study. *Psychol Med*. 2009;39(4):625-634. doi:10.1017/S0033291708003760

5. Hanssen M, Bak M, Bijl R, Vollebergh W, van Os J. The incidence and outcome of subclinical psychotic experiences in the general population. *Br J Clin Psychol*. 2005;44(Pt 2):181-191. doi:10.1348/014466505X29611

6. Pechey R, Halligan P. Prevalence and correlates of anomalous experiences in a large non-clinical sample. *Psychol Psychother*. 2012;85(2):150-162. doi:10.1111/j.2044-8341.2011.02024.x

7. Kendler KS, Gallagher TJ, Abelson JM, Kessler RC. Lifetime prevalence, demographic risk factors, and diagnostic validity of nonaffective psychosis as assessed in a US community sample. The National Comorbidity Survey. *Arch Gen Psychiatry*. 1996;53(11):1022-1031. doi:10.1001/archpsyc.1996.01830110060007

8. van Os J, Hanssen M, Bijl RV, Ravelli A. Strauss (1969) revisited: a psychosis continuum in the general population? *Schizophr Res*. 2000;45(1-2):11-20. doi:10.1016/s0920-9964(99)00224-8

9. van Os J, Linscott RJ, Myin-Germeys I, Delespaul P, Krabbendam L. A systematic review and meta-analysis of the psychosis continuum: evidence for a psychosis proneness-persistence-impairment model of psychotic disorder. *Psychol Med*. 2009;39(2):179-195. doi:10.1017/S0033291708003814

10. Dominguez MD, Wichers M, Lieb R, Wittchen HU, van Os J. Evidence that onset of clinical psychosis is an outcome of progressively more persistent subclinical psychotic experiences: an 8-year cohort study. *Schizophr Bull*. 2011;37(1):84-93. doi:10.1093/schbul/sbp022

11. Cougnard A, Marcelis M, Myin-Germeys I, et al. Does normal developmental expression of psychosis combine with environmental risk to cause persistence of psychosis? A psychosis proneness-persistence model. *Psychol Med*. 2007;37(4):513-527. doi:10.1017/S0033291706009731

12. Wiles NJ, Zammit S, Bebbington P, Singleton N, Meltzer H, Lewis G. Self-reported psychotic symptoms in the general population: results from the longitudinal study of the British National Psychiatric Morbidity Survey. *Br J Psychiatry*. 2006;188:519-526. doi:10.1192/bjp.bp.105.012179

13. Mackie CJ, Castellanos-Ryan N, Conrod PJ. Developmental trajectories of psychotic-like experiences across adolescence: impact of victimization and substance use. *Psychol Med*. 2011;41(1):47-58. doi:10.1017/S0033291710000449

14. Lee KW, Chan KW, Chang WC, Lee EH, Hui CL, Chen EY. A systematic review on definitions and assessments of psychotic-like experiences. *Early Interv Psychiatry.* 2016;10(1):3-16. doi:10.1111/eip.12228

15. McGorry PD, Phillips LJ, Yung AR. Recognition and treatment of the pre-psychotic phase of psychotic disorders: frontier or fantasy? In: Miller T, Mednick SA, McGlashan TH, Libiger J, Johannessen JO, eds. *Early Intervention in Psychotic Disorders.* Kluwer Academic, 2001:101-122.

16. Yung AR, McGorry PD, McFarlane CA, Jackson HJ, Patton GC, Rakkar A. Monitoring and care of young people at incipient risk of psychosis. *Schizophr Bull.* 1996;22(2):283-303. doi:10.1093/schbul/22.2.283

17. Yung AR, McGorry PD. The initial prodrome in psychosis: descriptive and qualitative aspects. *Aust N Z J Psychiatry.* 1996;30(5):587-599. doi:10.3109/00048679609062654

18. Häfner H, Löffler W, Maurer K, Hambrecht M, an der Heiden W. Depression, negative symptoms, social stagnation and social decline in the early course of schizophrenia. *Acta Psychiatr Scand.* 1999;100(2):105-118. doi:10.1111/j.1600-0447.1999.tb10831.x

19. Larsen TK, McGlashan TH, Moe LC. First-episode schizophrenia: I. Early course parameters. *Schizophr Bull.* 1996;22(2):241-256. doi:10.1093/schbul/22.2.241

20. Keshavan MS, Shrivastava A, Gangadhar BN. Early intervention in psychotic disorders: challenges and relevance in the Indian context. *Indian J Psychiatry.* 2010;52(Suppl 1):S153-S158. doi:10.4103/0019-5545.69228

21. McGorry PD, Yung A, Phillips L. Ethics and early intervention in psychosis: keeping up the pace and staying in step. *Schizophr Res.* 2001;51(1):17-29. doi:10.1016/s0920-9964(01)00235-3

22. Yung AR, Jackson HJ. The onset of psychotic disorder: clinical and research aspects. In: McGorry PD, Jackson HJ, eds. *The Recognition and Management of Early Psychosis: A Preventive Approach.* Cambridge University Press; 1999:27-50.

23. Beiser M, Erickson D, Fleming JA, Iacono WG. Establishing the onset of psychotic illness. *Am J Psychiatry.* 1993;150(9):1349-1354. doi:10.1176/ajp.150.9.1349

24. Häfner H, Maurer K. The prodromal phase of psychosis. In: Miller T, Mednick SA, McGlashan TH, Libiger J, Johannessen JO, eds. *Early Intervention in Psychotic Disorders.* Kluwer Academic; 1998:71-100.

25. Malla AK, Norman RM. Prodromal symptoms in schizophrenia. *Br J Psychiatry.* 1994;164(4):487-493. doi:10.1192/bjp.164.4.487

26. Parnas J. From predisposition to psychosis: progression of symptoms in schizophrenia. *Acta Psychiatr Scand Suppl.* 1999;395:20-29. doi:10.1111/j.1600-0447.1999.tb05979.x

27. Huber G. Das Konzept substratnaher Basissymptome und seine Bedeutung für Theorie und Therapie schizophrener Erkrankungen [The concept of substrate-close basic symptoms and its significance for the theory and therapy of schizophrenic diseases]. *Nervenarzt.* 1983;54(1):23-32.

28. Schultze-Lutter F. Subjective symptoms of schizophrenia in research and the clinic: the basic symptom concept. *Schizophr Bull.* 2009;35(1):5-8. doi:10.1093/schbul/sbn139

29. Yung AR, Nelson B. The ultra-high risk concept – a review. *Can J Psychiatry.* 2013;58(1):5-12. doi:10.1177/070674371305800103

30. Polari A, Lavoie S, Yuen HP, et al. Clinical trajectories in the ultra-high risk for psychosis population. *Schizophr Res.* 2018;197:550-556. doi:10.1016/j.schres.2018.01.022

31. Yung AR, Yuen HP, McGorry PD, et al. Mapping the onset of psychosis: the comprehensive assessment of at-risk mental states. *Aust N Z J Psychiatry*. 2005;39(11-12):964-971. doi:10.1080/j.1440-1614.2005.01714.x
32. Larsen TK, Friis S, Haahr U, et al. Early detection and intervention in first-episode schizophrenia: a critical review. *Acta Psychiatr Scand*. 2001;103(5):323-334. doi:10.1034/j.1600-0447.2001.00131.x
33. Klosterkötter J, Gross G, Huber G, Wieneke A, Steinmeyer EM, Schultze-Lutter F. Evaluation of the 'Bonn scale for the assessment of basic symptoms – BSABS' as an instrument for the assessment of schizophrenia proneness: a review of recent findings. *Neurol Psychiatry Brain Res*. 1997;5:137-150.
34. McGlashan TH, Miller TJ, Woods SW, Hoffman RE, Davidson L. Instrument for the assessment of prodromal symptoms and states. In Miller T, Mednick SA, McGlashan TH, Libiger J, Hohannessen JO, eds. *Early Intervention in Psychotic Disorders*. Kluwer Academic Publishers. 2001:135-149.
35. Woods SW, Walsh BC, Powers AR, McGlashan TH: Reliability, validity, epidemiology, and cultural variation of the Structured Interview for Psychosis-Risk Syndromes (SIPS) and the Scale of Psychosis-Risk Symptoms (SOPS). In: Li H, Shapiro DI, Seidman LJ, eds. *Handbook of Attenuated Psychosis Syndrome Across Cultures*. Springer; 2019:85-113.
36. McGorry PD, Nelson B, Amminger GP, et al. Intervention in individuals at ultra-high risk for psychosis: a review and future directions. *J Clin Psychiatry*. 2009;70(9):1206-1212. doi:10.4088/JCP.08r04472
37. Sandini C, Zöller D, Schneider M, et al. Characterization and prediction of clinical pathways of vulnerability to psychosis through graph signal processing. *Elife*. 2021;10:e59811. Published Sep 27, 2021. doi:10.7554/eLife.59811
38. Lam MM, Hung SF, Chen EY. Transition to psychosis: 6-month follow-up of a Chinese high-risk group in Hong Kong. *Aust N Z J Psychiatry*. 2006;40(5):414-420. doi:10.1080/j.1440-1614.2006.01817.x
39. Lam MML, Hung SF, Chen EYH. 2-year follow-up of a Chinese high risk group. *Early Interv Psychiatry*. 2008;2(Suppl. 1):A67–A136, PO237. doi:10.1111/j.1751-7893.2008.00097.x
40. Chang WC, Strauss GP, Ahmed AO, et al. The latent structure of negative symptoms in individuals with attenuated psychosis syndrome and early psychosis: support for the 5 consensus domains. *Schizophr Bull*. 2021;47(2):386-394. doi:10.1093/schbul/sbaa129
41. Chang WC, Lee HC, Chan SI, et al. Negative symptom dimensions differentially impact on functioning in individuals at-risk for psychosis. *Schizophr Res*. 2018;202:310-315. doi:10.1016/j.schres.2018.06.041
42. Lam M, Abdul Rashid NA, Lee SA, et al. Baseline social amotivation predicts 1-year functioning in UHR subjects: A validation and prospective investigation. *Eur Neuropsychopharmacol*. 2015;25(12):2187-2196. doi:10.1016/j.euroneuro.2015.10.007
43. Chan KN, Chang WC, Ng CM, et al. Sex differences in symptom severity, cognition and psychosocial functioning among individuals with at-risk mental state for psychosis. *Early Interv Psychiatry*. 2022;16(1):61-68. doi:10.1111/eip.13131

44. Chang WC, Ng CM, Chan KN, et al. Psychiatric comorbidity in individuals at-risk for psychosis: relationships with symptoms, cognition and psychosocial functioning. *Early Interv Psychiatry*. 2021 Jun;15(3):616-623.

45. Yung AR, McGorry PD. The prodromal phase of first-episode psychosis: past and current conceptualizations. *Schizophr Bull*. 1996;22(2):353-370. doi:10.1093/schbul/22.2.353

46. Ching EY, Lee EH, Hui CL, et al. Prodromal psychosis: a case series of ten symptomatic patients. *East Asian Arch Psychiatry*. 2015;25(1):35-41.

47. McGorry PD, Hickie IB, Yung AR, Pantelis C, Jackson HJ. Clinical staging of psychiatric disorders: a heuristic framework for choosing earlier, safer and more effective interventions. *Aust N Z J Psychiatry*. 2006;40(8):616-622. doi:10.1080/j.1440-1614.2006.01860.x

48. Fulford KWM, Jackson M. Spiritual experience and psychopathology. *Philosophy, Psychiatry, & Psychology*. 1997;4(1):41-65. *Project MUSE*, doi:10.1353/ppp.1997.0002.

49. Wüsten C, Schlier B, Jaya ES, et al. Psychotic experiences and related distress: a cross-national comparison and network analysis based on 7141 participants from 13 countries. *Schizophr Bull*. 2018;44(6):1185-1194. doi:10.1093/schbul/sby087

50. Zammit S, Kounali D, Cannon M, et al. Psychotic experiences and psychotic disorders at age 18 in relation to psychotic experiences at age 12 in a longitudinal population-based cohort study. *Am J Psychiatry*. 2013;170(7):742-750. doi:10.1176/appi.ajp.2013.12060768

51. Chan SKW, Lee KKW, Chan VHY, et al. The 12-month prevalence of psychotic experiences and their association with clinical outcomes in Hong Kong: an epidemiological and a 2-year follow up studies. *Psychol Med*. 2021;51(14):2501-2508. doi:10.1017/S0033291720001452

52. Lee KW, Chan S, Chang WC, Lee E, Hui CLM, Chen E. Persistence of psychotic-like experiences (PLES) in the general population of Hong Kong. The 4th Biennial Schizophrenia International Research Conference; Apr 5–9, 2014; Florence, Italy. *Schizophr Res*. 2014;153(suppl. 1):S337, poster no. T134. doi:10.1016/S0920-9964(14)70951-X

53. Lam BY, Hui CL, Lui SS, et al. LevelMind@JC hubs-a novel community-based youth mental wellness early intervention in Hong Kong: an evaluation of stakeholders' perceptions and experiences. *Early Interv Psychiatry*. 2022;16(5):533-543. doi:10.1111/eip.13192

54. Hui CL, Suen YN, Lam BY, et al. LevelMind@JC: development and evaluation of a community early intervention program for young people in Hong Kong. *Early Interv Psychiatry*. 2022;16(8):920-925. doi:10.1111/eip.13261

55. McGrath JJ, Saha S, Al-Hamzawi A, et al. Psychotic experiences in the general population: a cross-national analysis based on 31,261 respondents from 18 countries. *JAMA Psychiatry*. 2015;72(7):697-705. doi:10.1001/jamapsychiatry.2015.0575

56. Kelleher I, Keeley H, Corcoran P, et al. Clinicopathological significance of psychotic experiences in non-psychotic young people: evidence from four population-based studies. *Br J Psychiatry*. 2012;201(1):26-32. doi:10.1192/bjp.bp.111.101543

57. Murray GK, Jones PB. Psychotic symptoms in young people without psychotic illness: mechanisms and meaning. *Br J Psychiatry*. 2012;201(1):4-6. doi:10.1192/bjp.bp.111.107789

8

Can Early Intervention Improve Long-Term Outcomes? Evidence from Hong Kong

Background

The Aim of Early Intervention

The ultimate objective of early intervention is not limited to the early phase of psychotic disorders, but to improve their outcome in the long term (1). Negative long-term outcomes have been a major concern for health professionals and patients (2). Psychosis can lead to substantial functional impairments in both vocational and social domains (3). Symptomatic outcomes are also less satisfactory than commonly assumed (4). Despite the advent of modern psychopharmacology, relapse and residual and refractory psychotic symptoms continue to impact the daily experience of a large proportion of patients over long periods (5). In addition, psychotic disorders carry significant mortality. The lifetime suicide mortality is 5%–10% (6). Early non-suicidal deaths also contribute to the staggering overall reduction in life expectancy for psychosis patients by ten to twenty years (7).

Since it has been demonstrated that poor outcomes are associated with delay in treatment, and that focused treatment in the early years of a psychotic disorder can improve a number of symptomatic and functional outcomes (8, 9, 10, 11), it is reasonable to ask whether early psychosis work can make an impact on longer-term outcomes, beyond the initial years of the active programme. Researchers have proposed the 'critical period hypothesis', which stipulates that there is a critical time window in the early course of the disorder in which early outcome may disproportionately affect the longer course of the illness (12). This critical period hypothesis is an important rationale for focusing more resources on attaining better outcomes in the early stage of the disorder. It is, however, important not to fall into an 'all or nothing' fallacy. It is now known that multiple factors contribute to the pathogenesis of psychotic disorders, and it is unlikely that all contributory factors will be malleable to the same extent during the critical period. It is therefore an important empirical question to determine the extent to which early efforts to improve outcomes can be carried over to the long term.

The Challenges of Measuring Long-Term Outcomes

Evaluating the long-term outcome of any intervention is a particularly challenging exercise because, during the long-time frame required for long-term outcome studies, healthcare practices often change for the better. This may favour the ongoing recovery of patients who were not exposed to early interventions (10). Such improvement in the 'standard care' comparison group may mask the long-term impact of early intervention services. On a number of occasions, the improvement in generic services has actually been a consequence of the success of early psychosis work. For example, in Hong Kong, the early psychosis programme initiated the first comprehensive use of case management. As a result, case management was introduced into generic psychiatric services several years later, thus also benefiting the long-term outcome of patients who did not previously receive early psychosis intervention.

Because of the logistic challenge of long-term outcome studies, only a few datasets are available on the long-term outcomes of early intervention (EI) worldwide. Apart from Hong Kong, for example, the OPUS project in Denmark has generated ten-year outcome data. The OPUS project compared cohorts of patients who received EI with those who did not receive early intervention for two years (standard care or SC group) and then followed them up after the EI input had ceased, with both groups receiving standard care for up to ten years. They found that the EI group did better in terms of symptomatic and functional outcomes at two years, but this advantage became more diluted with time so that by five years much of the difference in outcomes had become statistically insignificant. At ten-year follow-up, only the 'living independently' factor was still superior in individuals who had received EI (13). Notably, this convergence in outcome has been attributable to both improvements in standard care with time, as well as a decline in the effect of EI over time. It is also important to point out that the case management input to both the EI and the SC group was intensive in the OPUS project, with caseloads of ten and 20 cases per case manager, respectively, ensuring at least monthly contact with patients (13). This level of case management is seldom met in locations with more limited mental health resources. For example, in Hong Kong caseloads have varied between 80 and over 100 patients per case manager in EI services, and in the SC group, few patients received any case management at all.

Outcomes of Early Intervention in Hong Kong

Long-Term Outcomes

Comparable data from Hong Kong in EI and SC groups have been reported in a series of follow-up studies. We found that EI was associated with better outcomes in functioning and mortality for up to ten years, with the difference still being discernible in year four to year ten (9). Significantly, early intervention has been able to reduce the ten-year suicide rate from 7% to 4%, mostly due to the reduction of early suicide in the EI group in the first three years (14). Patients who had received EI were also less likely to attempt suicide and required fewer and shorter hospitalisations compared to patients receiving standard care (15). Improvements in occupational functioning also persisted for up to ten years (11).

Hierarchical cluster analysis of longitudinal patterns in functioning has identified groups of patients with good functional outcomes that could be maintained over time (16). EI and SC groups were similar in premorbid functional levels. However, in the EI group, more people achieved good longitudinal functional outcomes. Conversely, a smaller proportion of people in the EI group attained poor functional outcomes. It is interesting to observe that for patients in the EI group whose outcome was poor at ten-year follow-up, an improved functional outcome was observed in the first three years, probably as a direct result of the EI input. However, the favourable outcomes subsequently declined. This is in contrast to the corresponding poor functional outcome group in SC, where no initial improvement took place. This suggests that EI produces two effects on functioning in different groups of patients: first, a persistent effect resulting in good outcomes in the longer term; and second, a temporary effect of improved functioning while EI lasted, but this was not sustained when the patients were stepped down to standard care. These observations suggest that even in a low-resource setting, EI can achieve long-term effects by enhancing recovery in the critical period in a significant proportion of patients. However, for other patients, the benefits of EI are evident only during the early phase of the illness. Thus, there are both critical period and non-critical period factors mediating the long-term effects of EI. It is also important to note that the relative proportion of critical period factors may be population-specific, depending on the genetic and epigenetic expression of psychosis in the population, environmental adversity as well as service factors such as caseload, training, and availability of pharmacological and non-pharmacological treatments. These longitudinal studies also highlighted one important phenomenon associated with long-term outcome studies comparing SC with EI, namely a 'ripple effect' of EI leading to improvements in the quality and intensity of standard care several years later. Such improvements in standard care are a desirable outcome, even if this complicates long-term studies by making the long-term effects of EI more difficult to discern.

Short and Intermediate Outcomes

Several studies undertaken in Hong Kong have also examined predictors of functional remission over the early course of the illness. These showed that female patients typically improved more rapidly during the first six months with subsequent stabilisation compared to males who experienced a more gradual improvement over 12 months (17).

For female patients, better premorbid psychosocial functioning was predictive of better functional outcomes at 12 months, and poor educational attainment was a predictor of poor outcomes for both genders. An interesting and important finding was that those patients who had good insight at baseline had poorer functioning at six months. This has been somewhat puzzling as other studies have shown a positive correlation between insight and functional outcome albeit usually over 12 months or more (18, 19). For most patients, significant symptom reduction likely occurs over the first six months, particularly with good medication and treatment adherence that is usually associated with good insight. As symptoms recede up to 50% of patients develop depressive symptoms including suicidal ideation (20). Better cognitive insight has been shown to be significantly associated with higher levels of depression (21). Depression is known to negatively affect psychosocial functioning and this might explain the finding of poorer functioning at six months. However, the relationship between insight and severity of depressive symptoms is possibly mediated by complex interactions between premorbid adjustment, ruminatory style, perception of illness, and recovery as well as stigma (21). In addition, negative symptoms may become more prominent after the initial acute psychotic episode subsides and it can prove challenging to differentiate the cognitive and biological symptoms that define depressive disorders and negative symptomatology. Consequently, adequate and timely identification and treatment of depressive symptoms are paramount in the early phase of remission.

Another important result was that male patients were more likely to have a less favourable outcome at 12 months, particularly those who had lower premorbid adjustment and functioning. This finding also has practical consequences for assessment in that EI services may need to offer earlier and more intensive psychosocial rehabilitation for patients with poor premorbid functioning.

Early intervention has played a critical role in improving short- to medium-term outcomes of patients with first-episode psychosis (FEP) over the last two decades. In Hong Kong, patients enrolled in the Early Assessment Service for Young People (EASY) were more likely to be in full-time employment or study, to have fewer days of hospitalisation, and to experience less severe positive and negative symptoms after three years of initial presentation. As already mentioned, EI treatment has also been associated with a reduced suicide rate during the first few years, fewer disengagements, and more patients experiencing a period of recovery when compared to standard care. Rates of relapse and duration of untreated psychosis (DUP) among young people, however, have only improved slightly with EI from a median of around 100 days to 90 days (22, 23, 24). In contrast, the DUP in adult-onset patients significantly reduced from a median of around 180 days to 93 days (25).

Early Intervention and Engagement

Chan et al. (2014) examined the disengagement of service users and reported that patients with fewer symptoms and those with poorer medication adherence were more likely to disengage (26). Overall, only 13% of patients dropped out of treatment completely. Around two-thirds of patients had achieved symptomatic remission in the month of disengagement. Close to 20% of individuals who had temporarily disengaged, returned to our service following a relapse and rehospitalisation. Younger age was associated with earlier disengagement (27). The results indicate that patients disengage when they believe to have recovered from their psychotic illness and no longer require treatment or when they consider interventions ineffective. Given that a substantial number of patients experience a relapse of their psychotic illness, the risk of disengagement requires attention. To address this challenge, ongoing efforts to engage patients and their carers are important in co-producing effective individualised treatment plans.

Extending Early Intervention

Chang et al. (2015, 2016) have also shown that extending EI from two years to three years improves functional outcomes of young people in the medium term, particularly for female patients, those with better baseline functioning and premorbid adjustment as well as less severe positive symptoms (28, 29). In addition, extended EI may alleviate motivational impairment, a major determinant of functional outcome (30).

Chang et al. (2017) followed up 160 youths who were either receiving 12 months of extended EI (EI for three years) or standard EASY care (EI for two years) (31). Although symptoms and psychosocial functioning continued to improve for patients who received three years of EI compared to those who received two years of EI, these improvements could not be sustained two years after the cessation of the extended EI service. Symptom severity, service use, and functional outcome were found to be similar between the groups. These findings raise important questions about the optimal duration of EI services. Firstly, the lack of sustained difference between the groups may be related to the dosage of intervention. It could be that more intensive input is required for consolidating the additional benefits that are gained in the third year over and above the benefits already acquired in the first two years. This approach may help a significant proportion of patients attain adequate functional outcomes in the long term. It might well be that a sub-group of patients who present with poorer functioning after the first two years of treatment require more intensive care for an extended period of time to attain sustained functional gains. More personalisation of care during the critical period of intervention should be explored. Stratification of patients according to predicted symptomatic and functional outcomes might also allow a timely implementation of sub-programmes to deal with their specific needs, such as comorbid mood or anxiety disorders, negative symptoms, treatment refractoriness, and relapse.

Reflections: The Innovative Potential of Early Intervention Programmes

Early intervention for psychosis in Hong Kong has aligned with the overall objectives of international EI programmes, namely that of improving outcomes of psychotic disorders through earlier detection, and the provision of specialised interventions in the early years of the disorder. The evaluation of EI programmes is complex when long-term outcomes are involved. EI programmes have triggered improvements in generic services that likely lead to improved outcomes in standard care over time, making it more difficult to demonstrate the long-term superiority of EI programmes. In Hong Kong, we observed a reduction in DUP, but mainly for adult-onset psychosis, i.e. after the age of 25, and not for young people. It could be that a median DUP of around three months for young people was already the shortest that could realistically be achieved by the approaches we adopted, whereas the medium DUP for adult patients was around six months. Our approach to shortening DUP was based on the observation that DUP was related to family knowledge of psychotic disorders. The reasons why we were not able to reduce the DUP in young people to under three months were not clear, particularly given the possibility that some programmes in other countries were able to reduce the DUP to less than one month. One possible difference is that, in Hong Kong, we had not yet conducted an extensive public education campaign for clinical high-risk groups. Promoting awareness of clinical high-risk states may enable more young people to contact the EI service. If they went on to develop psychosis, they would already be engaged with our service and be informed about how to seek early help.

The lack of a clear impact on DUP for young people has enabled us to review the therapeutic elements in the Hong Kong EI programme without having to control for the length of DUP. The remaining main therapeutic drive leading to enhanced outcomes was the phase-specific intervention provided by case managers in specialised EI teams. Our findings, that improvements are evident while early intervention is provided, are in line with EI studies from around the world. We have also shown that the benefits from EI can be sustained after care is stepped down.

Sustained improvement in functioning, as well as a reduction in hospitalisation and suicides, have been observed. These findings are important as they support the idea of investing resources to manage the critical initial years of a psychotic disorder. It is important to note that in several long-term outcome studies, sustained effects of EI are not consistently reported. The OPUS project in Denmark observed that the effect of EI declined after the service was withdrawn. The difference may well be related to a difference in the level of input both in the EI and in the standard care group. The caseload for EI case workers in the OPUS programmes has been around 10; while that for the EASY programme has been approximately 70. Casework is available for people in Denmark for standard care, while casework is available in Hong Kong only for a smaller number of patients with high clinical risks.

Our observations have been made using a historical control group matched for premorbid functioning. Even though the time lag between the EI and control cohort was only one year, it is possible that some uncontrolled variables differed. This possibility was less likely as apart from functioning, some other clinical features, such as the relapse rate, were comparable between the two groups. Another possible difference is that the OPUS study adopted a randomised controlled trial (RCT) design. Participation in an RCT might have selected a sample of patients with better insight and adherence, while the Hong Kong study was a cohort before and after study with a more real-life sample.

Apart from improved occupational functioning and reduction in hospitalisation, the EI cohort also had fewer completed suicides. From a health economic perspective, these improvements were achieved without a significant increase in health service costs in the EI group. This is largely due to savings in inpatient costs. Thus, we have established an EI model for psychotic disorders in Hong Kong that is effective in reducing suicide and enhancing functional outcomes, and is economically viable.

Additional EI studies have explored further opportunities to improve the outcomes of psychotic disorders. We have investigated the impact of increasing the duration of case management from two years to three years and have demonstrated with an RCT that additional functional enhancements could be achieved. This has led to the extension of the EI programme in Hong Kong to three years. We have also investigated the possibility of offering case management to adult-onset patients over the age of 25 years with a three-arm RCT including a control group with no case management, a two-year case management, and a four-year case management group. Compared with youth-onset patients, the baseline functional impairment is not as severe in adult-onset patients when compared to that of young people. Thus there is less room for improving outcomes. We found that intervention impacted those patients who had a longer DUP. Since it is known that longer DUP negatively affects outcome, the impact of intervention for the group with worse overall outcomes suggests that they may have more room for improvement given their poor initial outcomes. Our findings have prompted the development of EI services for adult-onset patients, and the data suggest that individualising interventions may allow more effective deployment of resources.

Stratification of patients according to predicted symptomatic and functional outcomes might allow a timely transfer of patients with good predicted outcomes to non-specialist psychiatric services with the option of re-referral to EI services if this is required. For some patients, this might mean a less than two-year EI programme and could thus free up resources to support those patients with less favourable outcomes. However, any transfer of care usually requires comprehensive planning to ensure good handover and ongoing therapeutic engagement to avoid disruption of psychiatric care.

Questions remain as to which components of the phase-specific EI constitute effective treatment elements, whether in the short, medium, or longer term. Effective engagement is likely to be one important factor, alongside developing meaningful goal-directed individualised treatment plans, early occupational and social rehabilitation, and engaging carers. Defining functional outcomes is necessarily value-driven, and adequate psychosocial functioning has often been defined in ways that depend on the overall employment situation in the community. During times of economic recession, accessing employment is significantly more challenging for everyone of working age. Individuals with severe and enduring mental illness are already at a disadvantage in most work environments and will be disproportionately affected by economic crises without this being a sensitive reflection of the extent of their recovery. In addition, in many societies, there has been a shift away from traditional working patterns, and a significant proportion of the workforce is now employed less than full-time either out of choice or necessity and often work from home. Also, socialisation for most young people has moved from solely face-to-face contact to predominantly online interactions, even more so since the beginning of the COVID-19 pandemic. These are important societal developments to take into account when assessing functioning with conventional rating scales and adaptations of instruments may be required to more closely reflect current societal circumstances. Otherwise, one may risk underestimating functional outcomes.

Enhancing outcomes for psychotic disorders is an endeavour that requires iterative cycles of improvements. Specialised early psychosis services are well-placed to take on this challenge because they are positioned to provide focused interventions with designated staff in specialised settings. It is likely that generic services will also benefit from the experience of early psychosis programmes resulting in the improvement of standard care. When comparable standards have been achieved in generic services, early psychosis services will likely seek new ways to further enhance outcomes beyond that of the improved standard services, thus driving innovation forward.

References

1. Bertolote J, McGorry P. Early intervention and recovery for young people with early psychosis: consensus statement. *Br J Psychiatry Suppl.* 2005;48:s116-s119. doi:10.1192/bjp.187.48.s116

2. Collins PY, Patel V, Joestl SS, et al. Grand challenges in global mental health. *Nature.* 2011;475(7354):27-30. Published Jul 6, 2011. doi:10.1038/475027a

3. Chang WC, Chu AOK, Kwong VWY, et al. Patterns and predictors of trajectories for social and occupational functioning in patients presenting with first-episode non-affective psychosis: a three-year follow-up study. *Schizophr Res.* 2018;197:131-137. doi:10.1016/j.schres.2018.01.021

4. Chan SK, Chen EY, Tang JY, et al. Early intervention versus standard care for psychosis in Hong Kong: a 10-year study. *Hong Kong Med J.* 2015;21 Suppl 2:19-22.

5. Hui CL, Tang JY, Leung CM, et al. A 3-year retrospective cohort study of predictors of relapse in first-episode psychosis in Hong Kong. *Aust N Z J Psychiatry.* 2013;47(8):746-753. doi:10.1177/0004867413487229

6. Dutta R, Murray RM, Hotopf M, Allardyce J, Jones PB, Boydell J. Reassessing the long-term risk of suicide after a first episode of psychosis. *Arch Gen Psychiatry.* 2010;67(12):1230-1237. doi:10.1001/archgenpsychiatry.2010.157

7. Hjorthøj C, Stürup AE, McGrath JJ, Nordentoft M. Years of potential life lost and life expectancy in schizophrenia: a systematic review and meta-analysis [published correction appears in *Lancet Psychiatry.* Sep 2017;4(9):e19]. *Lancet Psychiatry.* 2017;4(4):295-301. doi:10.1016/S2215-0366(17)30078-0

8. Chang WC, Hui CL, Tang JY, et al. Impacts of duration of untreated psychosis on cognition and negative symptoms in first-episode schizophrenia: a 3-year prospective follow-up study. *Psychol Med.* 2013;43(9):1883-1893. doi:10.1017/S0033291712002838

9. Chan SKW, Hui CLM, Chang WC, Lee EHM, Chen EYH. Ten-year follow up of patients with first-episode schizophrenia spectrum disorder from an early intervention service: predictors of clinical remission and functional recovery. *Schizophr Res.* 2019;204:65-71. doi:10.1016/j.schres.2018.08.022

10. Chan SKW, Chan HYV, Devlin J, et al. A systematic review of long-term outcomes of patients with psychosis who received early intervention services. *Int Rev Psychiatry.* 2019;31(5-6):425-440. doi:10.1080/09540261.2019.1643704

11. Chan SKW, Pang HH, Yan KK, et al. Ten-year employment patterns of patients with first-episode schizophrenia-spectrum disorders: comparison of early intervention and standard care services. *Br J Psychiatry.* 2020;217(3):491-497. doi:10.1192/bjp.2019.161

12. Birchwood M, Todd P, Jackson C. Early intervention in psychosis: the critical period hypothesis. *Br J Psychiatry Suppl.* 1998;172(33):53-59.

13. Secher RG, Hjorthøj CR, Austin SF, et al. Ten-year follow-up of the OPUS specialized early intervention trial for patients with a first episode of psychosis. *Schizophr Bull.* 2015;41(3):617-626. doi:10.1093/schbul/sbu15510.1093/schbul/sbu155. Epub Nov 7, 2014. PMID: 25381449; PMCID: PMC4393691.

14. Chan SKW, Chan SWY, Pang HH, et al. Association of an Early intervention service for psychosis with suicide rate among patients with first-episode

schizophrenia-spectrum disorders. *JAMA Psychiatry*. 2018;75(5):458-464. doi:10.1001/jamapsychiatry.2018.0185

15. Chan SK, So HC, Hui CL, et al. 10-year outcome study of an early intervention program for psychosis compared with standard care service. *Psychol Med*. 2015;45(6):1181-1193. doi:10.1017/S0033291714002220

16. Chan SKW, Chan HYV, Pang HH, et al. Ten-year trajectory and outcomes of negative symptoms of patients with first-episode schizophrenia spectrum disorders. *Schizophr Res*. 2020;220:85-91. doi:10.1016/j.schres.2020.03.061

17. Chong CS, Siu MW, Kwan CH, et al. Predictors of functioning in people suffering from first-episode psychosis 1 year into entering early intervention service in Hong Kong. *Early Interv Psychiatry*. 2018;12(5):828-838. doi:10.1111/eip.12374

18. Segarra R, Ojeda N, Peña J, et al. Longitudinal changes of insight in first episode psychosis and its relation to clinical symptoms, treatment adherence and global functioning: one-year follow-up from the Eiffel study. *Eur Psychiatry*. 2012;27(1):43-49. doi:10.1016/j.eurpsy.2010.06.003

19. Bergé D, Mané A, Salgado P, et al. Predictors of relapse and functioning in first-episode psychosis: a two-year follow-up study. *Psychiatr Serv*. 2016;67(2):227-233. doi:10.1176/appi.ps.201400316

20. Herniman SE, Allott K, Phillips LJ, et al. Depressive psychopathology in first-episode schizophrenia spectrum disorders: a systematic review, meta-analysis and meta-regression. *Psychol Med*. 2019;49(15):2463-2474. doi:10.1017/S0033291719002344

21. Belvederi Murri M, Respino M, Innamorati M, et al. Is good insight associated with depression among patients with schizophrenia? Systematic review and meta-analysis. *Schizophr Res*. 2015;162(1-3):234-247. doi:10.1016/j.schres.2015.01.003

22. Chen EY, Tang JY, Hui CL, et al. Three-year outcome of phase-specific early intervention for first-episode psychosis: a cohort study in Hong Kong. *Early Interv Psychiatry*. 2011;5(4):315-323. doi:10.1111/j.1751-7893.2011.00279.x

23. Chiu CPY, Chen EY, Tang J, et al. A case-controlled study on the outcome of an early intervention programme for psychosis (EASY). The 12th International Congress on Schizophrenia Research (ICOSR 2009); Mar 28–Apr 1, 2009; San Diego, CA. *Schizophr Bull*. 2009;35(suppl. 1):134. doi:10.1093/schbul/sbn173

24. Chiu CPY, Tang JYM, Chen EYH, et al. Outcome of an early intervention programme for psychosis (EASY). The 6th International Conference on Early Psychosis; Oct 20–22, 2008; Melbourne, Australia. *Early Interv Psychiatry*. 2008;2(suppl. S1): A112, abstract no. PO169. doi:10.1111/j.1751-7893.2008.00096.x

25. Chan SKW, Chau EHS, Hui CLM, Chang WC, Lee EHM, Chen EYH. Long term effect of early intervention service on duration of untreated psychosis in youth and adult population in Hong Kong. *Early Interv Psychiatry*. 2018;12(3):331-338. doi:10.1111/eip.12313

26. Chan TC, Chang WC, Hui CL, Chan SK, Lee EH, Chen EY. Rate and predictors of disengagement from a 2-year early intervention program for psychosis in Hong Kong. *Schizophr Res*. 2014;153(1-3):204-208. doi:10.1016/j.schres.2014.01.033

27. Lau KW, Chan SKW, Hui CLM, et al. Rates and predictors of disengagement of patients with first-episode psychosis from the early intervention service for psychosis

service (EASY) covering 15 to 64 years of age in Hong Kong. *Early Interv Psychiatry.* 2019;13(3):398-404. doi:10.1111/eip.12491

28. Chang WC, Kwong VW, Chan GH, et al. Prediction of functional remission in first-episode psychosis: 12-month follow-up of the randomized-controlled trial on extended early intervention in Hong Kong. *Schizophr Res.* 2016;173(1-2):79-83. doi:10.1016/j.schres.2016.03.016

29. Chang WC, Chan GH, Jim OT, et al. Optimal duration of an early intervention programme for first-episode psychosis: randomised controlled trial. *Br J Psychiatry.* 2015;206(6):492-500. doi:10.1192/bjp.bp.114.150144

30. Chang WC, Kwong VW, Chan GH, et al. Prediction of motivational impairment: 12-month follow-up of the randomized-controlled trial on extended early intervention for first-episode psychosis. *Eur Psychiatry.* 2017;41:37-41. doi:10.1016/j.eurpsy.2016.09.007

31. Chang WC, Kwong VWY, Lau ESK, et al. Sustainability of treatment effect of a 3-year early intervention programme for first-episode psychosis. *Br J Psychiatry.* 2017;211(1):37-44. doi:10.1192/bjp.bp.117.198929

PART III

PSYCHOPATHOLOGY AND CLINICAL PATHWAYS

9

Pharmacological Treatments: What They Can and Cannot Do

Background

Antipsychotic Medication: Efficacy and Adverse Effects

The mainstay of pharmacological treatment of psychotic disorders is antipsychotics. They remain the most important treatment modality to relieve positive symptoms. Antipsychotic medications were introduced in the 1950s (1). Clozapine was the first 'second-generation' medication to be studied in the early 1970s and was found to be superior to chlorpromazine and other antipsychotics without troublesome neurological side effects (2). However, due to alarming reports of agranulocytosis in a high number of patients resulting in several deaths in Finland, clozapine was withdrawn within two years following its introduction (3, 4). Later studies revealed clozapine to be associated with a 1–2% incidence of agranulocytosis, 20 times lower than in the Finnish sample, and it was slowly reintroduced for the treatment of treatment-resistant schizophrenia with mandatory blood monitoring (2, 5, 6, 7).

Several other second-generation antipsychotics (SGAs) were approved for the treatment of schizophrenia throughout the 1990s and early 2000s such as risperidone, olanzapine, quetiapine, and aripiprazole. SGAs have fewer extrapyramidal side effects compared to phenothiazines or butyrophenones. However, many patients experience metabolic side effects including significant weight gain, dyslipidaemia, hypertension, impaired blood glucose tolerance, and diabetes.

Over 60 compounds with antipsychotic properties are currently listed by the World Health Organization, most of them being first-generation antipsychotics (8). Other than clozapine, which remains superior in its efficacy to all other antipsychotics in refractory psychosis, there appears to be little difference in effectiveness between typical and atypical drugs. Most clinicians favour SGAs due to their more favourable side effect profile; however, as Leucht et al. (2021) pointed out recently, most first-generation antipsychotics have been under-studied (9).

Several large trials such as the European Union First Episode Schizophrenia Trial (EUFEST), Comparison of Antipsychotics in First Episode Psychosis (CAFE), and Centre for Intervention Development and Advanced Research (CEDAR) have studied the efficacy of antipsychotic medication in the treatment of first-episode psychosis (10, 11, 12). Monotherapy at low to moderate doses is efficacious in a significant proportion of cases (13, 14). For example, median doses of 2 mg haloperidol per day were sufficient to achieve remission with at least 60% D2/3 receptor occupancy (15). This dose was also found to be the threshold for Parkinsonian side effects in first-episode psychosis (FEP) (16).

At present, there is no clear evidence suggesting that any one antipsychotic is superior to any other apart from clozapine for refractory psychosis. However, some second-generation medications may have lower discontinuation rates compared to haloperidol (14, 17). Although first-generation agents are known to cause more troubling extrapyramidal side effects, SGAs may have more metabolic effects. Interestingly, Tiihonen et al. (2009) followed up patients with schizophrenia for up to 11 years and could not show higher mortality rates for SGA in the Finnish population. In fact, clozapine, an antipsychotic known to have significant metabolic side effects, was associated with substantially lower mortality than other medications (18). However, clozapine remains the medication of choice for treatment-refractory schizophrenia due to its side effect of potentially fatal agranulocytosis. It has been shown to have response rates of up to 80% if prescribed early in the course of the illness, but rates drop to around 30% when treatment is delayed by more than 2.8 years (19).

Antipsychotics and Treatment Refractoriness

For non-responders, antipsychotic polypharmacy has been increasingly used over the last 20 years based on receptor pharmacology, without there being sufficient evidence from preclinical research to support such practice (20). Randomised clinical trials have not shown significant benefits for most drug combinations other than possibly clozapine and aripiprazole (20, 21, 22). In a large observational study, Tiihonen et al. (2019) reported a 14%–23% lower risk of re-hospitalisation with a clozapine–aripiprazole combination compared to clozapine monotherapy (21). There have also been concerns that antipsychotic polypharmacy may lead to underutilisation of clozapine, delay effective treatment, and lead to higher healthcare-related costs. Honer and colleagues (2008) have called for translational research models to link preclinical, clinical, and health services trials to enhance the understanding of the clinical efficacy and effectiveness of antipsychotic combinations (20).

Current Recommendations for Prescribing Antipsychotics

Current recommendations emphasise choosing an antipsychotic agent in collaboration with the patient based on clinical features and side effect profiles (23). First-line treatment should be continued at adequate doses for at least six weeks and the response monitored using established clinical rating scales such as the Positive and Negative Syndrome Scale. In FEP, the aim is usually a 40% to 50% reduction in symptoms to promote functional recovery. Although current guidelines have been consistent in their recommendations of optimal dosing of antipsychotics, there remains controversy regarding the specific choice and duration of treatment (24).

Should a second antipsychotic fail to produce the desired reduction in symptomatology, then a trial of clozapine is warranted. Following a first episode of psychosis, maintenance treatment is usually offered for at least two years before considering withdrawal. Some evidence points towards continuing medication for three years for the best possible long-term outcomes (25). Clinical presentation at onset, insight, risk of relapse, and side effects will guide conversations about withdrawal of medication. Alongside medication psychological interventions such as family therapy and cognitive-behavioural therapy for psychosis (CBTp) should be offered where available (23). Short-term treatment response rates in FEP tend to be higher compared to chronic psychosis, however, have been shown to vary widely between 9.1% to 76.2% depending on the definition of outcomes, follow-up, and medication (26).

Pharmacological Interventions for Psychosis in Hong Kong

Antipsychotic Use in Hong Kong

In Hong Kong, the use of antipsychotic medication has been studied from various angles reflecting the clinical needs of patients with first-episode psychosis. Prescribing trends for antipsychotics among young people were examined between 2004 and 2015 showing an increase in prescriptions. However, prescription rates remained below those in the United States (27). The increase in antipsychotic prescribing was thought to be due to the expansion of early intervention programmes but may have also been due to the more widespread use of antipsychotics in treating other clinical conditions.

A more in-depth analysis of patients in the late 1990s and early 2000s revealed that the majority of FEP patients received first-generation antipsychotics during the first three years of their illness. If initial treatment was unsuccessful, either due to lack of response or intolerable side effects, then olanzapine and risperidone were most commonly prescribed (28). Nowadays, SGAs are routinely commenced as first-line treatment in Hong Kong, although haloperidol and some phenothiazines are widely used to manage acute agitation.

In a study of 285 adult FEP patients, amisulpride was found to be associated with better quality of life when compared with haloperidol, olanzapine, risperidone, quetiapine, and sulpiride. Patients taking haloperidol and risperidone were more likely to experience extrapyramidal side effects. Amisulpride was also associated with higher mental health component scores on the Medical Outcomes Study Short Form 12-Item Health Survey (SF-12) when compared to risperidone. This finding may be explained by the fact that amisulpride likely exerts its differential effects via selective action at limbic and cortical dopamine D2/3 receptors and 5-HT7A receptor antagonism. This selectivity may be associated with improved cognitive functioning and better quality of life due to fewer troublesome extrapyramidal, metabolic, endocrinological, and sexual side effects (29).

Antipsychotics have been shown to improve positive symptoms as early as two weeks into treatment, with more than two-thirds of symptom reduction at one year being observed within the first four weeks (30, 31). Chua et al. (2009) found that FEP patients treated with antipsychotic medication for three to four weeks had significantly greater grey matter volumes in the bilateral caudate nuclei and cingulate gyri, extending to the left medial frontal gyrus when compared to untreated individuals (32). Although it was a small study of 48 patients, the findings suggest that antipsychotics are associated with an increase in striatum volume within a short period of time and that these volume changes might be associated with clinical response (33, 34). The exact mechanism underlying these volume reversals is yet to be determined but is likely to be underpinned by neuroplastic changes in fronto-limbic circuitries (32).

The route of antipsychotic administration significantly affects outcomes. Administration of long-acting injectable antipsychotics (LAIAs) is associated with reduced rates of hospitalisation and relapse (35). Since evidence for the superior efficacy of LAIAs has been very limited in the Chinese population, Wei et al. (2022) examined case records of patients being prescribed either oral antipsychotics (OA) or LAIAs between 2004 and 2019. One-third of the over 70,000 individuals identified were prescribed both OAs and LAIAs. Long-acting injectables were associated with lower rates of all-cause and psychiatric hospitalisation as well as admission due to relapse of schizophrenia or cardiovascular and somatic disease. Those receiving LAIAs were less likely to attempt suicide and had fewer extrapyramidal side effects. The findings suggest a more favourable profile of LAIAs when compared to oral preparations, including improved physical and psychosis outcomes and fewer adverse side effects (36).

Side Effects of Antipsychotic Medication and Their Monitoring

The monitoring of metabolic side effects has been an integral part of prescribing recommendations over many years, in recognition of the fact that not only do antipsychotics increase cardiovascular risks but that psychosis patients have high rates of physical multimorbidity. In our patient population, Chan et al. (2021, 2022) demonstrated that the mortality rates of these patients are twice as high when compared to patients without physical comorbidities (37, 38). However, similar to findings in Western countries, only around half of patients on antipsychotic medication in Hong Kong receive regular blood tests for glucose and lipids, with young people being disproportionately disadvantaged. One of the reasons for the poor uptake of metabolic screening might be the prevalent belief in Chinese culture that invasive procedures such as phlebotomy are harmful to bodily integrity (39).

Antipsychotic-induced tardive dyskinesia and dystonia are probably one of the more under-studied side effects encountered by psychosis patients. Current treatment strategies are considered largely ineffective, although clozapine has been proposed as a potential option. When systematically reviewing the literature, most studies investigating the possible beneficial effect of clozapine were of inefficient quality. Nonetheless, the findings suggest that it may alleviate tardive dyskinesia and dystonia in the majority of schizophrenia spectrum disorders with an average dose of 355 mg/day. Wong et al. (2022) also established the effectiveness of clozapine at comparatively lower doses and faster response in treating tardive dyskinesia and dystonia in non-psychotic disorders (40).

Antipsychotics have also been associated with significant sexual dysfunction, a side effect that is often overlooked in clinical practice. Its importance has been neglected in most clinical studies (41). Prolactin-raising medications such as olanzapine, risperidone, haloperidol, and clozapine have rates of sexual side effects of up to 60% (42).

Attitudes, Adherence, and Discontinuation of Antipsychotic Medication

It has been a longstanding concern that patients with psychotic illnesses have difficulties in taking antipsychotic medication regularly, particularly as the risk of relapse is up to four times higher upon discontinuation of medication following the first episode (43). Non-adherence is as high as 41% and appears to be relatively stable over time (44, 45). This compares to around 25% of patients with non-psychiatric disorders not taking prescribed medication regularly (46). Individuals with FEP may be even more likely to discontinue medication and follow-up studies suggest that up to 75% of patients take their medication only intermittently after two years of discharge from hospital (47, 48, 49). It had been hoped that SGAs may improve adherence due to better tolerability and some studies suggest that this might be the

126 • *Psychosis and Schizophrenia in Hong Kong*

case (50, 51, 52). However, a systematic review did not show conclusive advantages of SGAs over first-generation antipsychotics (FGAs) (53).

Attitudes towards and knowledge of antipsychotic medication have been known to significantly affect adherence in addition to insight, substance use, the therapeutic relationship, effects of medication, and dosing interval (54, 55, 56, 57). We investigated which medication factors influenced medication adherence in a sample of 70 patients with first-episode psychosis in Hong Kong. Similar to Western studies, we reported non-adherence rates of almost 40% and found a positive association between patients knowing why they take medication and adherence. Only 48.6% of patients knew the name of their medication, 60% were aware of the type of drug they were taking, and 61.4% could state the dosage they had been prescribed. Knowledge of antipsychotic name, drug type, and dosage was not related to adherence (58). Poor medication knowledge was associated with being 30 years or older, low levels of education and negative family relationships, and having received treatment for less than four years (59). We also asked patients how they perceived the Chinese name for antipsychotic medication, literally translated as 'anti-psyche drug' (抗精神藥物). More than half of our sample reported a negative attitude towards the term and we suggested that renaming antipsychotic medication might reduce stigma (58).

Negative attitudes towards medication may also be driven by views in the general population, even in highly educated young people (58, 60). Among professionals caring for FEP patients, differences in opinions have become apparent in relation to perceived relapse risk (61). Nurses were more likely to perceive a higher risk of relapse compared to social workers. This finding was likely due to nursing staff being more involved in the treatment of acutely unwell patients, whereas social workers tend to offer long-term support to more stable patients in the community.

Psychiatrists equally focus on relapse risk when making treatment decisions; however, there appear to be marked differences in the views on medication discontinuation across the world, probably driven by varying cultural and societal norms. For example, like Western clinicians, psychiatrists in Asia endorsed maintenance treatment for at least one to two years following remission, but they were more conservative when considering the appropriateness of stopping medication (62).

Differences in professional attitudes may impact coherent service delivery and optimal timing of medication discontinuation. To mediate discussions around the discontinuation of maintenance treatment it is essential to consider patients' period of remission, perceived relapse risks, and perceived optimal duration of maintenance treatment (61). Consensus and consistency around treatment planning are extremely important, particularly as patients and caregivers very likely underestimate the chances of relapse or that stopping medication may lead to relapse (63). We also demonstrated a correlation between patients' knowledge of aetiology and medication adherence, the association being mediated by insight. Health beliefs centring on the psychosocial origin of psychosis were also elicited, reflecting beliefs on the aetiology of disease rooted in Chinese culture (64). However, a biological illness attribution is also prevalent in our patient population and is directly linked to medication adherence (65).

Another study examining adherence in Hong Kong showed lower discontinuation rates of 26%, likely due to the fact that the sample consisted of FEP and chronic psychosis patients (66). Younger patients, who did not perceive any benefits from medication and did not like taking regular antipsychotics, were more likely to stop taking it. Clinicians were relatively poor at detecting non-adherence, with a sensitivity of 0.33, but were better at excluding it (specificity of 0.84) (66). Although negative attitudes were found to be predictive of non-adherent behaviours, determinants driving attitudes and behaviour differed. Poorer insight, more severe general psychopathology, more psychiatric medication side effects, and poorer working memory and verbal comprehension sub-scores were associated with negative attitudes towards medication in adult-onset FEP. In contrast, more severe positive symptoms, inpatient treatment at the onset of illness, and poorer engagement in extended social networks were associated with non-adherent behaviours (67).

When non-adherent behaviours were broken down into intentional, i.e., deciding to stop medication, and non-intentional actions (i.e., forgetting to take prescribed antipsychotics), FEP patients were shown to be more likely to engage in either behaviour compared to individuals with chronic psychosis (68). Intentional and non-intentional non-adherence occurred relatively independently of one another in FEP and tended to converge for chronic patients. This finding gives rise to the possibility of effective intervention by supporting patients to remember to take their medication. Non-adherence was significantly associated with feelings of embarrassment about taking medication, something of which clinicians were usually not aware. Exploring feelings of shame and embarrassment in relation to antipsychotic medication might therefore help to detect non-adherence and open up conversations to mitigate negative attitudes and improve adherence (68).

Reflections: Antipsychotic Prescribing in Context

As has been shown, adherence behaviours and attitudes are likely to be affected by a multitude of factors related not only to objective measures of symptom control, the severity of illness, co-occurring difficulties, side effects, medication factors, and health service provision but also patients' subjective experience of taking medication as well as perceived benefits and side effects, health beliefs, therapeutic relationships, and attitudes within wider social networks. Addressing negative feelings associated with having to take long-term antipsychotic medication may not only improve adherence and thus outcomes, but may also help individuals come to

128 • *Psychosis and Schizophrenia in Hong Kong*

terms with having a chronic illness, make adjustments to their lives and improve self-esteem. Encouraging open conversations with patients and their carers, as well as among health professionals is vital to providing individualised and coherent treatment plans. Joint-decision making will need to take into account individual patient factors related to illness, co-occurring disorders and life circumstances, pharmacological properties of medication, as well as patients' wishes and values in relation to their subjective quality of life.

It is important to consider the use of medication in psychosis in a holistic framework. It is easy to fall into the dichotomy between mind and brain and to polarise psychological and biological factors in a disorder. Conventional clinical research approaches try to discriminate between empirical therapeutic components and placebo effects. Empirical therapeutic effects presumably relate to mechanistic changes. Placebo effects depict subjective expectations of the patient. Evidence-based medicine tends to make this distinction and then focuses only on empirical effects and discards placebo effects. These often-ignored data suggest that placebo effects can account for over one-third of the improvements seen in clinical trials. In real-life clinical situations, the psychological effects of expectation, as well as personal meaning related to medication are potentially important factors determining adherence. These processes are often lost in busy clinics run as 'pragmatic' operations. In these impersonal situations, the negative connotations of antipsychotic medications are often left unaddressed.

Undoubtedly, treatment recommendations and guidelines for first-episode psychosis will change in the future with the development of new antipsychotic agents and emerging evidence regarding other pharmacological and non-pharmacological interventions. Clinicians can increase their effectiveness by integrating psychological skills into prescription processes to counteract the negative associations with antipsychotic medication. At the same time, ongoing efforts will be required to increase knowledge of mental health conditions and their treatment in the general population to reduce prejudice and stigma and to aid the meaningful integration of those affected by psychosis into society.

References

1. López-Muñoz F, Alamo C, Cuenca E, Shen WW, Clervoy P, Rubio G. History of the discovery and clinical introduction of chlorpromazine. *Ann Clin Psychiatry.* 2005;17(3):113-135. doi:10.1080/10401230591002002
2. Ramachandraiah CT, Subramaniam N, Tancer M. The story of antipsychotics: past and present. *Indian J Psychiatry.* 2009;51(4):324-326. doi:10.4103/0019-5545.58304
3. Idänpään-Heikkilä J, Alhava E, Olkinuora M, Palva I. Letter: clozapine and agranulocytosis. *Lancet.* 1975;2(7935):611. doi:10.1016/s0140-6736(75)90206-8

4. Crilly J. The history of clozapine and its emergence in the US market: a review and analysis. *Hist Psychiatry*. 2007;18(1):39-60. doi:10.1177/0957154X07070335
5. Shopsin B, Klein H, Aaronsom M, Collora M. Clozapine, chlorpromazine, and placebo in newly hospitalized, acutely schizophrenic patients: a controlled, double-blind comparison. *Arch Gen Psychiatry*. 1979;36(6):657-664. doi:10.1001/archpsyc.1979.01780060047005
6. Stephens P. A review of clozapine: an antipsychotic for treatment-resistant schizophrenia. *Compr Psychiatry*. 1990;31(4):315-326. doi:10.1016/0010-440x(90)90038-t
7. Kane J, Honigfeld G, Singer J, Meltzer H. Clozapine for the treatment-resistant schizophrenic. A double-blind comparison with chlorpromazine. *Arch Gen Psychiatry*. 1988;45(9):789-796. doi:10.1001/archpsyc.1988.01800330013001
8. WHO Collaborating Centre for Drug Statistics Methodology. Online. Published Jan 23, 2023. Accessed Feb 27, 2023. https://www.whocc.no/atc_ddd_index/?code=N05A&showdescription=no
9. Leucht S, Huhn M, Davis JM. Should 'typical', first-generation antipsychotics no longer be generally used in the treatment of schizophrenia? *Eur Arch Psychiatry Clin Neurosci*. 2021;271(8):1411-1413. doi:10.1007/s00406-021-01335-y
10. Kahn RS, Fleischhacker WW, Boter H, et al. Effectiveness of antipsychotic drugs in first-episode schizophrenia and schizophreniform disorder: an open randomised clinical trial. *Lancet*. 2008;371(9618):1085-1097. doi:10.1016/S0140-6736(08)60486-9
11. McEvoy JP, Lieberman JA, Perkins DO, et al. Efficacy and tolerability of olanzapine, quetiapine, and risperidone in the treatment of early psychosis: a randomized, double-blind 52-week comparison. *Am J Psychiatry*. 2007;164(7):1050-1060. doi:10.1176/ajp.2007.164.7.1050
12. Robinson DG, Gallego JA, John M, et al. A randomized comparison of aripiprazole and risperidone for the acute treatment of first-episode schizophrenia and related disorders: 3-month outcomes. *Schizophr Bull*. 2015;41(6):1227-1236. doi:10.1093/schbul/sbv125
13. Agid O, Schulze L, Arenovich T, et al. Antipsychotic response in first-episode schizophrenia: efficacy of high doses and switching. *Eur Neuropsychopharmacol*. 2013;23(9):1017-1022. doi:10.1016/j.euroneuro.2013.04.010
14. Zhu Y, Li C, Huhn M, et al. How well do patients with a first episode of schizophrenia respond to antipsychotics: a systematic review and meta-analysis. *Eur Neuropsychopharmacol*. 2017;27(9):835-844. doi:10.1016/j.euroneuro.2017.06.011
15. Kapur S, Zipursky R, Jones C, Remington G, Houle S. Relationship between dopamine D(2) occupancy, clinical response, and side effects: a double-blind PET study of first-episode schizophrenia. *Am J Psychiatry*. 2000;157(4):514-520. doi:10.1176/appi.ajp.157.4.514
16. Miller JL, Ashford JW, Archer SM, Rudy AC, Wermeling DP. Comparison of intranasal administration of haloperidol with intravenous and intramuscular administration: a pilot pharmacokinetic study. *Pharmacotherapy*. 2008;28(7):875-882. doi:10.1592/phco.28.7.875
17. Zhang JP, Gallego JA, Robinson DG, Malhotra AK, Kane JM, Correll CU. Efficacy and safety of individual second-generation vs. first-generation

antipsychotics in first-episode psychosis: a systematic review and meta-analysis. *Int J Neuropsychopharmacol*. 2013;16(6):1205-1218. doi:10.1017/S1461145712001277

18. Tiihonen J, Lönnqvist J, Wahlbeck K, et al. 11-year follow-up of mortality in patients with schizophrenia: a population-based cohort study (FIN11 study). *Lancet*. 2009;374(9690):620-627. doi:10.1016/S0140-6736(09)60742-X

19. Yoshimura B, Yada Y, So R, Takaki M, Yamada N. The critical treatment window of clozapine in treatment-resistant schizophrenia: secondary analysis of an observational study. *Psychiatry Res*. 2017;250:65-70. doi:10.1016/j.psychres.2017.01.064

20. Honer WG, Procyshyn RM, Chen EY, MacEwan GW, Barr AM. A translational research approach to poor treatment response in patients with schizophrenia: clozapine-antipsychotic polypharmacy. *J Psychiatry Neurosci*. 2009;34(6):433-442.

21. Tiihonen J, Taipale H, Mehtälä J, Vattulainen P, Correll CU, Tanskanen A. Association of antipsychotic polypharmacy vs monotherapy with psychiatric rehospitalization among adults with schizophrenia. *JAMA Psychiatry*. 2019;76(5):499-507. doi:10.1001/jamapsychiatry.2018.4320

22. Honer WG, Thornton AE, Chen EY, et al. Clozapine alone versus clozapine and risperidone with refractory schizophrenia. *N Engl J Med*. 2006;354(5):472-482. doi:10.1056/NEJMoa053222

23. Barnes TR, Drake R, Paton C, et al. Evidence-based guidelines for the pharmacological treatment of schizophrenia: updated recommendations from the British Association for Psychopharmacology. *J Psychopharmacol*. 2020;34(1):3-78. doi:10.1177/0269881119889296

24. Hui CLM, Lam BST, Lee EHM, et al. A systematic review of clinical guidelines on choice, dose, and duration of antipsychotics treatment in first- and multi-episode schizophrenia. *Int Rev Psychiatry*. 2019;31(5-6):441-459. doi:10.1080/09540261.2019.1613965

25. Hui CLM, Lam BST, Lee EHM, et al. Perspective on medication decisions following remission from first-episode psychosis. *Schizophr Res*. 2020;225:82-89. doi:10.1016/j.schres.2020.02.007

26. Hardy KV, Ballon JS, Noordsy DL, Adelsheim S. *Intervening Early in Psychosis: A Team Approach*. American Psychiatric Association Publishing; 2019.

27. Lee EH, Hui CL, Lin J, Chang WC, Chan SK, Chen EY. Antipsychotic treatment of young Chinese individuals from 2004 to 2015: a population-based study in Hong Kong. *Am J Psychiatry*. 2016;173(9):939-940. doi:10.1176/appi.ajp.2016.16030258

28. Tang JYM, Chen EYH, Hui CLM, et al. The naturalistic use of antipsychotics in early psychosis in Hong Kong. The 6th International Conference on Early Psychosis; October 20–22, 2008; Melbourne, Australia. *Early Interv Psychiatry*. 2008;2(Suppl.1):A100. doi:10.1111/j.1751-7893.2008.00096.x

29. Lee EH, Hui CL, Lin JJ, et al. Quality of life and functioning in first-episode psychosis Chinese patients with different antipsychotic medications. *Early Interv Psychiatry*. 2016;10(6):535-539. doi:10.1111/eip.12246

30. Johnstone EC, Crow TJ, Frith CD, Carney MW, Price JS. Mechanism of the antipsychotic effect in the treatment of acute schizophrenia. *Lancet*. 1978;1(8069):848-851. doi:10.1016/s0140-6736(78)90193-9

Pharmacological Treatments • 131

31. Leucht S, Busch R, Hamann J, Kissling W, Kane JM. Early-onset hypothesis of antipsychotic drug action: a hypothesis tested, confirmed and extended. *Biol Psychiatry*. 2005;57(12):1543-1549. doi:10.1016/j.biopsych.2005.02.023

32. Chua SE, Deng Y, Chen EY, et al. Early striatal hypertrophy in first-episode psychosis within 3 weeks of initiating antipsychotic drug treatment. *Psychol Med*. 2009;39(5):793-800. doi:10.1017/S0033291708004212

33. Chua SE, Cheung C, Cheung V, et al. Cerebral grey, white matter and csf in never-medicated, first-episode schizophrenia. *Schizophr Res*. 2007;89(1-3):12-21. doi:10.1016/j.schres.2006.09.009

34. Deng MY, McAlonan GM, Cheung C, et al. A naturalistic study of grey matter volume increase after early treatment in anti-psychotic naïve, newly diagnosed schizophrenia. *Psychopharmacology (Berl)*. 2009;206(3):437-446. doi:10.1007/s00213-009-1619-z

35. Kishimoto T, Hagi K, Kurokawa S, Kane JM, Correll CU. Long-acting injectable versus oral antipsychotics for the maintenance treatment of schizophrenia: a systematic review and comparative meta-analysis of randomised, cohort, and pre-post studies. *Lancet Psychiatry*. 2021;8(5):387-404. doi:10.1016/S2215-0366(21)00039-0

36. Wei Y, Yan VKC, Kang W, et al. Association of long-acting injectable antipsychotics and oral antipsychotics with disease relapse, health care use, and adverse events among people with schizophrenia. *JAMA Netw Open*. 2022;5(7):e2224163. Published Jul 1, 2022. doi:10.1001/jamanetworkopen.2022.24163

37. Chan JKN, Wong CSM, Yung NCL, Chen EYH, Chang WC. Pre-existing chronic physical morbidity and excess mortality in people with schizophrenia: a population-based cohort study. *Soc Psychiatry Psychiatr Epidemiol*. 2022;57(3):485-493. doi:10.1007/s00127-021-02130-9

38. Chan JKN, Wong CSM, Or PCF, Chen EYH, Chang WC. Risk of mortality and complications in patients with schizophrenia and diabetes mellitus: population-based cohort study. *Br J Psychiatry*. 2021;219(1):375-382. doi:10.1192/bjp.2020.248

39. Lee EHM, Hui CLM, Law EYL, et al. Metabolic screening for patients with second-generation antipsychotic medication: a population-based study from 2004 to 2016. *Schizophr Res*. 2018;197:618-619. doi:10.1016/j.schres.2018.02.028

40. Wong J, Pang T, Cheuk NKW, Liao Y, Bastiampillai T, Chan SKW. A systematic review on the use of clozapine in treatment of tardive dyskinesia and tardive dystonia in patients with psychiatric disorders. *Psychopharmacology (Berl)*. 2022;239(11):3393-3420. doi:10.1007/s00213-022-06241-2

41. Just MJ. The influence of atypical antipsychotic drugs on sexual function. *Neuropsychiatr Dis Treat*. 2015;11:1655-1661. Published Jul 8, 2015. doi:10.2147/NDT.S84528

42. Serretti A, Chiesa A. A meta-analysis of sexual dysfunction in psychiatric patients taking antipsychotics. *Int Clin Psychopharmacol*. 2011;26(3):130-140. doi:10.1097/YIC.0b013e328341e434

43. Alvarez-Jimenez M, Priede A, Hetrick SE, et al. Risk factors for relapse following treatment for first episode psychosis: a systematic review and meta-analysis of longitudinal studies. *Schizophr Res*. 2012;139(1-3):116-128. doi:10.1016/j.schres.2012.05.007

44. Lacro JP, Dunn LB, Dolder CR, Leckband SG, Jeste DV. Prevalence of and risk factors for medication nonadherence in patients with schizophrenia: a comprehensive review of recent literature. *J Clin Psychiatry*. 2002;63(10):892-909. doi:10.4088/jcp.v63n1007

132　•　*Psychosis and Schizophrenia in Hong Kong*

45. Ascher-Svanum H, Faries DE, Zhu B, Ernst FR, Swartz MS, Swanson JW. Medication adherence and long-term functional outcomes in the treatment of schizophrenia in usual care. *J Clin Psychiatry*. 2006;67(3):453-460. doi:10.4088/jcp.v67n0317

46. DiMatteo MR. Evidence-based strategies to foster adherence and improve patient outcomes. *JAAPA*. 2004;17(11):18-21.

47. Perkins DO, Gu H, Weiden PJ, et al. Predictors of treatment discontinuation and medication nonadherence in patients recovering from a first episode of schizophrenia, schizophreniform disorder, or schizoaffective disorder: a randomized, double-blind, flexible-dose, multicenter study. *J Clin Psychiatry*. 2008;69(1):106-113. doi:10.4088/jcp.v69n0114.

48. Coldham EL, Addington J, Addington D. Medication adherence of individuals with a first episode of psychosis. *Acta Psychiatr Scand*. 2002;106(4):286-290. doi:10.1034/j.1600-0447.2002.02437.x

49. Leucht S, Heres S. Epidemiology, clinical consequences, and psychosocial treatment of nonadherence in schizophrenia. *J Clin Psychiatry*. 2006;67 Suppl 5:3-8.

50. Dolder CR, Lacro JP, Dunn LB, Jeste DV. Antipsychotic medication adherence: is there a difference between typical and atypical agents? [published correction appears in *Am J Psychiatry* Mar 2002;159(3):514]. *Am J Psychiatry*. 2002;159(1):103-108. doi:10.1176/appi.ajp.159.1.103

51. Ascher-Svanum H, Zhu B, Faries DE, Lacro JP, Dolder CR, Peng X. Adherence and persistence to typical and atypical antipsychotics in the naturalistic treatment of patients with schizophrenia. *Patient Prefer Adherence*. 2008;2:67-77. Published Feb 2, 2008. doi:10.2147/ppa.s2940

52. Al-Zakwani IS, Barron JJ, Bullano MF, Arcona S, Drury CJ, Cockerham TR. Analysis of healthcare utilization patterns and adherence in patients receiving typical and atypical antipsychotic medications. *Curr Med Res Opin*. 2003;19(7):619-626. doi:10.1185/030079903125002270

53. Shuler KM. Approaches to improve adherence to pharmacotherapy in patients with schizophrenia. *Patient Prefer Adherence*. 2014;8:701-714. Published May 14, 2014. doi:10.2147/PPA.S59371

54. Haddad PM, Brain C, Scott J. Nonadherence with antipsychotic medication in schizophrenia: challenges and management strategies. *Patient Relat Outcome Meas*. 2014;5:43-62. Published Jun 23, 2014. doi:10.2147/PROM.S42735

55. Czobor P, Van Dorn RA, Citrome L, Kahn RS, Fleischhacker WW, Volavka J. Treatment adherence in schizophrenia: a patient-level meta-analysis of combined CATIE and EUFEST studies. *Eur Neuropsychopharmacol*. 2015;25(8):1158-1166. doi:10.1016/j.euroneuro.2015.04.003

56. Day JC, Bentall RP, Roberts C, et al. Attitudes toward antipsychotic medication: the impact of clinical variables and relationships with health professionals. *Arch Gen Psychiatry*. 2005;62(7):717-724. doi:10.1001/archpsyc.62.7.717

57. Coleman CI, Limone B, Sobieraj DM, et al. Dosing frequency and medication adherence in chronic disease. *J Manag Care Pharm*. 2012;18(7):527-539. doi:10.18553/jmcp.2012.18.7.527

58. Lau KC, Lee EH, Hui CL, Chang WC, Chan SK, Chen EY. Psychosis patients' knowledge, adherence and attitudes towards the naming of antipsychotic medication in Hong Kong. *Early Interv Psychiatry*. 2015;9(5):422-427. doi:10.1111/eip.12169
59. Lau KC, Lee EH, Hui CL, Chang WC, Chan SK, Chen EY. Demographic correlates of medication knowledge in Hong Kong early psychosis patients. *Early Interv Psychiatry*. 2018;12(1):107-112. doi:10.1111/eip.12351
60. Chung KF, Chen EY, Liu CS. University students' attitudes towards mental patients and psychiatric treatment. *Int J Soc Psychiatry*. 2001;47(2):63-72. doi:10.1177/002076400104700206
61. Chan KK, Chin QP, Tang JY, et al. Perceptions of relapse risks following first-episode psychosis and attitudes towards maintenance medication: a comparison between nursing and social work professionals. *Early Interv Psychiatry*. 2011;5(4):324-334. doi:10.1111/j.1751-7893.2011.00268.x
62. Hui CL, Wong AK, Leung WW, et al. Psychiatrists' opinion towards medication discontinuation in remitted first-episode psychosis: A multi-site study of the Asian Network for Early Psychosis. *Early Interv Psychiatry*. 2019;13(6):1329-1337. doi:10.1111/eip.12765
63. Chan KW, Wong MH, Hui CL, Lee EH, Chang WC, Chen EY. Perceived risk of relapse and role of medication: comparison between patients with psychosis and their caregivers. *Soc Psychiatry Psychiatr Epidemiol*. 2015;50(2):307-315. doi:10.1007/s00127-014-0930-0
64. Chan KW, Hui LM, Wong HY, Lee HM, Chang WC, Chen YH. Medication adherence, knowledge about psychosis, and insight among patients with a schizophrenia-spectrum disorder. *J Nerv Ment Dis*. 2014;202(1):25-29. doi:10.1097/NMD.0000000000000068
65. Suen YN, Yeung ETW, Chan SKW, et al. Integration of biological and psychological illness attributional belief in association with medication adherence behaviour: a path analysis. *Early Interv Psychiatry*. 2021;15(6):1686-1695. doi:10.1111/eip.13114
66. Hui CL, Chen EY, Kan C, Yip K, Law C, Chiu CP. Anti-psychotics adherence among outpatients with schizophrenia in Hong Kong. *Keio J Med*. 2006;55(1):9-14. doi:10.2302/kjm.55.9
67. Hui CLM, Poon VWY, Ko WT, et al. Risk factors for antipsychotic medication non-adherence behaviors and attitudes in adult-onset psychosis. *Schizophr Res*. 2016;174(1-3):144-149. doi:10.1016/j.schres.2016.03.026
68. Hui CL, Chen EY, Kan CS, Yip KC, Law CW, Chiu CP. Detection of non-adherent behaviour in early psychosis. *Aust N Z J Psychiatry*. 2006;40(5):446-451. doi:10.1080/j.1440-1614.2006.01821.x

10

Relapse in Psychotic Disorders: Prediction, Prevention, and Management

Background

The consequences of relapse can be devastating for patients, particularly for young adults whose psychosocial, educational, occupational, sociocultural, and cognitive development will almost invariably be disrupted by the re-emergence of psychotic symptoms. In addition, healthcare and non-medical costs as well as productivity losses pose an enormous economic burden to the individual and society (1). It has been shown that with each subsequent episode of relapse patients tend to have a poorer response to treatment, take longer to recover, and experience more functional deterioration (2, 3, 4, 5). Patients with a relapsing course of illness are also less likely to marry or sustain long-term relationships. Repeated relapses are associated with an increased risk of suicide, particularly in previously high-functioning young men (6, 7). Stigma is also likely to be a significant factor affecting recovery and thus might be implicated more indirectly in the occurrence of relapse.

The Definition of Relapse

Relapse is defined as the re-emergence of psychotic symptoms following remission. Remission denotes the illness phase during which psychotic symptoms have subsided (1). In recognition of the fact that patients do not always fully remit from their psychotic episode, Johnstone (1992) proposed relapse type I and type II in psychosis, whereby type I is the reappearance of psychotic symptoms following their complete resolution and type II is defined as the exacerbation of existing and persistent psychotic symptoms (8). Relapse and exacerbation have been considered together, or separately, in different relapse studies.

More recently, efforts to define relapse have focused on ascertaining whether remission has been achieved as set out by the Schizophrenia Working Group (9). Remission is defined as 'an improvement in core signs and symptoms to an extent that any remaining symptoms are of such low intensity that they no longer interfere significantly with behaviour and are below the threshold typically utilised in justifying an initial diagnosis of schizophrenia'. Improvements were considered to last six months to meet the criteria of remission and symptom severity was suggested to be measured using the Positive and Negative Syndrome Scale (PANSS) rating of mild ≤ 3 or Brief Psychiatric Rating Scale (BPRS) ≤ 3 (9). It is important to clarify whether relapse refers specifically to positive symptoms, or whether it refers also to other symptom dimensions such as negative symptoms. As pointed out by Hui (2011), not all patients achieve remission and therefore Johnstone's delineation of relapse might be more clinically important (1, 8).

Although remission has been more clearly defined there is no consensus regarding a symptom threshold required for relapse. Csernansky et al. (2006) set multidimensional criteria including re-hospitalisation/need for care, an increase of PANSS total score by 25% from baseline when there are significant baseline symptoms (10). This definition would include exacerbation in patients who did not attain remission as defined in Johnstone type II. In contrast, in our studies, we have focused on the reappearance of even mild psychotic symptoms in patients who have been free from them (Johnstone type I).

The Assessment of Relapse

Several methods have been deployed to operationally define and measure relapse. The most commonly used rating scales are the PANSS, Clinical Global Impressions (CGI), and the BPRS. Researchers have also used other indicators of relapse such as re-hospitalisation. However, this outcome can also occur due to other co-occurring psychiatric conditions not directly associated with the re-emergence of psychotic symptoms, such as depression or high risk of suicide or homicide. Re-hospitalisation as a proxy measure also risks seriously underestimating relapse rates as most modern healthcare systems have well-developed community services and a significant proportion of patients will be supported by outreach or crisis teams when they experience an increase in psychotic symptoms. Nonetheless, re-hospitalisation remains an important measure as it incurs significant healthcare-related costs.

Rates and Predictors of Relapse in Psychotic Disorders

Relapse in schizophrenia has been studied extensively as a key process in the course of the disorder. Studies have varied in relapse definitions and duration of follow-up.

Before the advent of antipsychotic medication, remission only occurred in a minority of patients. Morgan and colleagues (2014) compared Manfred Bleuler's cohort study of 208 patients admitted between 1942 and 1943 in Switzerland and followed up for 20 to 22 years, with a ten-year follow-up of patients in the Aetiology and Ethnicity in Schizophrenia and Other Psychoses (AESOP) study and International Study on Schizophrenia (ISoS) (11, 12). They found that only 12% of patients manifested a relapsing–remitting course and good outcomes before the introduction of antipsychotic medication in Bleuler's study, compared with around 50% of patients who were likely to have received medication in the more recent AESOP and ISoS studies. In India, a 20-year follow-up of the Madras longitudinal study revealed that around 40% of patients relapsed with complete recovery in between, 44% relapsed with partial remission, and only 8% recovered without further relapse (13). Naturalistic studies have found a cumulative relapse rate of 70% to 82% up to five years following the first episode or admission for a psychotic disorder (14, 15).

Various predictors of relapse have been explored in first-episode psychosis. Interestingly, clinical and demographic variables appear to have little impact. On the other hand, medication non-adherence, persistent substance use, being criticised by carers, and poor premorbid adjustment significantly increased the risk of relapse (16, 17). Patients exposed to high levels of expressed emotion by carers were at higher risk of relapse early on in the remission phase, whereas warmth expressed towards patients conferred a protective effect (17).

Relapse in Psychotic Disorders in Hong Kong

Relapse Rates in First-Episode Psychosis

In naturalistic studies, a relapse rate of around 20% was observed at 12 months after the first episode, with the rate rising to nearly 60% after three years (18, 19). At ten years, only around 25% of patients had not relapsed (20, 21). Patients who relapsed early in the course of their disorder had significantly poorer longitudinal outcomes. They had more attempted suicides, higher rates of violent episodes, more frequent hospitalisations, and lower employment rates (21).

Chen et al. (2002) investigated potential predictors of relapse in first-episode psychosis patients over a 12-month period. Seventy male and 83 female patients were recruited from two regional acute hospitals. The mean age of onset was 31.8 years, and they had 10.5 years of education on average. Most patients received a clinical diagnosis of schizophrenia (62%), followed by schizophreniform disorder (23.3%) and other types of psychotic disorders (14.7%). In the sample, 20 patients (13.3%) suffered at least one relapse during the follow-up period. Age of onset was found to be the only significant predictive factor for relapse during the first year, with

Relapse in Psychotic Disorders • 137

patients who relapsed being on average ten years younger (22). Advanced paternal age, particularly over the age of 40 years, was also linked to a higher risk of relapse within the first year of illness (23).

Relapse and Early Discontinuation of Antipsychotic Medication in First-Episode Psychosis

One of the key questions about relapse is whether maintenance antipsychotics make a similar impact on relapse in different stages of the disorder. The beneficial effect of maintenance medication in preventing relapse was first demonstrated in chronic patients. The question is whether the same applies to first-episode patients who have experienced only a single episode of illness. This question has important clinical implications, as many first-episode patients do not expect to take maintenance medication in the long term. Several randomised controlled trials (RCTs) for first-episode patients demonstrated that stopping maintenance antipsychotics within a few months of the first episode would result in relapse. Thus, it was concluded that maintenance medication is required for at least several months. Clinical guidelines mostly advise antipsychotic medications to be carried on for at least 12 months following a first episode. However, it was still unknown whether stopping maintenance treatment after one year would be advisable.

We carried out a double-blind randomised study to address this question. We recruited 178 patients who had been diagnosed with first-episode schizophrenia or related psychotic disorders, who had attained clinical remission from psychotic symptoms, and who had already received more than one year of maintenance treatment. We randomly assigned them to either a gradual discontinuation (placebo) arm or a continued maintenance arm (with quetiapine) for the next 12 months. After one year, 79% in the discontinuation group experienced a relapse compared to 41% in the maintenance group (24, 25, 26).

In this study, we focused on Johnstone type I relapse. We recruited patients who had no positive symptoms at baseline, those with even mild positive symptoms were not included. We considered relapse as the reappearance of positive symptoms, including mild symptoms. From this perspective, it is important to note that at the screening of all first-episode patients after one year of treatment, only about one-third were found to have good positive symptom remission. A significant proportion of patients either had at least mild residual positive symptoms or had already relapsed within one year of treatment. Thus, this study addressed those with a very good initial outcome following treatment of the first episode of psychosis. Our findings confirmed that even for this group of patients, discontinuation of medication after maintenance treatment of around 20 months still resulted in nearly 80% of individuals relapsing within the next 12 months.

It is also important to note that the relapse we observed did not necessarily occur immediately following the gradual discontinuation of medication, i.e., it was not a withdrawal-related phenomenon, but was distributed with different time lags after discontinuation. In fact, as we followed the cohort after the 12 months of the double-blind period, several further relapses were taking place in the discontinuation group. The patient with the longest time lag relapsed around three years after medication discontinuation. Her relapse was triggered by a stock market downturn in which she sustained a significant loss. Therefore, we could not even assert that 20% of patients had no further relapses after discontinuing medication. Nonetheless, we established several characteristics associated with being symptom-free after ten years of follow-up such as being male, having a shorter duration of untreated psychosis and a diagnosis other than one on the schizophrenia spectrum, and having better functioning in the early phase of treatment (27). However, we also established that first-episode psychosis (FEP) patients who had fully responded to and continued maintenance therapy for at least three years after diagnosis were significantly more likely to remain well and were less likely to die by suicide at ten-year follow-up (28).

The Dilemma of Maintenance Treatment vs. Discontinuation of Antipsychotic Prescribing

The high rate of relapse for even this good prognosis group after more than one year of treatment was a disappointing message for many who had hoped that some patients may be able to come off medication without relapse following treatment of the first episode. It is indeed understandable from the perspective of patients. Patients were often young and had few other illness experiences. Those illnesses that are likely encountered at that age are most often one-off events, with full recovery, and do not need continued treatment, e.g., infections or bone fractures. Patients and carers commonly attribute a psychotic episode to being caused by external stress. Therefore, they often have difficulty appreciating the need for continued treatment. Subjectively, patients often underestimate their own chances of having a relapse. There is thus a need to provide a well-designed guided process whereby patients and carers would be able to make sense of what has happened during the psychotic episode and the implications of treatment. This process is complex and requires a dialogical approach rather than the delivery of one-way psychoeducational information.

The dilemma for a decision between maintenance treatment and discontinuation is a complex one, as one needs to balance the potential side effects of medication against the risk of relapse. One of the most important issues is that of cognitive function. While cognitive dysfunctions can be the results of psychotic disorders themselves, medications could either reduce cognitive dysfunctions, or increase them, depending on medication type, dose, and individual factors. We have shown in Chapter 14 that cognitive dysfunction is not well assessed in ordinary clinical settings. It is possible that patients may attribute any subjective experience of cognitive dysfunction to medications. This will increase the chance of non-adherence and intention to discontinue maintenance medication. Our double-blind randomised study offered an opportunity to investigate this problem. We measured cognition in participating patients before and after medication discontinuation and found that cognitive dysfunction remains an important feature in patients who had stopped medication and were thus on placebo. The same applies to other side effects, i.e., a significant level of side effects was reported even after patients had discontinued medication, suggesting a subjective expectation of side effects was part of the placebo response. However, metabolic side effects are expected to increase with long-term maintenance medication, even though our double-blind study of 12 months was perhaps not long enough to demonstrate a difference in metabolic side effects between the groups.

Predictors of Relapse in First-Episode Psychosis

Identifying predictors for relapse, or conversely, for non-relapse is important as it could guide clinicians and patients to a better-informed choice with more precise risk estimation. In our studies, significant predictors for relapse included patients being younger, having a longer duration of untreated psychosis (DUP), having a diagnosis of schizophrenia, premorbid schizoid or schizotypal traits, a history of smoking, lower cognitive functioning, more neurological soft signs, and a higher baseline spontaneous blink rate (18, 19, 20, 24, 25, 29, 30, 31).

However, the currently identified risk factors may not be sufficiently powerful to enable the discrimination into meaningfully distinctive groups regarding relapse risks. In addition, it is often difficult to identify early warning signs of the re-emergence of psychotic symptoms, particularly in low-resource settings. We have therefore developed an app called ReMind to improve the monitoring and detection of early relapse and to refine individual relapse indicators (32). We are hoping that ReMind will yield positive results in the near future.

Long-Term Effects of Early Medication Reduction or Discontinuation

One other important randomised study of medication reduction/discontinuation in the Netherlands suggested that despite having more initial relapses, in the longer term, i.e., after seven years, the medication reduction/discontinuation group had better functioning (33). We also investigated long-term outcomes with the cohort from our RCT relapse prevention study. We found that functional outcome was not different between the two groups after ten years, but that symptomatic outcomes were worse in the discontinuation group, with more patients becoming treatment-refractory or having died by suicide. This long-term follow-up study offers important insights into the impact of an early decision regarding medication discontinuation since the randomised study period was for 12 months from around month 20 of illness onset. Patients received the same treatment as usual after the study period, in which they and their clinician could choose between maintenance therapy or discontinuation at any time point in the ten-year follow-up period. The only difference was the choice of maintenance in around the third year following the first episode. Indeed, although more patients had a relapse in the discontinuation group during and immediately after the randomised study, the relapse rate between the two groups converged by year five. A review of the treatment pattern suggests that patients' choice of maintenance therapy roughly equalised in the two arms in the follow-up period. Therefore, the essential difference between the two arms is in the timing of the discontinuation, i.e., whether discontinuation was attempted relatively early (after 20 months) in the course of the disorder. Post-hoc analyses showed that poor outcomes related to early medication discontinuation were mediated by an early relapse at around year three. Indeed, for some of the patients who developed treatment refractoriness, this occurred one to two years after the first relapse. The emergence of treatment refractoriness following a first relapse has been supported by subsequent studies (34).

Our medication discontinuation study is different from the Dutch study in several aspects. First, we employed a narrower Johnstone type I conceptualisation of relapse and remission, while our Dutch colleagues used a broader mixed Johnstone type I and type II conceptualisation, i.e., they included patients who had mild psychotic symptoms in the study. Second, while we pursued to finely balance our patients' expectation to discontinue medication against the risk of relapse, the Dutch study aimed for dose reduction as well as discontinuation. In fact, most of their sample had a dose reduction rather than discontinuation. Third, although not mentioned in the report, Dutch patients may be expected to have had a higher level of comorbid substance use, e.g., cannabis, compared to the Hong Kong population. Thus, contributory factors and underlying aetiological factors such as the proportion of genetic factors involved may differ between the two patient populations. These differences may highlight some of the variations observed in the two studies. Our investigation showed that for a smaller group of FEP patients with complete remission of positive symptoms, early discontinuation of medication resulted in a poorer long-term outcome compared to continuation of maintenance medication, particularly for the risk of treatment refractoriness and suicide. The Dutch study revealed that for a wider group of patients, including those with mild residual psychotic symptoms, dose reduction can result in a better long-term functional outcome. Thus, the two sets of observations may not be in conflict (26, 33).

The Experience of Relapse

In qualitative interviews, patients reported that they were relying on their experience of the onset of psychosis to define relapse, i.e., they considered psychotic symptoms to signify the re-emergence of their illness but several also reported negative emotions and self-destructive behaviours to be early signs (35). Most patients thought that taking medication was the most important factor to prevent relapse and some felt that a relaxed state of mind, better living standards, healthy lifestyle choices, family support, and talking to others would contribute to remaining well. Views on antipsychotic medication differed – some patients thought they no longer required medication as they felt better, while others commented that antipsychotics had no effect on controlling symptoms over the long term. Not all patients were able to explain how medication helped to prevent relapse. One participant reported that antipsychotics gave her a sense of security, and another patient thought that medication reduced dopamine levels. Some had negative views of medication and one subject specifically talked about side effects affecting his social functioning (35).

From these interviews, it appears that patients tended to perceive relapse more broadly as affecting their perception of self and their relationships with other people, impacting perceived social support as well as the effects of medication. The re-emergence of psychotic symptoms played a less prominent role than in clinical perspectives on relapse.

Attitudes towards Maintenance Antipsychotic Treatment and Risk of Relapse

Maintenance of antipsychotic treatment and good medication adherence have been shown to be the most effective measures to reduce the risk of relapse (36, 37, 38). However, concerns about side effects in the long term have been voiced by patients and professionals alike (39, 40, 41, 42). Patients usually have to rely on the advice of healthcare professionals. It has been shown that clinicians' attitudes influence patients' perception of pharmacotherapy and risk of relapse (43, 44). Psychiatrists, for example, have tended to underestimate the relapse risk and overestimate the risk of adverse events and medication-related side effects (45, 46, 47, 48, 49). However, there is little data on the attitudes of other healthcare professionals such as nurses and social workers despite the fact that these clinicians usually provide the majority of clinical contacts, formulate individualised treatment plans, and deliver psychoeducation. We showed that social workers and nurses considered the remission period to be a significant predictor of perceived relapse risk after discontinuation of medication, i.e., a longer period of remission was associated with a lower perceived risk of relapse. The majority of the two professional groups considered the

142 • *Psychosis and Schizophrenia in Hong Kong*

importance of maintenance treatment to gradually decline as patients maintained remission for up to ten years (50).

Reflections: The Importance of Maintenance Treatment in Relapse Prevention

What has been shown in Hong Kong and internationally is that even with optimal psychopharmacological and psychosocial treatment, relapse is a common occurrence following a first episode of psychosis. Relapse has been considered to be an inherent feature of psychotic disorders since at least Kraepelin's first case series (51). Good adherence to medication regimes is the single most important factor to reduce the chance of future relapses. Clinicians in the Early Assessment Service for Young People (EASY) and Jockey Club Early Psychosis Project (JCEP) actively encourage patients' participation in discussions about their care and the purpose and role of maintenance medication. Relapse rates have been found to be similar in both programmes. In the initial stages, they were somewhat higher compared to 'treatment as usual' probably owing to the fact that prescribing was done more carefully and patients more often received lower doses of antipsychotics. Early intervention has not been able to reduce the time to the first relapse. However, patients who continued antipsychotic medication over several years of their illness were shown to have fewer relapses and hospitalisations after ten years of follow-up (52, 53).

There are many unanswered questions regarding the optimal length of treatment and maintenance dosing regimes. The early intervention teams in Hong Kong currently tailor pharmacotherapy using a collaborative and individualised approach, discussing in detail the anticipated benefits and risks of antipsychotic medication. We provide comprehensive psychoeducation bearing in mind potential differences in the perception of risks and relapse, and jointly agree on a slow reduction in medication where appropriate. We have also been mindful of the different perspectives of clinicians in our teams and encourage discussions about individualised care plans to ensure the delivery of coherent and effective early intervention.

There are many important questions surrounding relapse prevention. First of all, can we predict which patients will need long-term maintenance therapy in order to prevent relapse? From our long-term studies, it appears that only around 15% of patients remain well after discontinuation of medication. All other patients have a relapsing course of illness that will require maintenance medication to reduce the risk of recurrence. It is currently difficult to predict which patients will be able to discontinue medication without relapsing. Studies of relapse predictors have revealed that diagnosis, DUP and some neurocognitive markers may help to anticipate illness recurrence, but the level of precision has not yet reached a satisfactory level.

The most effective means of relapse prevention is maintenance antipsychotics. However, medications carry side effects as well as a contentious association with brain structural volume losses. Above all, medication also carries a negative association with the illness and may reinforce internalised stigma. Therefore, it is understandable that patients and clinicians contemplate the possibility of reducing and discontinuing medication.

The question has been raised whether having a relapse matters in the long term. There have been observations that despite an increased incidence of relapse patients who undergo medication dosage reductions fared better with regard to long-term functional outcomes. Nevertheless, these studies underscore the importance of psychopharmacological maintenance treatment. The question of whether reduced doses can help maintain recovery while lowering the risk of adverse side effects is an appealing one. Unfortunately, recent data suggest that after the first relapse, dose reduction is associated with an increased chance of a second relapse. Furthermore, after the second relapse, the preventative potential of antipsychotic maintenance treatment seems to be diminished leading to increased chances of further illness recurrence (34). The observation that relapses are associated with the need to increase subsequent medication dosage to control psychotic symptoms and the possible emergence of treatment-refractory states must be taken into consideration when dosage reduction or discontinuation is contemplated, alongside taking into account potential side effects and individual patient factors.

References

1. Hui CLM. Relapse in schizophrenia. *Medical Bulletin.* 2011;16(5):8-9.
2. Lieberman JA. Evidence for sensitization in the early stage of schizophrenia. *Eur Neuropsychopharmacology.* 1996;6(Suppl. 3):155.
3. Szymanski S, Lieberman JA, Alvir JM, et al. Gender differences in onset of illness, treatment response, course, and biologic indexes in first-episode schizophrenic patients. *Am J Psychiatry.* 1995;152(5):698-703. doi:10.1176/ajp.152.5.698
4. Lieberman J, Jody D, Geisler S, et al. Time course and biologic correlates of treatment response in first-episode schizophrenia. *Arch Gen Psychiatry.* 1993;50(5):369-376. doi:10.1001/archpsyc.1993.01820170047006
5. Wyatt RJ. Neuroleptics and the natural course of schizophrenia. *Schizophr Bull.* 1991;17(2):325-351. doi:10.1093/schbul/17.2.325
6. Dutta R, Murray RM, Allardyce J, Jones PB, Boydell J. Early risk factors for suicide in an epidemiological first episode psychosis cohort. *Schizophr Res.* 2011;126(1-3):11-19. doi:10.1016/j.schres.2010.11.021
7. Hor K, Taylor M. Suicide and schizophrenia: a systematic review of rates and risk factors. *J Psychopharmacol.* 2010;24(4 Suppl):81-90. doi:10.1177/1359786810385490
8. Johnstone EC. Relapse in schizophrenia: what are the major issues? In: Hawton K, ed. *Practical Problems in Clinical Psychiatry.* Oxford University Press; 1992:159-71.

9. Andreasen NC, Carpenter WT Jr, Kane JM, Lasser RA, Marder SR, Weinberger DR. Remission in schizophrenia: proposed criteria and rationale for consensus. *Am J Psychiatry*. 2005;162(3):441-449. doi:10.1176/appi.ajp.162.3.441

10. Csernansky JG, Mahmoud R, Brenner R; Risperidone-USA-79 Study Group. A comparison of risperidone and haloperidol for the prevention of relapse in patients with schizophrenia [published correction appears in *N Engl J Med* May 2, 2002;346(18):1424]. *N Engl J Med*. 2002;346(1):16-22. doi:10.1056/NEJMoa002028

11. Bleuler M. *The Schizophrenic Disorders: Long-Term Patient and Family Studies*. Yale University Press; 1978.

12. Morgan C, Lappin J, Heslin M, et al. Reappraising the long-term course and outcome of psychotic disorders: the AESOP-10 study [published correction appears in *Psychol Med*. Oct 2014;44(13):2727]. *Psychol Med*. 2014;44(13):2713-2726. doi:10.1017/S0033291714000282

13. Thara R. Twenty-year course of schizophrenia: the Madras Longitudinal Study. *Can J Psychiatry*. 2004;49(8):564-569. doi:10.1177/070674370404900808

14. The Scottish first episode schizophrenia study. VIII. Five-year follow-up: clinical and psychosocial findings. The Scottish Schizophrenia Research Group. *Br J Psychiatry*. 1992;161:496-500.

15. Robinson D, Woerner MG, Alvir JM, et al. Predictors of relapse following response from a first episode of schizophrenia or schizoaffective disorder. *Arch Gen Psychiatry*. 1999;56(3):241-247. doi:10.1001/archpsyc.56.3.241

16. Alvarez-Jimenez M, Priede A, Hetrick SE, et al. Risk factors for relapse following treatment for first episode psychosis: a systematic review and meta-analysis of longitudinal studies. *Schizophr Res*. 2012;139(1-3):116-128. doi:10.1016/j.schres.2012.05.007

17. Ma CF, Chan SKW, Chung YL, et al. The predictive power of expressed emotion and its components in relapse of schizophrenia: a meta-analysis and meta-regression. *Psychol Med*. 2021;51(3):365-375. doi:10.1017/S0033291721000209

18. Chen EY, Hui CL, Dunn EL, et al. A prospective 3-year longitudinal study of cognitive predictors of relapse in first-episode schizophrenic patients. *Schizophr Res*. 2005;77(1):99-104. doi:10.1016/j.schres.2005.02.020

19. Hui CL, Tang JY, Leung CM, et al. A 3-year retrospective cohort study of predictors of relapse in first-episode psychosis in Hong Kong. *Aust N Z J Psychiatry*. 2013;47(8):746-753. doi:10.1177/0004867413487229

20. Hui CL, Honer WG, Lee EH, et al. Predicting first-episode psychosis patients who will never relapse over 10 years. *Psychol Med*. 2019;49(13):2206-2214. doi:10.1017/S0033291718003070

21. Chan SKW, Chan HYV, Liao Y, et al. Longitudinal relapse pattern of patients with first-episode schizophrenia-spectrum disorders and its predictors and outcomes: A 10-year follow-up study. *Asian J Psychiatr*. 2022;71:103087. doi:10.1016/j.ajp.2022.103087

22. Chen EYH, Chan CK, Tso IF, et al. Predictors of relapse in first episode psychosis: 1-year follow up study in Hong Kong. The 11th Biennial Winter Workshop on Schizophrenia; Feb 24–Mar 1, 2002; Davos, Switzerland. *Schizophr Res*. 2002;53(3)(Suppl.):50, abstract A54. doi:10.1016/S0920-9964(01)00381-4

23. Hui CL, Chiu CP, Li YK, et al. The effect of paternal age on relapse in first-episode schizophrenia. *Can J Psychiatry*. 2015;60(8):346-353. doi:10.1177/070674371506000803

24. Hui CLM, Chen EYH, Lam M, et al. Predictors for relapse in a double-blind placebo-controlled discontinuation study of remitted first-episode psychosis patients. The 14th Biennial Winter Workshop on Schizophrenia and Bipolar Disorders; Feb 3–7, 2008; Montreux, Switzerland. *Schizophr Res.* 2008;98(Suppl.):13. doi:10.1016/j.schres.2007.12.020

25. Hui CL, Wong GH, Tang JY, et al. Predicting 1-year risk for relapse in patients who have discontinued or continued quetiapine after remission from first-episode psychosis. *Schizophr Res.* 2013;150(1):297-302. doi:10.1016/j.schres.2013.08.010

26. Chen EY, Hui CL, Lam MM, et al. Maintenance treatment with quetiapine versus discontinuation after one year of treatment in patients with remitted first episode psychosis: randomised controlled trial. *BMJ.* 2010;341:c4024. Published Aug 19, 2010. doi:10.1136/bmj.c4024

27. Hui CLM, Honer WG, Lee EHM, Chang WC, Chan SKW, Chen EYH. Factors Associated with successful medication discontinuation after a randomized clinical trial of relapse prevention in first-episode psychosis: a 10-year follow-up. *JAMA Psychiatry.* 2019;76(2):217-219. doi:10.1001/jamapsychiatry.2018.3120

28. Hui CLM, Honer WG, Lee EHM, et al. Long-term effects of discontinuation from antipsychotic maintenance following first-episode schizophrenia and related disorders: a 10-year follow-up of a randomised, double-blind trial. *Lancet Psychiatry.* 2018;5(5):432-442. doi:10.1016/S2215-0366(18)30090-7

29. Hui CLM, Chen EYH, Lam M, et al. Can we predict relapse in single episode psychosis patients with stable maintenance treatment for at least one year? The 6th International Conference on Early Psychosis; Oct 20–22, 2008; Melbourne, Australia. *Early Interv Psychiatry.* 2008;2(Suppl.1):A124.

30. Chen YH, Hui LM, Lam M, et al. A double-blind randomized placebo-controlled relapse prevention study in remitted first-episode psychosis patients following one year of maintenance therapy. The 14th Biennial Winter Workshop on Schizophrenia and Bipolar Disorders; Feb3–7, 2008; Montreux, Switzerland. In *Schizophr Res.* 2008;98(Suppl.):11-12. doi:10.1016/j.schres.2007.12.020

31. Chan KK, Hui CL, Lam MM, et al. A three-year prospective study of spontaneous eye-blink rate in first-episode schizophrenia: relationship with relapse and neurocognitive function. *East Asian Arch Psychiatry.* 2010;20(4):174-179.

32. Hui CL, Lam BS, Wong AK, et al. ReMind, a smartphone application for psychotic relapse prediction: A longitudinal study protocol. *Early Interv Psychiatry.* 2021;15(6):1659-1666. doi:10.1111/eip.13108

33. Wunderink L, Nieboer RM, Wiersma D, Sytema S, Nienhuis FJ. Recovery in remitted first-episode psychosis at 7 years of follow-up of an early dose reduction/discontinuation or maintenance treatment strategy: long-term follow-up of a 2-year randomized clinical trial. *JAMA Psychiatry.* 2013;70(9):913-920. doi:10.1001/jamapsychiatry.2013.19

34. Taipale H, Tanskanen A, Correll CU, Tiihonen J. Real-world effectiveness of antipsychotic doses for relapse prevention in patients with first-episode schizophrenia in Finland: a nationwide, register-based cohort study. *Lancet Psychiatry.* 2022;9(4):271-279. doi:10.1016/S2215-0366(22)00015-3

146 • *Psychosis and Schizophrenia in Hong Kong*

35. Hui CLM, Lo MCL, Chan EHC, et al. Perception towards relapse and its predictors in psychosis patients: A qualitative study. *Early Interv Psychiatry*. 2018;12(5):856-862. doi:10.1111/eip.12378

36. Coldham EL, Addington J, Addington D. Medication adherence of individuals with a first episode of psychosis. *Acta Psychiatr Scand*. 2002;106(4):286-290. doi:10.1034/j.1600-0447.2002.02437.x

37. Gitlin M, Nuechterlein K, Subotnik KL, et al. Clinical outcome following neuroleptic discontinuation in patients with remitted recent-onset schizophrenia. *Am J Psychiatry*. 2001;158(11):1835-1842. doi:10.1176/appi.ajp.158.11.1835

38. Whitehorn D, Richard JC, Kopala LC. Hospitalization in the first year of treatment for schizophrenia. *Can J Psychiatry*. 2004;49(9):635-638. doi:10.1177/070674370404900911

39. Hudson TJ, Owen RR, Thrush CR, et al. A pilot study of barriers to medication adherence in schizophrenia. *J Clin Psychiatry*. 2004;65(2):211-216. doi:10.4088/jcp.v65n0211

40. Perkins DO, Gu H, Weiden PJ, et al. Predictors of treatment discontinuation and medication nonadherence in patients recovering from a first episode of schizophrenia, schizophreniform disorder, or schizoaffective disorder: a randomized, double-blind, flexible-dose, multicenter study. *J Clin Psychiatry*. 2008;69(1):106-113. doi:10.4088/jcp.v69n0114

41. Robinson DG, Woerner MG, Alvir JM, Bilder RM, Hinrichsen GA, Lieberman JA. Predictors of medication discontinuation by patients with first-episode schizophrenia and schizoaffective disorder. *Schizophr Res*. 2002;57(2-3):209-219. doi:10.1016/s0920-9964(01)00312-7

42. Hui CL, Chen EY, Kan CS, Yip KC, Law CW, Chiu CP. Detection of non-adherent behaviour in early psychosis. *Aust N Z J Psychiatry*. 2006;40(5):446-451. doi:10.1080/j.1440-1614.2006.01821.x

43. Besenius C, Clark-Carter D, Nolan P. Health professionals' attitudes to depot injection antipsychotic medication: a systematic review. *J Psychiatr Ment Health Nurs*. 2010;17(5):452-462. doi:10.1111/j.1365-2850.2010.01550.x

44. Day JC, Bentall RP, Roberts C, et al. Attitudes toward antipsychotic medication: the impact of clinical variables and relationships with health professionals. *Arch Gen Psychiatry*. 2005;62(7):717-724. doi:10.1001/archpsyc.62.7.717

45. Heres S, Hamann J, Kissling W, Leucht S. Attitudes of psychiatrists toward antipsychotic depot medication. *J Clin Psychiatry*. 2006;67(12):1948-1953. doi:10.4088/jcp.v67n1216

46. Johnson DA, Rasmussen JG. Professional attitudes in the UK towards neuroleptic maintenance therapy in schizophrenia. The problem of inadequate prophylaxis. *Psychiatr Bull*. 1997;21:394-397.

47. Patel MX, Nikolaou V, David AS. Psychiatrists' attitudes to maintenance medication for patients with schizophrenia. *Psychol Med*. 2003;33(1):83-89. doi:10.1017/s0033291702006797

48. Simon AE, Lauber C, Ludewig K, Braun-Scharm H, Umbricht DS; Swiss Early Psychosis Project. General practitioners and schizophrenia: results from a Swiss survey. *Br J Psychiatry*. 2005;187:274-281. doi:10.1192/bjp.187.3.274

Relapse in Psychotic Disorders ⋅ 147

49. Kissling W. Compliance, quality assurance and standards for relapse prevention in schizophrenia. *Acta Psychiatr Scand Suppl*. 1994;382:16-24. doi:10.1111/j.1600-0447.1994.tb05860.x

50. Chan KK, Chin QP, Tang JY, et al. Perceptions of relapse risks following first-episode psychosis and attitudes towards maintenance medication: a comparison between nursing and social work professionals. *Early Interv Psychiatry*. 2011;5(4):324-334. doi:10.1111/j.1751-7893.2011.00268.x

51. Kraepelin E. *Einführung in Die Psychiatrische Klinik*. 4th ed. Vol 3. Verlag von Johann Ambrosius Barth; 1921.

52. Correll CU, Galling B, Pawar A, et al. Comparison of early intervention services vs treatment as usual for early-phase psychosis: a systematic review, meta-analysis, and meta-regression. *JAMA Psychiatry*. 2018;75(6):555-565. doi:10.1001/jamapsychiatry.2018.0623

53. Chan SKW, Chan HYV, Devlin J, et al. A systematic review of long-term outcomes of patients with psychosis who received early intervention services. *Int Rev Psychiatry*. 2019;31(5-6):425-440. doi:10.1080/09540261.2019.1643704

11

Treatment-Refractory States: An End-Game Scenario?

Background

The Definition and Prevalence of Treatment Resistance

Treatment resistance in psychotic disorders is generally defined as non-response to two different antipsychotics that have been administered at correct doses for a sufficient period of time and have been taken regularly (1). However, studies have varied widely in the operational use of the term 'treatment resistance' (2). In 2016, the Treatment Response and Resistance in Psychosis (TRRIP) Working Group undertook a systematic review of randomised clinical trials of antipsychotic medication in treatment-refractory schizophrenia and developed consensus operationalised criteria. These included current symptomatology determined by a standardised rating scale, moderate or worse functional impairment, having received treatment with two antipsychotics of adequate dose and duration, as well as adequate adherence that has been systematically monitored (2).

It is known that up to 30% of schizophrenia patients and 50% of first-episode psychosis (FEP) patients experience long-term incomplete remission or treatment resistance (3, 4, 5). A very recent meta-analysis by Siskind et al. (2021) reported a rate of treatment-resistant schizophrenia (TRS) of 22.8% in FEP patients and 24.4% among first-episode schizophrenia patients. Men were 1.57 times more likely to develop treatment resistance than women (6). Patients with TRS experience higher rates of unemployment, worse quality of life, and incur three- to eleven-fold higher direct healthcare costs (7, 8).

Predictive Factors of Treatment Resistance

Among the predictive factors for treatment resistance are lower premorbid functioning, lower level of education, negative symptoms during the first psychotic episode, comorbid substance use, younger age at onset, lack of early response, non-adherence to treatment, and longer duration of untreated psychosis. Gender and marital status were not shown to have a clear-cut association with treatment resistance (1). It appears that younger age at onset is the most consistent predictor of treatment resistance in FEP patients (9).

Legge et al. (2019) examined whether genetic liability for schizophrenia and/ or clinical characteristics measurable at illness onset could potentially predict a higher risk of treatment-resistant psychosis (TRP). In their sample of 1070 patients with schizophrenia or related disorders, younger age at onset, poor premorbid social adjustment, lower premorbid IQ, and cannabis use increased the risk of TRP. However, genetic liability for schizophrenia did not predict TRP (10). Similarly, a Danish population-based follow-up study did not find an association between polygenic risk scores for schizophrenia and TRS (11).

Treatment resistance may manifest from the first episode of psychosis, or may develop over time and might be preceded by relapses (12, 13, 14, 15, 16). For example, Lally and colleagues (2016) assessed clinical outcomes in a cohort of 246 FEP patients over the course of five years (13). They reported that 23% of participants were treatment-resistant from illness onset and that these patients were more likely to have an early age of contact with services. In their cohort, ethnicity and male gender were significantly associated with treatment resistance and early age of presentation.

Neurobiological Mechanisms in Treatment Resistance

It has been argued that outcomes for patients might be improved if TRS is identified earlier as it may allow for the timely prescription of clozapine, the only approved antipsychotic for the condition (17, 18). Several hypotheses have been put forward regarding the neurobiological mechanisms underlying TRS, including dopamine supersensitivity, hyperdopaminergic and normodopaminergic sub-types, glutamate dysregulation, inflammation and oxidative stress, and serotonin dysregulation (3). It has also been shown that abnormal presynaptic dopamine transmission usually seen in schizophrenia is absent in TRS. Instead, changes in anterior cingulate glutamate activity have been observed (19, 20). Furthermore, functional abnormalities of the N-methyl-D-aspartate (NMDA) receptor have been reported in schizophrenia (21). These findings might be unsurprising given the fact that dopaminergic antipsychotics do not produce an adequate treatment response in patients considered to be treatment-resistant. More recently, evidence is emerging for the role of

GABAergic dysfunction in the pathogenesis of schizophrenia (22, 23). Nasir and colleagues (2020) suggest that clozapine is a GABAB receptor agonist similar to baclofen after examining the X-ray crystal structure and molecular docking sites of the receptor and propose further exploration of their findings to support the development of biomarkers for TRS and more targeted treatments (22).

Are There Sub-types of Treatment Resistance?

Attempts have been made to differentiate sub-types of TRS according to neurodevelopmental or neurodegenerative considerations. It has been shown that patients who are treatment-resistant are more likely to have more severe positive and negative symptoms, lower premorbid psychosocial functioning, a higher frequency of obstetric complications and neurological soft signs, and are more vulnerable to tardive dyskinesia suggesting a neurodevelopmental component. A neurodegenerative hypothesis is supported by the correlation of duration of untreated psychosis (DUP) and treatment resistance, decreases in brain volumes as the disease progresses, and the link between an increase in treatment resistance with each subsequent relapse (24). However, it is doubtful that the two mechanisms exert their effects on the emergence of treatment resistance entirely independently. It seems more likely that both processes contribute, and that neurodevelopmental vulnerabilities precede and may potentiate the effects of neurodegenerative mechanisms.

Treatment Resistance and Clozapine

Up to 70% of patients with TRS are thought to respond to clozapine. However, more recent studies estimate that up to 60% of patients may not benefit (25, 26, 27). Moreover, it has been shown that only 30% of patients with TRS ever receive clozapine treatment and that clozapine initiation is often considerably delayed (28, 29). Until recently, it has not been possible to predict which patients will respond to clozapine (30). A recent meta-analysis by Okhuijsen-Pfeifer et al. (2020) reported that younger age, fewer negative symptoms at onset, and paranoid schizophrenia sub-types were associated with better response to clozapine in patients with an established diagnosis of schizophrenia (31). Interestingly, one study showed that clozapine-related elevated serum lipids were associated with improvements in schizophrenia symptoms. Whether the efficacy of clozapine is indeed associated with increased serum lipids will require verification (32).

Studies on Treatment-Refractory Psychosis in Hong Kong

Treatment-Resistant and Clozapine-Resistant Schizophrenia

We undertook a 12-year follow-up study of FEP patients to investigate early predictors of treatment-resistant schizophrenia and clozapine-resistant schizophrenia (CR-TRS) (33). Our team recruited 617 participants with first-episode schizophrenia-spectrum disorders from the Early Assessment Service for Young People (EASY) and matched them according to age, gender, and diagnosis with patients receiving standard care. 15% of our cohort were estimated to be treatment-resistant. Younger age of onset, poorer premorbid social adjustment during adulthood, longer duration of the first episode, a greater number of relapses, and a higher antipsychotic dose in the first 24 months were associated with earlier TRS. Of those patients who were treatment-resistant, 25% were resistant to clozapine. These patients had poorer premorbid social adjustment in late adolescence and a longer delay before clozapine initiation compared with non-CR-TRS. CR-TRS had poorer clinical and functional outcomes at 12-year follow-up. However, TRS patients on clozapine had a lower mortality rate compared with non-TRS patients. We also showed that specialist early intervention (EI) did not alter the development of TRS, but patients in the EI group had a shorter delay to clozapine initiation.

Our relatively low rate of TRS may reflect a relatively low prevalence of substance misuse (8.4%) in our sample compared to around 30% in most other published studies, as well as a narrower definition of TRS based on the TRRIP criteria (13, 34). Other factors to consider might be the fact that the majority of FEP patients reside with family in Hong Kong and thus may perceive to have better psychosocial support when family members are well-trained to provide care.

Psychotic disorders have a considerable genetic variance and polygenic mechanisms are thought to be relevant in TRS (35). Genetic polymorphisms in Chinese patients may differ from those of other ethnicities affecting treatment response partly mediated by pharmacokinetic and pharmacodynamic mechanisms. For example, clinical practice has shown that patients of Asian descent often respond to much smaller doses of clozapine to reach clinically significant plasma levels.

Given that a significant proportion of patients do not respond to clozapine we participated in a multinational trial comparing the effectiveness of clozapine augmentation with risperidone (36). A total of 68 patients who were already taking clozapine were randomly assigned to receive either risperidone or placebo for eight weeks. The mean total score for the severity of symptoms decreased in both groups and there was no statistically significant difference in symptomatic benefit between augmentation with risperidone and placebo at the end of the study.

The Management of Treatment-Refractory Psychosis

Perhaps the most important aspect of TRP is its ongoing careful management. Before a diagnosis of TRS is reached, other psychiatric conditions such as schizoaffective disorder or affective psychosis should be excluded as well as any underlying physical health conditions, whether these might be nutritional deficiencies, endocrine disorders, metabolic diseases, neurological disorders, or infectious disorders (37). A careful medication and substance use history will also need to be taken and a full physical examination and investigations including blood tests, neuroimaging, and drug screening should be carried out.

Exploring medication adherence will likely involve talking to relatives, counting the number of tablets taken by the patient, and monitoring drug levels. In addition, a review of antipsychotic dosing is vital to determine whether an adequate dose has been prescribed for at least four to six weeks before assuming that a patient is treatment-resistant. Patients who smoke are likely to require a higher dose of medication due to the fact that polycyclic hydrocarbons in cigarettes induce hepatic cytochrome P450 enzymes, which metabolise haloperidol, olanzapine, and clozapine, resulting in lower serum levels.

Genetic testing might be helpful if a patient is suspected to be a rapid metaboliser of antipsychotics such as haloperidol, zuclopenthixol, risperidone, thioridazine, and perphenazine. Particularly, patients from Saudi Arabia or Ethiopia may carry a duplication in the CYP2D6 gene and would therefore be more likely to be rapid metabolisers. Clozapine is also an option at this point. Reaching an adequate serum level of at least 250 ng/ml and closely monitoring for agranulocytosis, lipid disturbance, seizure, and other side effects cannot be overstated (37). One may add that given our findings and evidence from two other studies of an association between delay in clozapine prescribing and clozapine resistance, it is important to consider timely assessments of whether patients are treatment-resistant and to offer clozapine without delay (32, 38, 39). Despite its efficacy, clinicians remain hesitant to commence clozapine due to concerns about the need for frequent blood monitoring, its tolerability, and potential complications (40).

Augmentation might be necessary to improve response to antipsychotic treatment. Lamotrigine, valproate, and eicosapentaenoic acid, an omega-3 polyunsaturated fatty acid, may be tried. Non-pharmacological strategies such as counselling, psychological support, psychoeducation, and social rehabilitation should be offered alongside pharmacological treatment. Electroconvulsive therapy has also been used in cases of TRS and some benefits have been observed although more systematic data are lacking regarding its efficacy. Other physical treatments, such as repetitive transcranial magnetic stimulation (rTMS), have been found to reduce symptoms in patients with treatment-resistant auditory hallucinations; however, good-quality data has not been available to support its widespread clinical use.

A Case Study of Treatment-Refractory Psychosis

We followed the illness course of a young woman with schizophrenia with repeated clinical evaluations and imaging using Tc-99m hexamethylpropylene amine oxime single photon emission computed tomography (HMPAO SPECT) (41). Aged 19, the patient presented with a six-month history of auditory and visual hallucinations, persecutory delusions, and delusions of control. She was right-handed, did not have any neurological or physical illness, and did not use substances. Premorbidly, she had been well adjusted, was studying, achieving average academic grades, and led an active social life. Physical examination, laboratory investigations, electrophysiological studies, and neuroimaging did not show any abnormalities. She was diagnosed with paranoid schizophrenia by two senior psychiatrists. The young woman was followed up over the course of five years, at months 6, 10, 40, 44, 56, and 66 from illness onset. Her symptoms were assessed using the Brief Psychiatric Rating Scale (BPRS) and High Royds Evaluation of Negativity Scale. In addition, her cognition was tested and serial brain SPECT was carried out.

In her first episode, the patient responded well to haloperidol after two weeks and achieved full remission. Her antipsychotic medication was changed to sulpiride as she was experiencing extrapyramidal side effects while taking haloperidol. She was working as a secretary and remained asymptomatic for almost four years while taking maintenance medication. Her relapse at 44 months had been precipitated by non-adherence. After three weeks of treatment with sulpiride, her symptoms subsided, there were no residual negative symptoms or functional impairment, and she could return to her employment as a secretary. Six months later, she again relapsed. This time, she presented with blunted affect, impoverishment of thought, social withdrawal, and poor volition. She had cognitive deficits and was no longer able to carry out her job. She failed to respond to two conventional antipsychotics. Clozapine was commenced, her psychotic symptoms subsided, and her cognitive function normalised after two months of treatment. Despite the longer duration of her third episode and the emergence of negative symptoms, she recovered her psychosocial functioning and continued to work as a secretary. Brain SPECT imaging revealed under-activity in the left temporal area in the course of our patient's illness despite intermittent remission of symptoms. Bilateral prefrontal under-activity became evident as negative symptoms, executive neurocognitive dysfunction, and treatment refractoriness emerged.

This case study illustrates very well the relapsing and remitting course of schizophrenia and the development of treatment resistance over time. One might wonder whether TRS would have emerged if the young woman had continued taking her medication following her first episode and whether maintenance medication may have protected her from developing negative symptoms and cognitive impairment by reducing her risk of relapse. We postulated that left temporal under-activity reflects an underlying disease process. Other neuroimaging case studies have reported different patterns of brain metabolic activities over time. However, consistent with other studies, was the reduction in prefrontal activity with the emergence of negative symptoms, cognitive dysfunction, and treatment resistance. As our patient responded to clozapine, activity in the right prefrontal lobe normalised. Whether persistent changes in activity in the left anterior temporal lobe and possibly in the left prefrontal lobe represent neurobiological correlates for the emergence of treatment-resistant states and increase the risk of further relapses is an interesting question and warrants further exploration (41).

Reflections: The Challenges of Managing Treatment-Refractory Psychosis

Before the advent of antipsychotic medication, the outcome of psychotic states was mostly chronic with persistent psychotic symptoms, and patients with spontaneous remission were few. Antipsychotic treatment has enabled the control of psychotic symptoms in most patients. However, some patients do not respond to the usual antipsychotic medication.

Most antipsychotics work by blocking dopamine D2 receptors. Failure to respond to antipsychotics suggests that the pathogenetic pathway may involve systems other than the dopamine system. A treatment-refractory status can be present at first presentation, but it could also arise in the course of the illness. The fact that some patients are treatment-responsive and after several years become treatment-refractory implies that neurobiological changes occur in the interim period. While the underlying mechanisms have not yet been clarified, this observation does suggest that important changes can occur in brain systems subsequent to the onset of the disorder.

The emergence of treatment refractoriness can be associated with episodes of relapse. In our case study, we observed that there had been good clinical remission following the first episode and after the first relapse. However, following medication discontinuation leading to the second relapse in the fourth year of illness, the brain activation pattern as detected by a SPECT scan changed from a primarily temporal activation pattern to a frontal hypofunction pattern. At the same time, the patient experienced cognitive impairment and treatment refractoriness. Of course, this is not a controlled study, but one might be very tempted to pose the question of whether this state would have developed had the medication not been discontinued. There is some preliminary evidence showing possible clinical illness progression in patients experiencing a relapse of their psychotic illness, although good-quality larger-scale data are currently lacking (16, 42). Should further research support these findings, then stratification of patients at high risk of relapse and strengthening medication adherence will be of paramount importance to reduce the risk of relapse and prevent a deteriorating course.

When we take a broader multidimensional perspective of psychotic disorders, it is important to recognise that although the key feature of psychotic disorders is psychotic episodes, there are other dimensions of the disorder such as cognitive dysfunction that affect functional outcomes. Dopamine dysregulation has been considered the final common pathway converging towards the expression of psychotic disorders. Antipsychotic medications target downstream dopamine receptors and are effective in achieving symptomatic relief. However, they may not be effective in addressing the upstream cause of dopamine dysregulation, hence the need for long-term treatment for the majority of patients. It is also important to be aware that other dimensions of the disorder such as cognitive dysfunction, including motivational impairments are not addressed by antipsychotic medications, and sometimes may even be aggravated by them. Treatment-refractory psychosis, in which psychotic symptoms become unresponsive to antipsychotic medication, reflects an important process whereby a non-dopamine mediated pathway contributes to the maintenance of symptoms. Importantly, such a pathway may be expressed at the onset of the disorder, or as a progressive process subsequent to the first episode. There is evidence that this process may be facilitated by relapses. Hence the window of freedom from psychotic symptoms provided by antipsychotic medication is not unconditionally secured. While a major factor in relapse is the discontinuation of maintenance medication, there are also cases where treatment refractoriness develops despite maintenance medication. There is evidence that the emergence of treatment refractoriness is associated with brain processes that also result in the appearance of neurocognitive symptoms such as cognitive dysfunction or neurological signs. While the freedom from psychotic features may not necessarily guarantee good functioning, the presence of significant symptoms is mostly associated with poor functioning. Apart from the optimal treatment of psychotic symptoms, there is a large treatment gap for non-dopamine-related dimensions of psychotic disorders.

References

1. Bozzatello P, Bellino S, Rocca P. Predictive factors of treatment resistance in first episode of psychosis: a systematic review. *Front Psychiatry*. 2019;10:67. Published Feb 26, 2019. doi:10.3389/fpsyt.2019.00067
2. Howes OD, McCutcheon R, Agid O, et al. Treatment-resistant schizophrenia: Treatment Response and Resistance in Psychosis (TRRIP) Working Group Consensus Guidelines on Diagnosis and Terminology. *Am J Psychiatry*. 2017;174(3):216-229. doi:10.1176/appi.ajp.2016.16050503

3. Potkin SG, Kane JM, Correll CU, et al. The neurobiology of treatment-resistant schizophrenia: paths to antipsychotic resistance and a roadmap for future research. *NPJ Schizophr.* 2020;6(1):1. Published Jan 7, 2020. doi:10.1038/s41537-019-0090-z

4. Meltzer HY. Treatment-resistant schizophrenia – the role of clozapine. *Curr Med Res Opin.* 1997;14(1):1-20. doi:10.1185/03007999709113338

5. Huber CG, Naber D, Lambert M. Incomplete remission and treatment resistance in first-episode psychosis: definition, prevalence and predictors. *Expert Opin Pharmacother.* 2008;9(12):2027-2038. doi:10.1517/14656566.9.12.2027

6. Siskind D, Orr S, Sinha S, et al. Rates of treatment-resistant schizophrenia from first-episode cohorts: systematic review and meta-analysis. *Br J Psychiatry.* 2022;220(3):115-120. doi:10.1192/bjp.2021.61

7. Iasevoli F, Giordano S, Balletta R, et al. Treatment resistant schizophrenia is associated with the worst community functioning among severely-ill highly-disabling psychiatric conditions and is the most relevant predictor of poorer achievements in functional milestones. *Prog Neuropsychopharmacol Biol Psychiatry.* 2016;65:34-48. doi:10.1016/j.pnpbp.2015.08.010

8. Kennedy JL, Altar CA, Taylor DL, Degtiar I, Hornberger JC. The social and economic burden of treatment-resistant schizophrenia: a systematic literature review. *Int Clin Psychopharmacol.* 2014;29(2):63-76. doi:10.1097/YIC.0b013e32836508e6

9. Smart SE, Kępińska AP, Murray RM, MacCabe JH. Predictors of treatment resistant schizophrenia: a systematic review of prospective observational studies. *Psychol Med.* 2021;51(1):44-53. doi:10.1017/S0033291719002083

10. Legge SE, Dennison CA, Pardiñas AF, et al. Clinical indicators of treatment-resistant psychosis. *Br J Psychiatry.* 2020;216(5):259-266. doi:10.1192/bjp.2019.120

11. Wimberley T, Gasse C, Meier SM, Agerbo E, MacCabe JH, Horsdal HT. Polygenic risk score for schizophrenia and treatment-resistant schizophrenia. *Schizophr Bull.* 2017;43(5):1064-1069. doi:10.1093/schbul/sbx007

12. Demjaha A, Lappin JM, Stahl D, et al. Antipsychotic treatment resistance in first-episode psychosis: prevalence, subtypes and predictors. *Psychol Med.* 2017;47(11):1981-1989. doi:10.1017/S0033291717000435

13. Lally J, Ajnakina O, Di Forti M, et al. Two distinct patterns of treatment resistance: clinical predictors of treatment resistance in first-episode schizophrenia spectrum psychoses. *Psychol Med.* 2016;46(15):3231-3240. doi:10.1017/S0033291716002014

14. Robinson DG, Woerner MG, Alvir JM, et al. Predictors of treatment response from a first episode of schizophrenia or schizoaffective disorder. *Am J Psychiatry.* 1999;156(4):544-549. doi:10.1176/ajp.156.4.544

15. Altamura AC, Bassetti R, Cattaneo E, Vismara S. Some biological correlates of drug resistance in schizophrenia: a multidimensional approach. *World J Biol Psychiatry.* 2005;6 Suppl 2:23-30. doi:10.1080/15622970510030027

16. Takeuchi H, Siu C, Remington G, et al. Does relapse contribute to treatment resistance? Antipsychotic response in first- vs. second-episode schizophrenia. *Neuropsychopharmacology.* 2019;44(6):1036-1042. doi:10.1038/s41386-018-0278-3

17. Yada Y, Yoshimura B, Kishi Y. Correlation between delay in initiating clozapine and symptomatic improvement. *Schizophr Res.* 2015;168(1-2):585-586. doi:10.1016/j.schres.2015.07.045

18. Kane JM, Agid O, Baldwin ML, et al. Clinical guidance on the identification and management of treatment-resistant schizophrenia. *J Clin Psychiatry*. 2019;80(2):18com12123. Published Mar 5, 2019. doi:10.4088/JCP.18com12123

19. Demjaha A, Murray RM, McGuire PK, Kapur S, Howes OD. Dopamine synthesis capacity in patients with treatment-resistant schizophrenia. *Am J Psychiatry*. 2012;169(11):1203-1210. doi:10.1176/appi.ajp.2012.12010144

20. Demjaha A, Egerton A, Murray RM, et al. Antipsychotic treatment resistance in schizophrenia associated with elevated glutamate levels but normal dopamine function. *Biol Psychiatry*. 2014;75(5):e11-e13. doi:10.1016/j.biopsych.2013.06.011

21. Veerman SR, Schulte PF, de Haan L. The glutamate hypothesis: a pathogenic pathway from which pharmacological interventions have emerged. *Pharmacopsychiatry*. 2014;47(4-5):121-130. doi:10.1055/s-0034-1383657

22. Nair PC, McKinnon RA, Miners JO, Bastiampillai T. Binding of clozapine to the GABAB receptor: clinical and structural insights. *Mol Psychiatry*. 2020;25(9):1910-1919. doi:10.1038/s41380-020-0709-5

23. O'Connor WT, O'Shea SD. Clozapine and GABA transmission in schizophrenia disease models: establishing principles to guide treatments. *Pharmacol Ther*. 2015;150:47-80. doi:10.1016/j.pharmthera.2015.01.005.

24. Woolfolk R, Allen L, ed. *Mental Disorders – Theoretical and Empirical Perspectives*. INTECH, Institute for New Technologies, Maastricht, Netherlands; 2013.

25. Meltzer HY. Treatment of the neuroleptic-nonresponsive schizophrenic patient. *Schizophr Bull*. 1992;18(3):515-542. doi:10.1093/schbul/18.3.515

26. Farooq S, Agid O, Foussias G, Remington G. Using treatment response to subtype schizophrenia: proposal for a new paradigm in classification. *Schizophr Bull*. 2013;39(6):1169-1172. doi:10.1093/schbul/sbt137

27. Siskind D, Siskind V, Kisely S. Clozapine response rates among people with treatment-resistant schizophrenia: data from a systematic review and meta-analysis. *Can J Psychiatry*. 2017;62(11):772-777. doi:10.1177/0706743717718167

28. Farooq S, Taylor M. Clozapine: dangerous orphan or neglected friend? *Br J Psychiatry*. 2011;198(4):247-249. doi:10.1192/bjp.bp.110.088690

29. Doyle R, Behan C, O'Keeffe D, et al. Clozapine use in a cohort of first-episode psychosis. *J Clin Psychopharmacol*. 2017;37(5):512-517. doi:10.1097/JCP.0000000000000734

30. Samanaite R, Gillespie A, Sendt KV, McQueen G, MacCabe JH, Egerton A. Biological predictors of clozapine response: a systematic review. *Front Psychiatry*. 2018;9:327. Published Jul 26, 2018. doi:10.3389/fpsyt.2018.00327

31. Okhuijsen-Pfeifer C, Sterk AY, Horn IM, Terstappen J, Kahn RS, Luykx JJ. Demographic and clinical features as predictors of clozapine response in patients with schizophrenia spectrum disorders: a systematic review and meta-analysis. *Neurosci Biobehav Rev*. 2020;111:246-252. doi:10.1016/j.neubiorev.2020.01.017

32. Procyshyn RM, Wasan KM, Thornton AE, et al. Changes in serum lipids, independent of weight, are associated with changes in symptoms during long-term clozapine treatment. *J Psychiatry Neurosci*. 2007;32(5):331-338.

33. Chan SKW, Chan HYV, Honer WG, et al. Predictors of treatment-resistant and clozapine-resistant schizophrenia: a 12-year follow-up study of first-episode schizophrenia-spectrum disorders. *Schizophr Bull*. 2021;47(2):485-494. doi:10.1093/schbul/sbaa145

34. Wimberley T, Støvring H, Sørensen HJ, Horsdal HT, MacCabe JH, Gasse C. Predictors of treatment resistance in patients with schizophrenia: a population-based cohort study [published correction appears in *Lancet Psychiatry*. Apr 2016;3(4):320]. *Lancet Psychiatry*. 2016;3(4):358-366. doi:10.1016/S2215-0366(15)00575-1

35. Ruderfer DM, Fanous AH, Ripke S, et al. Polygenic dissection of diagnosis and clinical dimensions of bipolar disorder and schizophrenia. *Mol Psychiatry*. 2014;19(9):1017-1024. doi:10.1038/mp.2013.138

36. Honer WG, Thornton AE, Chen EY, et al. Clozapine alone versus clozapine and risperidone with refractory schizophrenia. *N Engl J Med*. 2006;354(5):472-482. doi:10.1056/NEJMoa053222

37. Lam PTC. Treatment resistance in schizophrenia. *Medical Bulletin*. 2008;13(2):16-18.

38. Shah P, Iwata Y, Brown EE, et al. Clozapine response trajectories and predictors of non-response in treatment-resistant schizophrenia: a chart review study. *Eur Arch Psychiatry Clin Neurosci*. 2020;270(1):11-22. doi:10.1007/s00406-019-01053-6

39. Shah P, Iwata Y, Plitman E, et al. The impact of delay in clozapine initiation on treatment outcomes in patients with treatment-resistant schizophrenia: a systematic review. *Psychiatry Res*. 2018;268:114-122. doi:10.1016/j.psychres.2018.06.070

40. Zheng S, Lee J, Chan SKW. Utility and barriers to clozapine use: a joint study of clinicians' attitudes from Singapore and Hong Kong. *J Clin Psychiatry*. 2022;83(4):21m14231. Published May 18, 2022. doi:10.4088/JCP.21m14231

41. Chen RY, Chen E, Ho WY. A five-year longitudinal study of the regional cerebral metabolic changes of a schizophrenic patient from the first episode using Tc-99m HMPAO SPECT. *Eur Arch Psychiatry Clin Neurosci*. 2000;250(2):69-72. doi:10.1007/s004060070036

42. Emsley R, Chiliza B, Asmal L. The evidence for illness progression after relapse in schizophrenia. *Schizophr Res*. 2013;148(1-3):117-121. doi:10.1016/j.schres.2013.05.016

12

Ideas of Reference: Complexities in the Most Common Symptom in Psychosis

Background

Definitions of Ideas and Delusions of Reference and the Historical Context

Ideas and delusions of reference (I/DOR) are defined as a spurious sense of self-reference in otherwise neutral events in one's immediate environment. Examples include attaching specific self-referential meanings to objects or events, feelings of being talked about, or perceiving mass media as having hidden meanings with personal significance. These phenomena have been described in some of the earliest texts on mental disorders in the West (1). Kraepelin, Jaspers, and Schneider described similar phenomena and considered them an integral part of delusional perception and content (2, 3, 4). Kretschmer coined the term 'sensitiver Beziehungswahn' ('sensitive delusion of reference') and postulated that it constitutes a separate entity characterised by genetic predisposition, psychopathological exhaustibility, and a psycho-reactive origin. He proposed the presence of sensitive character traits, a shameful experience of one's own insufficiencies, and distinct environmental effects as specific psychological factors leading to the emergence of sensitive delusions of reference (5). The content and affect of the delusion were supposedly centred on the pathogenic experience and the symptoms took an exaggerated form of the sensitive character traits. Kretschmer differentiated four sub-types – acute dissociative delusions of short duration, systematic paranoid states, erratic delusions that emerge briefly from highly neurotic states, and relational neuroses. Prognosis varied widely, in its milder form symptoms were fully reversible. Personality was thought to remain unchanged with lively psychological reactivity. Kretschmer was heavily criticised by his contemporaries most notably Eugen Kahn calling his work 'speculative, poetic, confused' although he conceded that as a symptom complex one may encounter sensitive delusions of reference in a number of psychiatric conditions (6).

Ideas and Delusions of Reference as Phenomenological Entities

Self-referential ideas have also been described in social anxiety in the form of feelings of being talked about negatively, laughed at, or watched. These ideas are usually less pervasive and held to be true to a lesser degree. Ideas of reference (IOR) and delusions of reference (DOR) have often been lumped together despite probably being phenomenologically separate entities in both form and content. Some researchers proposed that I/DOR lie on a continuum from mild – as might be seen in social anxiety – to severe in psychotic illness. However, DOR tend to have more bizarre content and are held with unreasonable conviction as compared to IOR encountered in low self-esteem and are often accompanied by physical symptoms of anxiety. Another difficulty is that delusions by definition are necessarily self-referential in nature and therefore conceptual boundaries between DOR and other types of delusions, particularly persecutory delusions and erotomania, have been blurred (7).

The Measurement of Ideas and Delusions of Reference

Kendler et al. (1989) reported on their difficulty in defining and assessing IOR when they developed the Structural Interview for Schizotypy to assess schizotypy in relatives of schizophrenia patients (8). They found that although the symptom was a strong discriminator between non-schizophrenia relatives of patients with the disorder versus other healthy control subjects, the symptom was also considered a normal reaction when individual experiences were contextualised. In addition to IOR being more common in relatives of schizophrenia patients, I/DOR has also been recognised to be a prodromal and early relapse sign (9, 10).

Efforts have been made over several decades to standardise assessment tools to capture this phenomenologically diverse symptom. Research teams have conceptualised I/DOR in different ways including how to best assess severity and pervasiveness. Particularly self-rating scales have been beset with issues regarding their sensitivity and specificity of assessed items due to patients' varying levels of insight, suspiciousness, selection of individual questions, and assessment of context. This, together with difficulties in clearly defining the symptom, has impacted the validity and reliability of proposed assessment schedules (8, 11).

Despite these difficulties, it is estimated that up to 70% of recent-onset schizophrenia patients experience IOR and/or DOR (12). Overall, the lifetime prevalence of ideas of reference is estimated to be 0.4% (13).

Ideas and Delusions of Reference in Psychosis in Hong Kong

The Development of the Ideas of Reference Interview Scale

In Hong Kong, our team developed an interview-based instrument, the Ideas of Reference Interview Scale (IRIS), to provide clearer definitions and standardise the assessment of I/DOR to enable more refined research into neurocognitive mechanisms underlying this phenomenon (14). We undertook a comprehensive literature review to delineate symptoms in I/DOR and their definitions in diagnostic criteria. We then carried out in-depth interviews with patients who had experienced I/DOR. This allowed the extraction of common themes and the development of a 15-item scale covering a range of self-referential experiences. To describe I/DOR phenomena in their social contexts, the IRIS assesses the extent to which information is specifically targeting or referring to oneself. Patients are assessed as to whether their subjective sense of self-referential information matches objective evaluation by a trained interviewer. The discrepancy between subjective and objective assessment is encoded on a 5-point scale. The questionnaire was validated in 137 subjects with remitted schizophrenia spectrum disorder and IRIS was found to have good internal consistency, inter-rater reliability, and divergent validity with other symptoms. IRIS correlated satisfactorily with the I/DOR item or sub-scale on the Scale for the Assessment of Positive Symptoms and the Schizotypal Personality Questionnaire.

The Prevalence of Ideas and Delusions of Reference and Their Association with Anxiety Symptoms

We reported a point prevalence of 31.4% for I/DOR in our sample. The most commonly reported phenomena were 'being talked about/laughed at' (73%), 'being followed' (30%), 'being gazed upon' (29%), and 'being depicted in mass media' (28%). I/DOR were associated with auditory hallucinations, persecutory delusions, and circumstantiality. Impersistence at work/school, an inability to feel intimacy or closeness, and depression were also correlated with I/DOR, however, insight was not (15). 14% of our stabilised patients still reported I/DOR phenomena. The results were very similar to the findings of the two-year follow-up study of the World Health Organization International Pilot Study of Schizophrenia (IPSS), in which 18% of patients were experiencing these symptoms (16). Perhaps unsurprisingly, patients with I/DOR were 3.8 times more likely to be socially anxious (17).

We explored the association between IOR and social anxiety further using the Leibowitz Social Anxiety Scale (LSAS) (18). We observed that close to half of outpatients met the criteria for social anxiety disorder (SAD) and that symptomatic patients were significantly more likely to have a comorbid diagnosis of SAD and had more severe symptoms of anxiety. Social anxiety was also associated with several positive symptoms. Patients with existing I/DOR were more likely to be socially anxious and scored higher on LSAS than those who no longer or had never experienced I/DOR. There appears to be a direct link between negative symptoms and IOR to social anxiety, although other factors likely play a role in the development and maintenance of social anxiety in patients with psychosis. Interestingly, insight was not shown to be directly related to social anxiety (19).

Delusions of Reference, the Default Mode Network, and Theory of Mind

It has been hypothesised that DOR at the cognitive level might be related to excessive use of an internally generated, top-down processing strategy and that this might be mediated via hyperactivity and hyperconnectivity in the default mode network (DMN) of the brain (20). The DMN is considered to be most active when individuals are not engaging in tasks demanding attention. It has also been implicated in self-focused attention and 'stimulus-independent thoughts', as well as baseline monitoring and automatic attention to salient environmental stimuli. Anomalies in the DMN such as the connectivity between brain regions implicated in DMN and inactivation or suppression of the network have been reported in schizophrenia and a link with positive symptoms such as IOR has been suggested (21, 22, 23).

We utilised game theory to investigate the relationship between theory of mind (ToM) deficits and DOR, and observed that schizophrenia patients showed significant ToM impairments compared to controls. However, mentalising deficits were only observed for those patients who had DOR (24). I/DOR may also be associated with heightened attentional shifts towards subjects' own names. Our preliminary findings await further evaluation to ascertain whether these shifts are due to general or specific distractibility related to self-referential information (25).

Delusions of Reference and Neurobiological Correlates

Other neurocognitive models have proposed aberrant salience and associative learning to be involved in the formation of DOR leading to the ascription of personal meaning to neutral or irrelevant stimuli. The dopaminergic system in mesocorticolimbic areas might be implicated in salience attribution through disrupted prediction-error signalling and some researchers believe that delusions are the result of patients trying to make sense of these anomalous experiences (26, 27). It has also been shown that the caudate nucleus has a prominent role in perception and prediction-error coding, associative learning and working memory, and is the primary target of the cognitive/limbic association cortex (28, 29, 30, 31). In a collaboration with the Central South University in Changsha, Hunan, we hypothesised that abnormalities in the caudate nucleus would be associated with DOR and constitute part of its neuroanatomical substrate (32). We demonstrated that patients with DOR had reduced grey matter density in the caudate nucleus compared with patients without DOR and healthy controls. Other brain areas such as the thalamus, and left anterior and posterior cerebellar lobes also showed significant differences between groups. These results suggest that DOR might be the result of the cortico-striato-pallido-thalamic (CSPT) circuitry failing to filter irrelevant incoming information, which may then lead to aberrant salience or prediction-error abnormalities (32).

A more recent study showed that cortical midline structures (CMS) including the ventro- and dorsomedial prefrontal cortex, anterior and posterior cingulate cortex, precuneus, sub-cortical structures such as the ventral striatum, as well as ventral temporal cortices, are involved in processing self-relevant information (33). Larivière et al. (2017) proposed two functionally distinct CMS networks and demonstrated that non-delusional patients had muted activity in the posterior CMS network, whereas delusional patients showed hyperactivity in the anterior CMS network. In addition, activity in the anterior CMS network was positively associated with the intensity of delusion of reference suggesting that hyperactivity in this network may underlie this psychopathology (33).

Delusions of Reference and Gaze Perception

We undertook a study on self-referential gaze perception (SRGP) in schizophrenia patients with DOR (34). All symptomatic patients showed higher rates of unambiguous SRGP, those with more severe DOR had more unambiguous SRGP bias. General cognition also appeared to be implicated in gaze perception. It might very well be that patients with psychotic symptoms hypermentalise gaze perception towards themselves and that patients with prominent DOR display more profound bias in gaze perception. It is an interesting question how gaze perception relates to ToM in patients with prominent DOR and it remains to be seen as to how these deficits potentially interact.

Population-Level Stressors and Ideas and Delusions of Reference

The role of environmental stressors or life events in the formation of I/DOR has been difficult to study as most research efforts have focused on patients who have an established diagnosis of psychosis. Thus, factors implicated in the development of I/DOR have been assessed retrospectively. Environmental events and vulnerable personality traits are difficult to disentangle, as individuals with traits prone to IOR may perceive and report more environmental events. However, we undertook a prospective study in 2020, at the height of the social unrest in Hong Kong, to understand the nature of potentially shared population-level stressors leading to the formation of ideas of reference (35). We distinguished two different levels of ideas of reference, namely attenuated IOR, the experience of feeling particularly referred to within a group, and exclusive IOR, the experience of feeling exclusively referred to while others were not. Those who had event-based ruminations were more likely to have attenuated and exclusive IOR. Traumatic events, such as being attacked or having experienced sexual violence, being arrested, and being verbally abused, were significant predictors for attenuated IOR. On the other hand, education level significantly predicted exclusive IOR. Rumination significantly mediated between traumatic events and IOR severity. It is likely that attenuated and exclusive IOR lie on a continuum. However, further studies will need to elucidate whether subjects exposed to traumatic events and having ruminations move along a continuum, particularly when they are exposed to differing levels of environmental stressors. The study perhaps also highlights an opportunity for preventative intervention to address ruminative tendencies in those who have experienced a high level of distressing events. How an individual's resilience and susceptibility to experiencing ideas of reference might be mediated by distinct personality traits is an interesting area of study, a subject explored in depth by Kretschmer at the beginning of the twentieth century.

Reflections: The Unique Nature of Ideas and Delusions of Reference

One might wonder why we focus on one particular symptom among the many psychotic symptoms reported in schizophrenia. Ideas of reference are the most commonly described symptom of the disorder. In contrast to other psychotic symptoms, the distribution of ideas of reference also appears to fall much more on a continuum in the general population. The transdiagnostic presence of ideas of reference in normally developing individuals, as psychotic-like experiences, as part of schizotypal traits, and in mood disorders also makes them a good candidate to study transitions between diagnostic boundaries.

Unlike other delusions, DOR are unique in that they are not defined by their content. Instead, they are specified by a spurious association with information in the environment. The occurrence of ideas of reference suggests to us that there is an underlying mechanism in healthy individuals, not yet fully explored in cognitive neuroscience, which deals with the handling of self-related information. Insights gained from the clinical phenomenon may facilitate an understanding of how healthy subjects deal with filtering relevant social information. Observations from neuroimaging studies have gained some ground with the discovery that midline brain structures, thought to represent the DMN, are implicated in self-cognition.

Ideas of reference are important clinically because they may cause substantial social disability. They are often confused with social anxiety and may negatively impact the course of psychotic disorders. It is not uncommon that patients following recovery from their psychotic illness continue to harbour self-referential ideas. Eliciting I/DOR can be challenging because patients might feel intensely embarrassed or ashamed, particularly when these involve sexual themes. Increased sensitivity to spurious self-related information may indeed produce widespread difficulties in work and school situations and lead to increasing social isolation and relapse of psychosis. Whether psychological interventions such as cognitive-behavioural therapy might have a role in managing I/DOR and associated distress, and to what extent antipsychotic medication can alleviate self-referential symptoms effectively will require further systematic study.

It is also important to bear in mind that the assessment of self-referential ideas is necessarily more complicated and involves an in-depth exploration of contextual factors to avoid misdiagnosis. This can be challenging in clinical settings where resources are limited. Psychotic presentations with predominantly DOR symptomatology may have a more favourable prognosis, although given their rarity and the paucity of data their status as a possibly separate illness entity remains unclear.

References

1. Burton R. *The anatomy of melancholy: what it is, with all the kinds, causes, symptomes, prognostickes, & seuerall cures of it: in three partitions, with their severall sections, members & subsections philosophically, medicinally, historically opened & cut vp* / by Democritus Junior; with a satyricall preface, conducing to the following discourse. 3rd ed. Iohn Lichfield, for Henry Cripps; 1628.
2. Kraepelin E. *Manic-Depressive Insanity and Paranoia*. E&S Livingstone; 1921/1989.
3. Jaspers K. *General Psychopathology*. 7th ed. Manchester University Press; 1946/1963.
4. Schneider K. The concept of delusion. In: Hirsch S, Shepherd M, eds. *Themes and Variations in European Psychiatry*. John Wright & Sons Ltd; 1949/1974:33-39.
5. Kretschmer E. Zusammenfassung und Abgrenzung. In: *Der Sensitive Beziehungswahn*. Springer; 1950. doi:10.1007/978-3-642-49690-5_10
6. Priwitzer M. *Ernst Kretschmer und das Wahnproblem*. Doctoral dissertation. Medizinischen Fakultät, Eberhard-Karls-Universität; 2004.
7. Oyebode F, Sims ACP. *Sims' Symptoms in the Mind: An Introduction to Descriptive Psychopathology*. Saunders/Elsevier; 2008.
8. Kendler KS, Lieberman JA, Walsh D. The Structured Interview for Schizotypy (SIS): a preliminary report. *Schizophr Bull*. 1989;15(4):559-571. doi:10.1093/schbul/15.4.559
9. Yung AR, Yuen HP, McGorry PD, et al. Mapping the onset of psychosis: the comprehensive assessment of at-risk mental states. *Aust N Z J Psychiatry*. 2005;39(11-12):964-971. doi:10.1080/j.1440-1614.2005.01714.x
10. Birchwood M, Smith J, Macmillan F, et al. Predicting relapse in schizophrenia: the development and implementation of an early signs monitoring system using patients and families as observers, a preliminary investigation. *Psychol Med*. 1989;19(3):649-656. doi:10.1017/s0033291700024247
11. Lenzenweger MF, Bennett ME, Lilenfeld LR. The referential thinking scale as a measure of schizotypy: scale development and initial construct validation. *Psychol Assess*. 1997;9:452-463, doi:10.1037/1040-3590.9.4.452

12. World Health Organization. *Schizophrenia: A Multinational Study. World Health Organization.* Geneva; 1973.
13. McGrath JJ, Saha S, Al-Hamzawi A, et al. Psychotic experiences in the general population: a cross-national analysis based on 31,261 respondents from 18 countries. *JAMA Psychiatry.* 2015;72(7):697-705. doi:10.1001/jamapsychiatry.2015.0575
14. Wong GH, Hui CL, Tang JY, et al. Screening and assessing ideas and delusions of reference using a semi-structured interview scale: a validation study of the Ideas of Reference Interview Scale (IRIS) in early psychosis patients. *Schizophr Res.* 2012;135(1-3):158-163. doi:10.1016/j.schres.2011.12.006
15. Wong GHY, Chiu CPY, Law CW, Chen EYH. Themes and prevalence of ideas/delusions of reference in early psychosis. The 14th Biennial Winter Workshop on Schizophrenia and Bipolar Disorders; Feb 3–7, 2008; Montreux, Switzerland. In *Schizophr Res.* 2008;98(suppl.):181-182. doi:10.1016/j.schres.2007.12.427
16. World Health Organization. *Schizophrenia: An International Follow-Up Study.* John, Wiley and Sons; 1979.
17. Wong GHY, Hui CLM, Chiu CPY, Chen EYH. Subthreshold symptom: ideas of reference. The 6th International Conference on Early Psychosis, Oct 20–22, 2008; Melbourne, Australia. In *Early Interv Psychiatry.* 2008;2(suppl. 1):A77. doi:10.1111/j.1751-7893.2008.00096.x
18. Wong GHY, Chiu CPY, Law CW, Chen EYH. Social anxiety and ideas/delusions of reference in early psychosis. The 14th Biennial Winter Workshop on Schizophrenia and Bipolar Disorders, Feb 3–7, 2008 Montreux, Switzerland. In *Schizophr Res.* 2008;98(suppl.):182-183. doi:10.1016/j.schres.2007.12.429
19. Wong GH. Social anxiety within a network of mild delusional ideations, negative symptoms and insight in outpatients with early psychosis: a psychopathological path analysis. *Anxiety Stress Coping.* 2020;33(3):342-354. doi:10.1080/10615806.2020.1723007
20. Wong GHY, Tao H, He Z, et al. Delusions of reference, excessive top-down processing, and default mode network in first-episode schizophrenia. The 2nd Biennial Schizophrenia International Research Conference; Apr 10–14, 2010; Florence, Italy. In *Schizophr Res.* 2010;117(2-3):491. doi:10.1016/j.schres.2010.02.931
21. Hu ML, Zong XF, Mann JJ, et al. A review of the functional and anatomical default mode network in schizophrenia. *Neurosci Bull.* 2017;33(1):73-84. doi:10.1007/s12264-016-0090-1
22. Wang H, Zeng LL, Chen Y, Yin H, Tan Q, Hu D. Evidence of a dissociation pattern in default mode subnetwork functional connectivity in schizophrenia. *Sci Rep.* 2015;5:14655. Published Sep 30, 2015. doi:10.1038/srep14655
23. Zhou L, Pu W, Wang J, et al. Inefficient DMN suppression in schizophrenia patients with impaired cognitive function but not patients with preserved cognitive function. *Sci Rep.* 2016;6:21657. Published Feb 17, 2016. doi:10.1038/srep21657
24. Chan KKS, Wong GHY, Hui CLM, et al. Game theoretical approach to theory of mind deficits in schizophrenic patients with delusion(s) of reference. The 2nd Biennial Schizophrenia International Research Conference; Apr 10–14, 2010; Florence, Italy. In *Schizophr Res.* 2010;117(2-3):286. doi:10.1016/j.schres.2010.02.471

25. Tang LS, Wong GH, Chen EY. Increased distractibility to own name in psychotic patients with ideas and delusions of reference. *Cogn Neuropsychiatry*. 2016;21(2):107-115. doi:10.1080/13546805.2015.1137212

26. Kapur S. Psychosis as a state of aberrant salience: a framework linking biology, phenomenology, and pharmacology in schizophrenia. *Am J Psychiatry*. 2003;160(1):13-23. doi:10.1176/appi.ajp.160.1.13

27. Corlett PR, Honey GD, Aitken MR, et al. Frontal responses during learning predict vulnerability to the psychotogenic effects of ketamine: linking cognition, brain activity, and psychosis. *Arch Gen Psychiatry*. 2006;63(6):611-621. doi:10.1001/archpsyc.63.6.611

28. Levy R, Friedman HR, Davachi L, Goldman-Rakic PS. Differential activation of the caudate nucleus in primates performing spatial and nonspatial working memory tasks. *J Neurosci*. 1997;17(10):3870-3882. doi:10.1523/JNEUROSCI.17-10-03870.1997

29. Williams ZM, Eskandar EN. Selective enhancement of associative learning by microstimulation of the anterior caudate. *Nat Neurosci*. 2006;9(4):562-568. doi:10.1038/nn1662

30. Schiffer AM, Schubotz RI. Caudate nucleus signals for breaches of expectation in a movement observation paradigm. *Front Hum Neurosci*. 2011;5:38. Published Apr 8, 2011. doi:10.3389/fnhum.2011.00038

31. Alexander GE, Crutcher MD, DeLong MR. Basal ganglia-thalamocortical circuits: parallel substrates for motor, oculomotor, "prefrontal" and "limbic" functions. *Prog Brain Res*. 1990;85:119-146.

32. Tao H, Wong GH, Zhang H, et al. Grey matter morphological anomalies in the caudate head in first-episode psychosis patients with delusions of reference. *Psychiatry Res*. 2015;233(1):57-63. doi:10.1016/j.pscychresns.2015.04.011

33. Larivière S, Lavigne KM, Woodward TS, Gerretsen P, Graff-Guerrero A, Menon M. Altered functional connectivity in brain networks underlying self-referential processing in delusions of reference in schizophrenia. *Psychiatry Res Neuroimaging*. 2017;263:32-43. doi:10.1016/j.pscychresns.2017.03.005

34. Chan SKW, Liu T, Wong AOY, et al. Self-referential gaze perception of patients with schizophrenia and its relationship with symptomatology and cognitive functions. *Schizophr Res*. 2021;228:288-294. doi:10.1016/j.schres.2020.12.034

35. Wong SMY, Hui CLM, Wong CSM, et al. Induced ideas of reference during social unrest and pandemic in Hong Kong. *Schizophr Res*. 2021;229:46-52. doi:10.1016/j.schres.2021.01.027

13

Mortality and Suicide: Silent Killers in Psychosis

Background

Risk Factors for Suicide and Attempted Suicide

It has been shown that fleeting suicidal ideation, serious and persistent ideation, planning, suicide attempts, and suicide exist on a continuum of risk (1, 2). Sociodemographic factors such as age, gender, and marital and socioeconomic status are correlated with suicidal behaviours (3). A psychiatric diagnosis is considered the most important risk factor, and depression and anxiety have been shown to precede suicidal ideation and behaviour (4, 5, 6). In a systematic review, Hawton et al. (2013) reported that male gender, a family history of psychiatric disorder, previously attempted suicide, more severe depression, hopelessness, and co-occurring disorders such as anxiety and substance and alcohol use were significantly associated with suicide in patients with depression (7). Risk factors for suicide in schizophrenia patients include a previous history of depression, previous suicide attempts, drug misuse, agitation or motor restlessness, fear of mental disintegration, poor treatment adherence, and recent loss. Interestingly, a reduced risk of suicide was associated with hallucinations (8). Negative life events have also been found to be important mediators of suicide risk, particularly with more serious suicidal ideation and behaviours (9, 10). A sexual abuse history was moderately elevated in those who attempted suicide (11).

Theoretical Considerations

Several theoretical frameworks have been proposed to conceptualise interactions between life experiences and the risk of suicide, such as the diathesis-stress paradigm or the interpersonal theory of suicide (12, 13, 14). These hypotheses were developed in recognition of the fact that even the most severe stress does not result in suicidal ideation in all exposed individuals. It is now assumed that a vulnerability predisposes the individual to suicidal behaviour when stress is encountered (12). Chu et al. (2017) found that a sense of thwarted belongingness and perceived burdensomeness was significantly associated with suicidal ideation (14). Stress-related biomarkers have been associated with suicidal behaviour. For example, aberrant stress cortisol levels and inflammatory cytokines are present in suicidal individuals. A recent network meta-analysis of putative stress mediators suggests that a genetic stress susceptibility with downstream cortisol axis dysfunction and anomalous interaction with the inflammatory system may leave the individual physiologically susceptible and unable to cope with environmental stressors (15).

Protective Factors

Research on protective factors has been more limited. Social support has emerged as one of the strongest factors. More recently, internet support has also been identified as a potential protective factor (16). In addition, self-esteem, resilience, access to mental health services, and a positive attitude towards services were inversely related to suicidal ideation (17). Reasons for living, moral objections to suicide, and survival and coping beliefs may also protect against suicidal ideation and attempts (18).

Interactions between risk and protective factors are often complex at individual and population levels and effective suicide prevention efforts require addressing multiple factors simultaneously. Evidence for restricting access to lethal means, with regard to control of analgesics and hot spots for suicide by jumping, has strengthened in recent years. School-based programmes are effective in reducing suicide attempts and suicidal ideation, and so are effective pharmacological and psychological treatments for depression. However, there is insufficient evidence for screening in primary care, general public education, and media guidelines (19).

Suicide and Preventative Efforts in East Asia

Research on suicidal behaviour and suicide prevention has mainly focused on Western populations. It is, however, estimated that at least 60% of all suicides worldwide occur on the Asian continent (20). Population-based studies show that up to 97% of those who had died by suicide had a diagnosable mental disorder and that only 35% to 40% of suicides were associated with a diagnosis of depression. It also appears that demographic and sociocultural risk factors and methods of suicide differ substantially (20, 21). For example, Yip et al. (2000) showed that male suicide rates in China between 1991 and 1996 were lower than that of females and that rural suicide rates for both genders were higher than for their urban counterparts.

170 • *Psychosis and Schizophrenia in Hong Kong*

The elderly and women aged 20–29 years had the highest suicide rates (22). This contrasts with findings in Western cultures where male suicide rates are four times higher than that of women, although women are more likely to attempt suicide (23, 24). When broken down by age, Southeast Asia has the highest male suicide rate in the 15–29 age group compared to the 45–59 age group in European males. Southeast Asian adolescent and young adult females also had high suicide rates, with South Korea having some of the highest female suicide rates in the world (23). Concerted efforts to reduce suicide rates have been lacking in many Asian countries. Existing evidence suggests that restricting access to strong pesticides, provision of crisis counselling services, improving access to mental health services, and promoting responsible media reporting are effective in suicide prevention and should be incorporated into culturally sensitive local programmes (21).

Suicide and Mortality in Hong Kong

The Prevalence of Suicide and Its Clinical and Psychosocial Predictors in Hong Kong

In Hong Kong, changes in the epidemiological profile of suicides over time have been reported (25). Between 1981 and 2001 the suicide rate increased from 9.6 to 15 per 100,000, rising from 2% to 3% of all deaths during that time. Suicide ranked ninth and sixth among the leading causes of death in 1981 and 2001, respectively. Charcoal burning as a method of suicide increased significantly from 6% before 1998 to over 28% in 2001 and likely contributed to the increase in suicide rates. The late 1990s and early 2000s brought the Asian financial crisis and the severe acute respiratory syndrome (SARS) outbreak. Charcoal burning was perceived to be an easy and painless escape and was often romanticised by the media as a dignified way to die leaving the body intact with a rosy glow.

The rise in suicide rates in Hong Kong led to an urgent need to explore risk factors for suicidal ideation, behaviours, suicides and suicide attempts in order to guide effective intervention programmes in the city. To better understand the relationship between socioeconomic and psychological factors and their association with suicidal ideation a population-based survey among adults aged 20 to 59 years was carried out (26). Almost 30% of the Hong Kong population had lifetime suicidal ideation; 6% considered suicide in the previous year; 1.9% had planned suicide; and it was estimated that 1.4% had attempted suicide. Only 0.1% of those who had attempted suicide had come to medical attention. Suicidal ideation and behaviour decreased with age and were more prevalent among women. Breaking up from a stable relationship in the past year, higher distress, hopelessness, and reluctance to seek help from family and friends were associated with past-year suicidal ideation. Reasons for living were found to moderate the effect of perceived stress on suicidal ideation.

In the 1990s, suicide rates of young people in Hong Kong were lower than that of adolescents in the Western world (27, 28). Nonetheless, suicide was the leading cause of death among young people aged 15 to 24. In addition, those young people who had died by suicide had fewer depressive and antisocial symptoms, and were less likely to have a diagnosis of substance use disorders compared to their Western counterparts. However, they were more likely to have psychotic symptoms (29). When data on suicidality was examined among adolescents as part of the Youth Sexuality Survey in the early 2000s, 17.8% of all students reported having considered suicide in the previous year, 5.4% had planned to end their life, 8.4% attempted suicide at least once, and 1.2% of students required medical intervention following at least one attempt (30). Risk factors associated with suicidality were being female, having poor self-rated health, an unhappy or average family life, using inhalants and alcohol, body image difficulties, and early onset of sexual activity.

The Detailed Study of Suicide

Hong Kong experienced a further sharp rise in suicide rates to 18.6 per 100,000 in 2003 (31). To gain a better understanding of the clinical and psychosocial factors associated with suicide in youth and adult populations, we used a case-control psychological autopsy method (32). Of the 150 suicide cases studied, the male-to-female ratio in the sample was 1.78:1, very similar to a previous study (33). The mean age of the sample was 38.7 years, ranging from 16 to 59 years. Almost half died by jumping from a height, one-third by charcoal burning, 12.7% by hanging, and almost 10% used multiple means to kill themselves. The majority of cases died at home, almost half left at least one suicide note, and around 50% implicitly or explicitly expressed a suicide plan. 45% of the cases died within a month of their relatives becoming aware of their suicidal thoughts.

Those who had died by suicide were more likely to have never married, have lower educational attainment, live alone, be unemployed, receive less income, have unmanageable debts, and have experienced negative expressed emotions and physical abuse at home. By contrast, a wide social network and accessible support were more prevalent in the control group. For male suicides, the impact of unemployment was apparent across different age groups and most prominent in 20 to 24-year-olds. The suicide cases had also experienced more intense negative life stressors in their relationships, work/school, and physical health in the year prior to their death, particularly more intense relationship problems in the final month. Psychiatric illness was also more frequent in the suicide group, with mood disorders being the most commonly diagnosed illnesses. Seventeen (31.5%) women and 19 (19.8%) men who had died by suicide, but none in the control group, had suffered a psychotic disorder. Of those who had psychiatric illnesses, almost 30% had comorbid diagnoses, whereas there were only two cases in the control group. However, less than half of the diagnosable suicide cases had ever been in contact with psychiatric services and only 48.7% had ever sought emotional treatment. The suicide and control groups also differed significantly in other clinical and psychological features. The deceased were more likely to have attempted suicide before, to have received emotional and psychiatric treatment, and to have a chronic physical health problem compared to the control subjects. Those who had died by suicide were also more likely to have experienced an impulsive state in the last week before death and have compulsive buying habits. Other risk factors independently associated with suicide included never having married and living alone, and it appears that the presence of non-disease related social risk factors such as unemployment and unmanageable debt, a past suicide attempt, and current major depressive disorder conveyed the highest risk of suicide (34, 35, 36). Conversely, in a sample of unemployed individuals, those who had died by suicide were more likely to be male, to have a psychiatric disorder, to have attempted suicide previously, and to be less adept at social problem-solving (37). By contrast, those who had acquired social problem-solving skills and led a healthy lifestyle were half as likely to be at risk of suicide (32).

There had been concerns among psychiatrists that with the reduction of psychiatric beds during the 2000s, acutely suicidal patients may not receive adequate care and suicides would rise further as a result. However, an association between suicide and the number of psychiatric beds available was not observed, probably due to an accompanying improved provision of community mental healthcare (36).

Differential Psychiatric and Psychosocial Correlates in Suicide Sub-types

Circumstances of death to define sub-types of those who had died by suicide were also explored and psychiatric and psychosocial correlates of such clusters were investigated (38). Two sub-groups were identified; the first group was associated with suicide by charcoal burning, no psychiatric illness, indebtedness, better problem-solving ability, chronic work or school stress, and higher suicide intent. The second group was more likely to have jumped from a height, to have been diagnosed with a psychotic disorder, to have received psychiatric treatment, to have suffered acute stress, and to have lower suicide intent. Charcoal burning emerged as a suicide method in Hong Kong at the end of the twentieth century and soon became the second most common suicide method after jumping from a height for people under 65 years. Further analysis of persons dying by carbon monoxide poisoning showed that the method was more prevalent in the 31–45 age group, in those who were married or divorced and had unmanageable debts (39, 40). Schizophrenia spectrum disorders were less commonly found in those who died by charcoal burning (40).

Suicide in Psychotic Disorders

It has been estimated that the lifetime risk of suicide in schizophrenia is around 5% and that 25% to 50% of patients attempt suicide in their lifetime (41, 42, 43). A meta-analysis of 96 studies identified several continuous and categorical risk factors for suicidal ideation, suicide attempts, and suicide in this population. Depressive symptoms, the general score on the Positive and Negative Syndrome Scale (PANSS), and the number of hospitalisations were significantly higher in patients with suicidal ideation (44). Those who attempted suicide were more likely to be white, have a history of alcohol, tobacco or substance use, a family history of psychiatric illness or suicide, physical comorbidity, and a history of depression or current depressive symptoms. Male gender, history of attempted suicide, younger age, higher IQ, poor adherence to treatment, and hopelessness were factors more consistently associated with suicide (44).

First-episode psychosis (FEP) is also correlated with a higher risk of suicidal behaviour even in the longer term, probably mediated via the presence of depressive symptoms (45). Those deemed at high risk of psychosis have also been shown to have a high prevalence of recent suicidal ideation, lifetime self-harm, and lifetime suicide attempts. Risk factors associated with self-harm and attempted suicide were comorbid psychiatric difficulties, mood variability, and a family history of psychiatric problems (46).

Suicide in Psychosis and Its Predictors in Hong Kong

In Hong Kong, suicide rates and their predictors in young people with first-episode psychosis during their initial three years of treatment were examined. Around 10% to 25% of patients had attempted suicide prior to treatment, and over 40% reported suicidal ideation, with just over 1% ending in suicide (47, 48, 49). More than half of the suicidal behaviours occurred in the first year of follow-up. Jumping from a height was the most common suicide method. A history of substance use, a pretreatment suicide attempt, and poorer baseline social functioning were identified as independent predictors of suicidal behaviours (47, 48). Those with suicidal ideation were more likely to feel hopeless, to have lower levels of internal control, to have a greater belief in external locus of control, to make more suicide attempts, to have better affect reactivity, and to have a greater depressive symptom severity when compared to psychosis patients without suicidal thoughts. Suicidal ideation was associated with higher levels of insight, impulsivity, tendencies to be more pessimistic and fearful of social disapproval, and less use of survival and coping beliefs as reasons for living (49, 50).

Mortality Other Than Suicide

We followed up a cohort of FEP patients for 13 years (51). The mean age of onset was around 30.2 years. At follow-up, the average age was 45 years. Out of 153 patients, 14 (9.2%) had died during the follow-up period and only half were related to suicide or suspected suicide. The remaining deaths were due to a variety of physical conditions. This observation corroborates international studies that suggest that psychosis patients have a significant reduction in life expectancy. The actual physical illnesses leading to death were diverse. This finding indicates that psychosis patients are either prone to a range of physical illnesses or are less likely to receive timely help for physical ill health or both. In psychosis, diverse genetic factors implicated in the illness are not only confined to the brain but, for example, affect immune and inflammatory systems. This suggests that we should not rule out a more systemic involvement of other organ systems in psychosis. While there has been increasing awareness of metabolic conditions related to long-term antipsychotic treatments, there may still be a failure to detect and manage other physical illnesses once they emerge. There may be a reduced ability of patients to be aware of physical symptoms and seek help. There is also a possibility that clinicians are less sensitive to physical complaints in a patient with a psychotic disorder. Studies have revealed that primary care physicians are less likely to order investigations or make specialist referrals for a patient with a mental health diagnosis (52). Clinician training to deploy appropriate indices of suspicion for psychotic patients with physical symptoms is thus required.

The Impact of Early Intervention on Suicide

With the introduction of the Early Assessment Service for Young People (EASY), we hoped to improve symptomatic outcomes for youth with FEP with a focus on alleviating psychotic symptoms, providing comprehensive psychoeducation to the general public and systematically researching its effectiveness.

We followed patients who had completed treatment at the EASY service for 12 years to examine suicide rates and risk factors for early and late suicide, using a historical control study design (53). Suicide rates were 7.5% in the standard care group and significantly lower at 4.4% in the early intervention (EI) group. Patients in the EI group had significantly better survival, with the maximum effect observed in the first three years. The number of suicide attempts was a predictor of early suicide, while a different set of predictors was identified for later suicides: premorbid occupational impairment, number of relapses, and poor adherence during the initial three years.

Reflections: The Role of Early Intervention Programmes in Suicide Prevention and Reducing Mortality

Setting up effective systems for screening and intervention is one of the most challenging endeavours in the field of suicide prevention research. Focusing on the early psychosis population offers an opportunity to engage a group of patients with relatively high suicide risk. Psychotic disorders carry a lifetime suicide mortality of 5% to 10%, and most suicides occur within the first few years following the onset of the illness. It is therefore strategically important to strengthen the components of early psychosis programmes that have the potential to reduce suicide. One of the challenges in such an initiative is to detect suicidal tendencies early enough to implement preventative interventions. It is known that for patients who are admitted to hospital during their first episode, the period after discharge is of particularly high risk. Therefore, for inpatients, it is important to identify those who might be at risk and intervene before they are discharged. Empathic understanding of patients' experiences and insight into clinical risk factors as well as a comprehensive psychosocial formulation are important processes in the evaluation of risk.

Our research efforts have highlighted a multitude of risk factors for suicide or suicidal behaviours and have shown that EI contributed to effective suicide prevention. Within the EASY service, particular attention has been paid to comprehensive clinical and actuarial risk assessment. There has also been increasing awareness of the potentially devastating effects of the nature of psychotic illnesses. Casework efforts for patients and their relatives have focused on fostering an understanding of the illness, a realistic appreciation of outcomes, the importance of treatment adherence, maintaining a positive outlook, and taking a proactive approach to managing the condition.

Non-suicide-related mortality in psychosis is an area of increasing concern. Physical illness in psychosis patients may be due to shared vulnerability, the impact of psychosis on lifestyle, as well as side effects of treatments for psychosis. Presentation of physical symptoms may be complicated by difficulties in detection by patients, as well as difficulties in communication. Clinicians involved in the care of psychosis patients should also have an appropriate index of suspicion for emerging physical conditions and support individuals to access physical healthcare in a timely fashion.

References

1. Burless C, De Leo D. Methodological issues in community surveys of suicide ideators and attempters. *Crisis*. 2001;22(3):109-124. doi:10.1027//0227-5910.22.3.109
2. Beautrais AL. Suicides and serious suicide attempts: two populations or one? *Psychol Med*. 2001;31(5):837-845. doi:10.1017/s0033291701003889

3. Kjøller M, Helweg-Larsen M. Suicidal ideation and suicide attempts among adult Danes. *Scand J Public Health*. 2000;28(1):54-61. doi:10.1177/140349480002800110

4. Jacobs DG, Brewer M, Klein-Benheim M. Suicide assessment: an overview and recommended protocol. In: Jacobs DG, ed. *The Harvard Medical School Guide to Suicide Assessment and Intervention*. Jossey-Bass; 1999:3-39.

5. Goldney RD, Wilson D, Dal Grande E, Fisher LJ, McFarlane AC. Suicidal ideation in a random community sample: attributable risk due to depression and psychosocial and traumatic events. *Aust N Z J Psychiatry*. 2000;34(1):98-106. doi:10.1046/j.1440-1614.2000.00646.x

6. Sareen J, Cox BJ, Afifi TO, et al. Anxiety disorders and risk for suicidal ideation and suicide attempts: a population-based longitudinal study of adults. *Arch Gen Psychiatry*. 2005;62(11):1249-1257. doi:10.1001/archpsyc.62.11.1249

7. Hawton K, Casañas I Comabella C, Haw C, Saunders K. Risk factors for suicide in individuals with depression: a systematic review. *J Affect Disord*. 2013;147(1-3):17-28. doi:10.1016/j.jad.2013.01.004

8. Hawton K, Sutton L, Haw C, Sinclair J, Deeks JJ. Schizophrenia and suicide: systematic review of risk factors. *Br J Psychiatry*. 2005;187:9-20. doi:10.1192/bjp.187.1.9

9. Liu RT, Miller I. Life events and suicidal ideation and behavior: a systematic review. *Clin Psychol Rev*. 2014;34(3):181-192. doi:10.1016/j.cpr.2014.01.006

10. Howarth EJ, O'Connor DB, Panagioti M, Hodkinson A, Wilding S, Johnson J. Are stressful life events prospectively associated with increased suicidal ideation and behaviour? A systematic review and meta-analysis. *J Affect Disord*. 2020;266:731-742. doi:10.1016/j.jad.2020.01.171

11. May AM, Klonsky ED. What distinguishes suicide attempters from suicide ideators? A meta-analysis of potential factors. *Clinical Psychology: Science and Practice*. 2016;23(1): 5-20. doi:10.1037/h0101735

12. van Heeringen K. Stress–Diathesis Model of Suicidal Behavior. In: Dwivedi Y, ed. *The Neurobiological Basis of Suicide*. CRC Press/Taylor & Francis; 2012. PMID: 23035289

13. Schotte DE, Clum GA. Problem-solving skills in suicidal psychiatric patients. *J Consult Clin Psychol*. 1987;55(1):49-54. doi:10.1037//0022-006x.55.1.49

14. Chu C, Buchman-Schmitt JM, Stanley IH, et al. The interpersonal theory of suicide: A systematic review and meta-analysis of a decade of cross-national research. *Psychol Bull*. 2017;143(12):1313-1345. doi:10.1037/bul0000123

15. Thomas N, Armstrong CW, Hudaib AR, Kulkarni J, Gurvich C. A network meta-analysis of stress mediators in suicide behaviour. *Front Neuroendocrinol*. 2021;63:100946. doi:10.1016/j.yfrne.2021.100946

16. McClatchey K, Murray J, Chouliara Z, Rowat A. Protective factors of suicide and suicidal behavior relevant to emergency healthcare settings: a systematic review and narrative synthesis of post-2007 reviews. *Arch Suicide Res*. 2019;23(3):411-427. doi:10.1080/13811118.2018.1480983

17. Holman MS, Williams MN. Suicide risk and protective factors: a network approach. *Arch Suicide Res*. 2022;26(1):137-154. doi:10.1080/13811118.2020.1774454

18. Bakhiyi CL, Calati R, Guillaume S, Courtet P. Do reasons for living protect against suicidal thoughts and behaviors? A systematic review of the literature. *J Psychiatr Res*. 2016;77:92-108. doi:10.1016/j.jpsychires.2016.02.019

19. Zalsman G, Hawton K, Wasserman D, et al. Suicide prevention strategies revisited: 10-year systematic review. *Lancet Psychiatry.* 2016;3(7):646-659. doi:10.1016/S2215-0366(16)30030-X

20. Vijayakumar L. Suicide and mental disorders in Asia. *Int Rev Psychiatry.* 2005;17(2):109-114. doi:10.1080/09540260500074735

21. Wei KC, Chua HC. Suicide in Asia. *Int Rev Psychiatry.* 2008;20(5):434-440. doi:10.1080/09540260802397446

22. Yip PS, Callanan C, Yuen HP. Urban/rural and gender differentials in suicide rates: east and west. *J Affect Disord.* 2000;57(1-3):99-106. doi:10.1016/s0165-0327(99)00058-0

23. Värnik P. Suicide in the world. *Int J Environ Res Public Health.* 2012;9(3):760-771. doi:10.3390/ijerph9030760

24. Weissman MM, Bland RC, Canino GJ, et al. Prevalence of suicide ideation and suicide attempts in nine countries. *Psychol Med.* 1999;29(1):9-17. doi:10.1017/s0033291798007867

25. Yip PS, Law CK, Law YW. Suicide in Hong Kong: epidemiological profile and burden analysis, 1981 to 2001. *Hong Kong Med J.* 2003;9(6):419-426.

26. Liu KY, Chen EY, Chan CL, et al. Socio-economic and psychological correlates of suicidality among Hong Kong working-age adults: results from a population-based survey. *Psychol Med.* 2006;36(12):1759-1767. doi:10.1017/S0033291706009032

27. Yip PS. Suicides in Hong Kong, Taiwan and Beijing. *Br J Psychiatry.* 1996;169(4):495-500. doi:10.1192/bjp.169.4.495

28. Yip PS. Suicides in Hong Kong, 1981-1994. *Soc Psychiatry Psychiatr Epidemiol.* 1997;32(5):243-250. doi:10.1007/BF00789036

29. Yip PSF, Ho TP, Hung SF, et al. *Youth Suicides in Hong Kong.* Befrienders International; 1998.

30. Yip PS, Liu KY, Lam TH, Stewart SM, Chen E, Fan S. Suicidality among high school students in Hong Kong, SAR. *Suicide Life Threat Behav.* 2004;34(3):284-297. doi:10.1521/suli.34.3.284.42772

31. C&SD. Hong Kong in Figures. Census and Statistics Department: Hong Kong SAR. www.info.gov.hk/censtatd/eng/hkstat/index.html. Published 2005. Accessed Feb 23, 2023.

32. Chen EY, Chan WS, Wong PW, et al. Suicide in Hong Kong: a case-control psychological autopsy study. *Psychol Med.* 2006;36(6):815-825. doi:10.1017/S0033291706007240

33. Liu KY, Chen EY, Cheung AS, Yip PS. Psychiatric history modifies the gender ratio of suicide: an East and West comparison. *Soc Psychiatry Psychiatr Epidemiol.* 2009;44(2):130-134. doi:10.1007/s00127-008-0413-2

34. Wong PW, Chan WS, Chen EY, Chan SS, Law YW, Yip PS. Suicide among adults aged 30-49: a psychological autopsy study in Hong Kong. *BMC Public Health.* 2008;8:147. Published May 1, 2008. doi:10.1186/1471-2458-8-147

35. Chan SS, Chiu HF, Chen EY, et al. Population-attributable risk of suicide conferred by axis I psychiatric diagnoses in a Hong Kong Chinese population. *Psychiatr Serv.* 2009;60(8):1135-1138. doi:10.1176/ps.2009.60.8.1135

36. Lee EHM, Hui CLM, Chan PY, Chang WC, Chan SKW, Chen EYH. Suicide rates, psychiatric hospital bed numbers, and unemployment rates from 1999 to 2015:

a population-based study in Hong Kong. *Am J Psychiatry.* 2018;175(3):285-286. doi:10.1176/appi.ajp.2017.17070766

37. Chan WS, Yip PS, Wong PW, Chen EY. Suicide and unemployment: what are the missing links? *Arch Suicide Res.* 2007;11(4):327-335. doi:10.1080/13811110701541905

38. Chen EY, Chan WS, Chan SS, et al. A cluster analysis of the circumstances of death in suicides in Hong Kong. *Suicide Life Threat Behav.* 2007;37(5):576-584. doi:10.1521/suli.2007.37.5.576

39. Chan KP, Yip PS, Au J, Lee DT. Charcoal-burning suicide in post-transition Hong Kong. *Br J Psychiatry.* 2005;186:67-73. doi:10.1192/bjp.186.1.67

40. Chan SS, Chiu HF, Chen EY, et al. What does psychological autopsy study tell us about charcoal burning suicide – a new and contagious method in Asia? *Suicide Life Threat Behav.* 2009;39(6):633-638. doi:10.1521/suli.2009.39.6.633

41. Palmer BA, Pankratz VS, Bostwick JM. The lifetime risk of suicide in schizophrenia: a reexamination. *Arch Gen Psychiatry.* 2005;62(3):247-253. doi:10.1001/archpsyc.62.3.247

42. Hor K, Taylor M. Suicide and schizophrenia: a systematic review of rates and risk factors. *J Psychopharmacol.* 2010;24(4 Suppl):81-90. doi:10.1177/1359786810385490

43. Meltzer HY. Treatment of suicidality in schizophrenia. *Ann N Y Acad Sci.* 2001;932:44-60. doi:10.1111/j.1749-6632.2001.tb05797.x

44. Cassidy RM, Yang F, Kapczinski F, Passos IC. Risk factors for suicidality in patients with schizophrenia: a systematic review, meta-analysis, and meta-regression of 96 studies. *Schizophr Bull.* 2018;44(4):787-797. doi:10.1093/schbul/sbx131

45. McGinty J, Sayeed Haque M, Upthegrove R. Depression during first episode psychosis and subsequent suicide risk: A systematic review and meta-analysis of longitudinal studies. *Schizophr Res.* 2018;195:58-66. doi:10.1016/j.schres.2017.09.040

46. Taylor PJ, Hutton P, Wood L. Are people at risk of psychosis also at risk of suicide and self-harm? A systematic review and meta-analysis. *Psychol Med.* 2015;45(5):911-926. doi:10.1017/S0033291714002074

47. Chen SM, Chang WC, Hui CLM, Chan KW, Lee HME, Chen EYH. Prediction of suicidal behaviours in young people presenting with first-episode psychosis in Hong Kong: a 3-year follow up study. The 4th Biennial Schizophrenia International Research Conference, Florence, Italy, Apr 5–9, 2014. In *Schizophr Res.* 2014;153(Suppl. 1):S190, poster no. M3. doi:10.1016/S0920-9964(14)70553-5

48. Chang WC, Chen ES, Hui CL, Chan SK, Lee EH, Chen EY. Prevalence and risk factors for suicidal behavior in young people presenting with first-episode psychosis in Hong Kong: a 3-year follow-up study. *Soc Psychiatry Psychiatr Epidemiol.* 2015;50(2):219-226. doi:10.1007/s00127-014-0946-5

49. Chang WC, Chen ES, Hui CL, Chan SK, Lee EH, Chen EY. The relationships of suicidal ideation with symptoms, neurocognitive function, and psychological factors in patients with first-episode psychosis. *Schizophr Res.* 2014;157(1-3):12-18. doi:10.1016/j.schres.2014.06.009

50. Heidi C, Chen EY, Chan CK, et al. A comparison of psychological profiles between suicide ideators and non-ideators among psychiatric patients: a preliminary report. The 9th International Congress on Schizophrenia Research, Colorado Springs,

CO., Mar 29–Apr 2, 2003. In *Schizophr Res.* 2003;60(Suppl 1):337. doi:10.1016/S0920-9964(03)80327-4

51. Tang JY, Chang WC, Hui CL, et al. Prospective relationship between duration of untreated psychosis and 13-year clinical outcome: a first-episode psychosis study. *Schizophr Res.* 2014;153(1-3):1-8. doi:10.1016/j.schres.2014.01.022

52. Roberts L, Roalfe A, Wilson S, Lester H. Physical health care of patients with schizophrenia in primary care: a comparative study. *Fam Pract.* 2007;24(1):34-40. doi:10.1093/fampra/cml054

53. Chan SKW, Chan SWY, Pang HH, et al. Association of an early intervention service for psychosis with suicide rate among patients with first-episode schizophrenia-spectrum disorders. *JAMA Psychiatry.* 2018;75(5):458-464. doi:10.1001/jamapsychiatry.2018.0185

PART IV

NEUROCOGNITIVE DYSFUNCTIONS

14

Cognitive Dysfunctions: The Hidden Impediments of Psychosis

Background

Historical Context

Up to 80% of persons with schizophrenia experience cognitive dysfunction that significantly affects their clinical and functional outcomes (1). Emil Kraepelin was the first to describe significant cognitive decline in what he called 'dementia praecox' in his psychiatric textbook *Psychiatrie. Ein Lehrbuch für Studierende und Ärzte*, published in 1899 (2). He described the illness as akin to having 'an orchestra without a conductor' (3). Dementia praecox was characterised by a progressive deterioration of intellectual functioning, particularly in the domains of attention, memory, and goal-directed behaviour (2). In 1908, Eugen Bleuler introduced the term 'the schizophrenias' to replace dementia praecox during a lecture at a meeting of the German Psychiatric Association in Berlin (4). Bleuler did not consider cognitive decline to be inevitable but regarded another aspect of cognition to be a central feature of psychotic disorders, namely 'the splitting of the different psychic functions' (5). The prominence of cognitive dysfunction in psychosis diminished as the name 'dementia praecox' was replaced by 'the schizophrenias' (6, 7).

The interest in cognitive dysfunctions was revisited when the research team around Professors Tim Crow, Eve Johnstone, Chris Frith, and David Owens recognised that chronic patients at Northwick Park Hospital presented with significant cognitive difficulties such as being unable to correctly identify even their own age despite being fully orientated (8, 9). This discovery led to intensified efforts to study cognition in schizophrenia with almost 30,000 scientific articles having been published on the topic over the last 30 years.

184 • *Psychosis and Schizophrenia in Hong Kong*

Research Paradigms

With the identification of an increasing range of cognitive impairments, research paradigms have shifted from the initial search for a single, defining, schizophrenia-specific cognitive dysfunction, to describing a profile of impairments across different brain systems, as well as to organising types of dysfunctions identified in order to map them onto genes. We have pointed out that research in identifying specific cognitive features of psychosis may have been hindered by approaching the illness narrowly from a neuropsychological perspective, assuming that any cognitive dysfunction thus identified has to be a deficit, i.e., a reduction of a normal cognitive function. This approach might have inadvertently limited efforts to account for the complex inter-relationships between cognition and aberrant symptoms such as auditory hallucinations or delusions (10). In addition, despite more than a decade of research, cognitive 'endophenotypes' have not yet proven to be a fruitful concept to delineate specific clinical or cognitive sub-categories that tidily map onto genes. However, given the fact that approximately one-third of the human genome encodes brain-related information, it is likely that even very circumscribed cognitive capacities are driven by multiple genes. In addition, the susceptibility to psychosis appears to be determined by a multitude of genetic variants, ranging from single nucleotide polymorphisms to copy number variants with pleiotropic effects on diagnosis and personality traits (11, 12, 13, 14, 15, 16, 17). This likely further impedes the identification of useful clinical and cognitive 'endophenotypes'.

Another important limitation was that human cognition has been studied as an input–output system based on the computational processing of neutral contents (10). Only more recently efforts have been made to investigate emotionally and meaning-laden content to reflect the social nature of cognition in everyday life. Evolutionary psychology theories could be employed in this context to further our understanding of selection pressures for socially relevant cognitions (10).

The Emergence of Cognitive Dysfunction in Psychosis

Despite the ongoing challenges in characterising the cognitive profiles of people with psychotic illnesses, important information has been obtained, for example in the timing of the emergence of cognitive dysfunctions. It has been shown that deficits are present in almost all cognitive domains (18). It appears that general cognition, as well as specific sub-domains such as attention, memory, reasoning, executive functions, and processing speed, are impaired prior to the onset of a psychotic disorder. Individuals who develop psychosis several years later already perform less well academically in their secondary education compared to their peers (19, 20, 21). Those at clinically high risk of psychosis have poorer executive functioning, attention, general intelligence level, processing speed, verbal fluency, and visual, verbal and working memory, but seem less impaired than subjects with first-episode psychosis (FEP) (22). Also, Catalan et al. (2021) reported that high-risk individuals who went on to develop a psychotic illness were more cognitively impaired than those who did not, suggesting that poorer neurocognitive function may predict a transition to psychosis (18, 22). Another study suggests that cognitive impairments progress from the prodromal period to FEP (23).

Aetiology and Course of Cognitive Impairments

There have been two main hypotheses regarding the aetiology and progression of cognitive deficits in psychosis. The neurodevelopmental position suggests that these deficits arise during early brain development and remain stable over the course of the illness (24). The neurodegenerative hypothesis considers ongoing mechanisms that contribute to a further decline in cognitive functioning after illness onset (25). Overall, evidence increasingly suggests that a progressive decline in IQ, verbal knowledge, and memory of variable severity can occur after onset (26, 27, 28). However, longer-term studies have been beset by a number of difficulties including limited duration of follow-up, the presence of age-related changes, the use of control groups, and other patient-related confounding factors (18). Also, it remains unclear to what extent cognitive difficulties arise as a result of psychosis *per se* or co-occurring physical ill health such as metabolic syndrome, smoking, substance use, or other lifestyle factors (18).

There has been a longstanding debate about whether antipsychotic medication may negatively impact cognitive ability in FEP. Fatouros-Bergman et al. (2014) showed in their meta-analysis that drug-naïve FEP patients had similar cognitive deficits compared to those treated with an antipsychotic (29). However, individual antipsychotic medications may be associated with cognitive dysfunction. Medications that produce extrapyramidal side effects likely impact all cognitive functions that require speed and flexibility, those with anticholinergic side effects probably affect memory-related functions, at least in the short term. The potential long-term cognitive effects of antipsychotic treatment are less clear.

Progressive changes in brain structure seem to occur in the course of a psychotic disorder. In their meta-analysis, Haijma et al. (2013) showed that brain grey matter volume is reduced at illness onset and continues to decrease as the illness progresses (30). A longer duration of illness and a greater number of hospital admissions also appear to be associated with cortical volume changes (18).

Neurocomputational Frameworks as a Means to Integrate Complex Data

More recent neurocomputational frameworks have conceptualised schizophrenia as a cognitive brain disorder. Computational modelling has been used to help understand data from basic neurobiology, functional imaging studies, phenomenology, and cognitive neurosciences. In this framework, psychosis is viewed to result from maladaptive inferences due to reduced precision in the encoding of prior beliefs relative to incoming sensory data. Neurochemically, in addition to the classic dopamine hypothesis, several neurotransmitters are thought to mediate aberrant encoding in psychosis, particularly involving glutaminergic pathways, N-methyl-D-aspartate (NMDA) receptors and GABAergic neurons (31, 32). Whether computational frameworks will allow for greater integration of preclinical and clinical data and can account for the clinical heterogeneity of psychosis remains to be seen (31).

Social Cognition in Psychosis

The importance of social cognition in psychosis has been increasingly recognised. Social cognition refers to the perception and interpretation of socially relevant information, understanding the intentions and motivations of others, as well as recognising and managing one's own emotional states. They are thought to be essential in successfully navigating social interactions, and initiating and maintaining adaptive social behaviours (33, 34). Some studies have shown that social cognition may mediate the effects of neurocognition on outcomes (35, 36). Impairments in several domains have been identified in psychosis, namely social perception, emotion processing, theory of mind, and attributional bias (37). These deficits are present in at-risk states and in FEP, and seem to remain stable over the course of the illness (38, 39, 40). People with schizophrenia across the world appear to show a similar range and severity of difficulties in all social cognitive domains (34).

Studies on Cognitive Functioning in Hong Kong

The investigation of cognitive dysfunction in Hong Kong started with explorations of potential associations between symptoms and cognition. In the following section we will present the results of a selection of studies from a larger body of work our team has undertaken to illustrate different aspects of cognitive impairments encountered in psychosis utilising a variety of innovative approaches.

Symptomatology and Cognitive Dysfunction

We investigated the relationship between cognitive dysfunction and negative symptoms after establishing the reliability and validity of the High Royds Evaluation of Negativity Scale, a simple and efficient measure to assess negative symptoms in schizophrenia. We then showed that negative symptoms were significantly correlated with deficits in general verbal ability and more specifically with semantic fluency (41). We reported the slow and partial recovery of cognitive performance following FEP in non-semantic cognitive domains (42).

Our team observed, using neurological soft signs as a measure of neurocognitive function, that patients with schizophrenia showed progressive deterioration in neurological soft signs such as motor coordination, sensory integration, and disinhibition over the course of three years despite stability in symptom profile and medication (43). This was one of the first longitudinal studies that demonstrated a decline in neurocognitive function.

Executive Dysfunction

Executive dysfunction has been shown to be associated with clinical outcomes early in the course of psychosis. It may be progressive as demonstrated by the fact that individuals with FEP have fewer circumscribed reinforcement learning deficits compared to chronic patients and greater deficits in random number generation (44, 45, 46, 47, 48). The exact underlying neurobiological mechanisms pertaining to executive dysfunction require further investigation, nevertheless, it is clear that in psychosis localised and circumscribed brain injury is unlikely (49). Moreover, specific executive functioning impairments in the domain of sustained attention were observed in medication-naïve young people with first-episode schizophrenia when compared to matched healthy controls. These deficits were correlated with negative but not positive symptoms (50, 51).

Insight may be affected by executive dysfunction in adult FEP patients, and improved cognitive flexibility appears to facilitate better insight during the early course of psychosis. However, other factors, such as the presence of psychotic symptoms, likely play a greater role in whether patients are aware of being ill and understand the associated consequences and the need to take medication (52, 53).

To gain a more detailed understanding of the effects of executive dysfunction on daily life, we used a test capturing day-to-day executive difficulties patients experience in problem-solving (54). The Modified Six Elements Test (MSET) requires patients to structure each given task prior to completion and has been shown to be more sensitive than other tests to elicit frontal lobe dysfunction in brain injury and schizophrenia (50, 55, 56). Schizophrenia patients had impairments in executive functioning at illness onset compared to matched healthy controls. The cognitive difficulties persisted following clinical stabilisation over the course of three years. However, scores on more conventional executive function tests such as the modified Wisconsin Card Sorting Test (WCST) improved. In addition, it could be shown that better executive functioning predicted improved negative and positive symptoms after three years. The same cohort of patients also completed another measure of executive functioning, namely the Hayling Sentence Completion Test (HSCT). At illness onset, patients had deficits in semantic inhibition, an important capacity in efficient verbal communication and interpersonal functioning. In contrast to executive functioning, semantic inhibition gradually improved over the course of three years but did not predict changes in positive or negative symptoms (57).

The Complexities of Assessing Cognitive Functioning

A variety of neurocognitive tests have been developed over the years to assess specific cognitive functions. However, one has to bear in mind that test batteries were based on a variety of theoretical models such as Luria's model of mental processing or the supervisory attentional system to conceptualise executive dysfunction. Most tests correlate poorly with real-life functioning and fail to take into account the psychosocial realities of those affected by cognitive impairments (58). Also, test results usually reflect a composite of different cognitive domains despite this not necessarily being explicated by test batteries (47, 49, 59). For example, the Tower of Hanoi task, a simple mathematical puzzle to assess planning and problem-solving abilities, requires intact visual and auditory working memory as well as reasoning skills (59). These complex interactions between various cognitive domains thus make it necessary to employ a number of different cognitive test batteries to be able to differentiate the contribution of each sub-domain, and their effect on each other as well as on symptomatology and function. A similar difficulty has been encountered in elucidating theory of mind (ToM) deficits in psychosis due to the fact that conventional ToM tasks focus on third-person perspectives and fail to capture the demands placed upon individuals in their daily lives. We believe that using game theoretical paradigms may avoid these pitfalls as they require the direct involvement of the first person and situate the participant's interpersonal reasoning within an interactive context (60).

It is likely that performance in cognitive function tests, such as the WCST, requires the integrity of multiple sub-components of more basic modules such as attention, working memory, and set-shifting. Deficits in any of the sub-modules will compromise the overall test results. One approach is to focus on the more basic sub-modules, i.e., tasks that are simpler and do not have many components. In this direction, we have studied early visual processing with the attentional blink paradigm. This refers to the phenomenon that if a visual stimulus is presented in a rapid sequence, the registration of an earlier signal will inhibit the processing of signals that immediately follow within a time window, so that the subject is unaware of the later signals. This is called the attentional blink window. We demonstrated that the attentional blink window is increased in schizophrenia. This finding is noteworthy in the context of other findings that reported a weakening of attentional control in schizophrenia (61, 62).

Self-Monitoring and the Experience of Passivity Phenomena

Another approach to cognitive studies is to target functions that may provide an account of symptoms in psychosis. Self-monitoring of motor action is an important process that may be relevant to the sense of agency, which in turn might be associated with the psychotic experience of passivity (63). We reported on the use of a simple and novel motor memory paradigm to elicit internal predictive representations in patients with and without passivity experiences and hallucinations (64). Healthy participants and patients without passivity experiences replicated more accurately in the active compared with the passive conditions. Individuals with passivity experiences were less precise in the voluntary active condition compared with the passive tactile condition. The results suggest that patients with passivity experiences have deficits in self-monitoring systems independently of their cognitive abilities or ability to perform self-monitoring tasks.

Deficits in Verbal Working Memory

We also investigated specific aspects of verbal working memory after deficits had been shown in the encoding and semantic organisation of persons with schizophrenia. An auditory serial recall task containing word lists with low semantic coherence and either syntactically familiar or unfamiliar structure was employed to elicit patients' ability to process syntactic information compared to matched healthy controls. Individuals with schizophrenia performed significantly worse on the test compared to controls and appeared to have particular difficulty in utilising syntactic information to facilitate recall. We postulated that this might be based on difficulties processing syntactic information or using syntactic cues to aid recall (65). In contrast, prose memory appears to be better preserved when patients are presented with syntactically and semantically congruent information (66).

Reflections on Cognitive Deficits in Psychosis

What emerges from the discussion of a selection of studies carried out in Hong Kong, as well as other studies in the field, is that in schizophrenia, cognitive dysfunction occurs at both a global level and at the level of more specific cognitive deficits. These deficits occur along differing trajectories and without consistent association with psychotic symptoms.

Cognitive dysfunction in psychosis gives us important information about the condition. It is a clear signal that psychosis cannot be explained by a simple psychodynamic account without reference to concurrent changes in brain systems. Instead, the existence of widespread cognitive dysfunction indicates that brain systems involved in these functions are implicated in psychosis. This insight has led to intensive research efforts to try to grasp the core cognitive abnormality in schizophrenia, in the hope that this will point towards a single or a small number of key abnormal brain mechanisms. This endeavour has generated important knowledge about psychotic disorders. In particular, it could be shown that not only general cognition is disrupted, but also that a number of distinct and specific functions are more selectively affected in psychosis. Importantly, the data indicates that psychotic disorders can neither be traced to a single location in the brain, nor to a single brain system. Rather, evidence points towards the existence of both generic and specific neurocognitive processes suggesting multiple levels of pathogenesis being implicated in psychotic disorders. These observations contributed to the recently developed polygenic and multifactorial pathogenesis model of psychosis.

Exploring individual cognitive functioning often requires costly assessment time and expertise and is therefore not routinely available in most clinical settings. Nevertheless, they constitute an essential component of psychotic disorders and are relevant not only to our understanding of the condition but also have significant clinical implications. While not all patients are aware of their cognitive deficits, some patients do report subjective changes in their cognitive abilities. Subjective awareness of cognitive dysfunction does not always align perfectly with objective measures. For example, patients with impaired insight may be unaware of their cognitive impairments, while those with depressed mood may overestimate their cognitive difficulties (67). Despite these caveats, cognitive dysfunction is extremely relevant to the assessment and management of psychosis.

We cannot ignore the fact that patients frequently notice changes in their cognitive abilities such as a slowing in their processing speed, long after their psychotic symptoms have resolved. If clinicians fail to facilitate conversations about these changes, and in the absence of explicit information, patients often, unsurprisingly, attribute their difficulties entirely to antipsychotic medication. This can be an important cause of treatment non-adherence. Nevertheless, clinicians often have difficulties initiating discussions about cognitive dysfunction due to a dearth of resources to facilitate comprehensive cognitive assessments, as well as a lack of knowledge about the complex nature and course of cognitive impairment in psychosis.

As we have seen in our work and that of others, cognitive dysfunction is a core feature of psychotic disorders. It emerges during early neurodevelopment, further declines in the prodromal phase of the disorder, and is exacerbated in the acute psychotic phase. Following treatment of the first episode, cognition improves to a certain extent but can be affected by several antipsychotic medications. Lack of stimulation and negative symptoms also compound cognitive dysfunction. Antipsychotic medication may not be effective for cognitive dysfunction, but cognitive remediation and exercise interventions do appear to have a beneficial effect.

Satisfactory cognitive ability is the most important factor determining functional outcomes in psychosis. In clinical consultations, professionals often focus on symptom control and more general psychosocial functioning. The failure to appreciate and address the impact of cognitive deficits may not only affect the therapeutic relationship and adherence to medication but may also lead to the withholding of effective treatment strategies such as cognitive remediation and exercise interventions. It is therefore paramount to gain an understanding of cognitive ability at onset and during the course of psychosis – bearing in mind that the majority of patients will experience at least subtle cognitive deficits, only some of which will improve – and to offer psychological, occupational, physical, and social interventions whenever these are available.

References

1. McEvoy JP. The costs of schizophrenia. *J Clin Psychiatry*. 2007;68 Suppl 14:4-7.
2. Kraepelin E. *Psychiatrie: ein Lehrbuch für Studierende und Aerzte*. J.A. Barth; 1899.
3. Kraepelin E. *Dementia Praecox and Paraphrenia*. Robert E. Krieger Publishing Co. Inc.; 1919, 1971.
4. Kyziridis TC. Notes on the history of schizophrenia. *German J Psychiatry*. 2005;8:42–8.
5. Bleuler E. *Dementia Praecox: Or the Group of Schizophrenias*. International Universities Press; 1911.
6. Schneider K. *Clinical Psychopathology*. 5th ed. Grune & Stratton; 1959.
7. Jablensky A. The diagnostic concept of schizophrenia: its history, evolution, and future prospects. *Dialogues Clin Neurosci*. 2010;12(3):271-287. doi:10.31887/DCNS.2010.12.3/ajablensky
8. Johnstone EC, Crow TJ, Frith CD, Husband J, Kreel L. Cerebral ventricular size and cognitive impairment in chronic schizophrenia. *Lancet*. 1976;2(7992):924-926. doi:10.1016/s0140-6736(76)90890-4
9. Johnstone EC, Owens DG, Gold A, Crow TJ, MacMillan JF. Institutionalization and the defects of schizophrenia. *Br J Psychiatry*. 1981;139:195-203. doi:10.1192/bjp.139.3.195
10. Chen EY, Wong GH, Hui CL, et al. Phenotyping psychosis: room for neurocomputational and content-dependent cognitive endophenotypes? *Cogn Neuropsychiatry*. 2009;14(4-5):451-472. doi:10.1080/13546800902965695
11. So HC, Chen EY, Sham PC. Genetics of schizophrenia spectrum disorders: looking back and peering ahead. *Ann Acad Med Singap*. 2009 May;38(5):436-439.
12. Wong EH, So HC, Li M, et al. Common variants on Xq28 conferring risk of schizophrenia in Han Chinese. *Schizophr Bull*. 2014;40(4):777-786. doi:10.1093/schbul/sbt104
13. So HC, Chen RY, Chen EY, Cheung EF, Li T, Sham PC. An association study of RGS4 polymorphisms with clinical phenotypes of schizophrenia in a Chinese population. *Am J Med Genet B Neuropsychiatr Genet*. 2008;147B(1):77-85. doi:10.1002/ajmg.b.30577
14. Bigdeli TB, Ripke S, Bacanu SA, et al. Genome-wide association study reveals greater polygenic loading for schizophrenia in cases with a family history of illness. *Am J Med Genet B Neuropsychiatr Genet*. 2016;171B(2):276-289. doi:10.1002/ajmg.b.32402

15. So HC, Fong PY, Chen RY, et al. Identification of neuroglycan C and interacting partners as potential susceptibility genes for schizophrenia in a Southern Chinese population. *Am J Med Genet B Neuropsychiatr Genet.* 2010;153B(1):103-113. doi:10.1002/ajmg.b.30961

16. Chan RC, Chen RY, Chen EY, et al. The differential clinical and neurocognitive profiles of COMT SNP rs165599 genotypes in schizophrenia. *J Int Neuropsychol Soc.* 2005;11(2):202-204. doi:10.1017/s1355617705050241

17. Garcia-Barceló MM, Miao X, Tang CS, et al. No NRG1 V266L in Chinese patients with schizophrenia. *Psychiatr Genet.* 2011;21(1):47-49. doi:10.1097/YPG.0b013e328341355b

18. Harvey PD, Bosia M, Cavallaro R, et al. Cognitive dysfunction in schizophrenia: an expert group paper on the current state of the art. *Schizophr Res Cogn.* 2022;29:100249. Published Mar 22, 2022. doi:10.1016/j.scog.2022.100249

19. Sheffield JM, Karcher NR, Barch DM. Cognitive deficits in psychotic disorders: a lifespan perspective. *Neuropsychol Rev.* 2018;28(4):509-533. doi:10.1007/s11065-018-9388-2

20. Woodberry KA, Giuliano AJ, Seidman LJ. Premorbid IQ in schizophrenia: a meta-analytic review. *Am J Psychiatry.* 2008;165(5):579-587. doi:10.1176/appi.ajp.2008.07081242

21. Dickson H, Hedges EP, Ma SY, et al. Academic achievement and schizophrenia: a systematic meta-analysis. *Psychol Med.* 2020;50(12):1949-1965. doi:10.1017/S0033291720002354

22. Catalan A, Salazar de Pablo G, Aymerich C, et al. Neurocognitive functioning in individuals at clinical high risk for psychosis: a systematic review and meta-analysis [published online ahead of print, Jun 16, 2021]. *JAMA Psychiatry.* 2021;78(8):859-867. doi:10.1001/jamapsychiatry.2021.1290

23. Simon AE, Cattapan-Ludewig K, Zmilacher S, et al. Cognitive functioning in the schizophrenia prodrome. *Schizophr Bull.* 2007;33(3):761-771. doi:10.1093/schbul/sbm018

24. Zipursky RB, Reilly TJ, Murray RM. The myth of schizophrenia as a progressive brain disease. *Schizophr Bull.* 2013;39(6):1363-1372. doi:10.1093/schbul/sbs135

25. Monji A, Kato TA, Mizoguchi Y, et al. Neuroinflammation in schizophrenia especially focused on the role of microglia. *Prog Neuropsychopharmacol Biol Psychiatry.* 2013;42:115-121. doi:10.1016/j.pnpbp.2011.12.002

26. Bora E, Murray RM. Meta-analysis of cognitive deficits in ultra-high risk to psychosis and first-episode psychosis: do the cognitive deficits progress over, or after, the onset of psychosis? *Schizophr Bull.* 2014;40(4):744-755. doi:10.1093/schbul/sbt085

27. Zanelli J, Mollon J, Sandin S, et al. Cognitive change in schizophrenia and other psychoses in the decade following the first episode [published correction appears in *Am J Psychiatry.* Dec 1, 2019;176(12):1051]. *Am J Psychiatry.* 2019;176(10):811-819. doi:10.1176/appi.ajp.2019.18091088

28. Fett AJ, Velthorst E, Reichenberg A, et al. Long-term changes in cognitive functioning in individuals with psychotic disorders: findings from the Suffolk County Mental Health Project. *JAMA Psychiatry.* 2020;77(4):387-396. doi:10.1001/jamapsychiatry.2019.3993

29. Fatouros-Bergman H, Cervenka S, Flyckt L, Edman G, Farde L. Meta-analysis of cognitive performance in drug-naïve patients with schizophrenia. *Schizophr Res.* 2014;158(1-3):156-162. doi:10.1016/j.schres.2014.06.034

30. Haijma SV, Van Haren N, Cahn W, Koolschijn PC, Hulshoff Pol HE, Kahn RS. Brain volumes in schizophrenia: a meta-analysis in over 18 000 subjects. *Schizophr Bull.* 2013;39(5):1129-1138. doi:10.1093/schbul/sbs118

31. Sterzer P, Adams RA, Fletcher P, et al. The predictive coding account of psychosis. *Biol Psychiatry.* 2018;84(9):634-643. doi:10.1016/j.biopsych.2018.05.015

32. Valton V, Romaniuk L, Douglas Steele J, Lawrie S, Seriès P. Comprehensive review: computational modelling of schizophrenia. *Neurosci Biobehav Rev.* 2017;83:631-646. doi:10.1016/j.neubiorev.2017.08.022

33. Penn DL, Sanna LJ, Roberts DL. Social cognition in schizophrenia: an overview. *Schizophr Bull.* 2008;34(3):408-411. doi:10.1093/schbul/sbn014

34. Weinreb S, Li F, Kurtz MM. A meta-analysis of social cognitive deficits in schizophrenia: does world region matter? *Schizophr Res.* 2022;243:206-213. doi:10.1016/j. schres.2022.04.002

35. Schmidt SJ, Mueller DR, Roder V. Social cognition as a mediator variable between neurocognition and functional outcome in schizophrenia: empirical review and new results by structural equation modeling. *Schizophr Bull.* 2011;37 Suppl 2(Suppl 2):S41-S54. doi:10.1093/schbul/sbr079

36. Halverson TF, Orleans-Pobee M, Merritt C, Sheeran P, Fett AK, Penn DL. Pathways to functional outcomes in schizophrenia spectrum disorders: Meta-analysis of social cognitive and neurocognitive predictors. *Neurosci Biobehav Rev.* 2019;105:212-219. doi:10.1016/j.neubiorev.2019.07.020

37. Pinkham AE, Penn DL, Green MF, Buck B, Healey K, Harvey PD. The social cognition psychometric evaluation study: results of the expert survey and RAND panel. *Schizophr Bull.* 2014;40(4):813-823. doi:10.1093/schbul/sbt081

38. Shakeel MK, Lu L, Cannon TD, et al. Longitudinal changes in social cognition in individuals at clinical high risk for psychosis: an outcome based analysis. *Schizophr Res.* 2019;204:334-336. doi:10.1016/j.schres.2018.08.032

39. Healey KM, Bartholomeusz CF, Penn DL. Deficits in social cognition in first episode psychosis: a review of the literature. *Clin Psychol Rev.* 2016;50:108-137. doi:10.1016/j. cpr.2016.10.001

40. McCleery A, Lee J, Fiske AP, et al. Longitudinal stability of social cognition in schizophrenia: a 5-year follow-up of social perception and emotion processing. *Schizophr Res.* 2016;176(2-3):467-472. doi:10.1016/j.schres.2016.07.008

41. Chen EY, Lam LC, Chen RY, Nguyen DG. Negative symptoms, neurological signs and neuropsychological impairments in 204 Hong Kong Chinese patients with schizophrenia. *Br J Psychiatry.* 1996;168(2):227-233. doi:10.1192/bjp.168.2.227

42. Tso IF, Chan RCK, Chen EYH, et al. A. 251. Longitudinal profiles of neurocognitive function in first-episode psychosis. XIth Biennial Winter Workshop on Schizophrenia; Feb 24–Mar 1; Davos, Switzerland. *Schizophr Res.* 2002;53(3)(suppl. 1):1-269. doi. org/10.1016/S0920-9964(01)00381-4.

194 • *Psychosis and Schizophrenia in Hong Kong*

43. Chen EY, Kwok CL, Au JW, Chen RY, Lau BS. Progressive deterioration of soft neurological signs in chronic schizophrenic patients. *Acta Psychiatr Scand.* 2000;102(5):342-349. doi:10.1034/j.1600-0447.2000.102005342.x

44. Tso F, Chen EYH, Chan RCK et al. A. 252. Cognitive predictors of clinical outcome in early course of psychosis. The 11th Biennial Winter Workshop on Schizophrenia; Feb 24–Mar 1; Davos, Switzerland. *Schizophr Res.* 2002;53(3)(suppl. 1):1-269. doi.org/10.1016/S0920-9964(01)00381-4.

45. Chang WC, Waltz JA, Gold JM, Chan TCW, Chen EYH. Mild reinforcement learning deficits in patients with first-episode psychosis. *Schizophr Bull.* 2016;42(6):1476-1485. doi:10.1093/schbul/sbw060

46. Chan CT [陳緻韻]. *Reward Learning Impairments in Patients with First-Episode Schizophrenia-Spectrum Disorder.* Thesis. Pokfulam, Hong Kong SAR: University of Hong Kong; 2015. Retrieved from http://dx.doi.org/10.5353/th_b5435664

47. Chan RC, Chen EY, Cheung EF, Cheung HK. Executive dysfunctions in schizophrenia. Relationships to clinical manifestation. *Eur Arch Psychiatry Clin Neurosci.* 2004;254(4):256-262. doi:10.1007/s00406-004-0492-3

48. Chan KK, Hui CL, Tang JY, et al. Random number generation deficit in early schizophrenia. *Percept Mot Skills.* 2011;112(1):91-103. doi:10.2466/02.15.19.22. PMS.112.1.91-103

49. Chan RC, Chen EY, Cheung EF, Chen RY, Cheung HK. Problem-solving ability in chronic schizophrenia: a comparison study of patients with traumatic brain injury. *Eur Arch Psychiatry Clin Neurosci.* 2004;254(4):236-241. doi:10.1007/s00406-004-0486-1

50. Chan RC, Chen EY, Law CW. Specific executive dysfunction in patients with first-episode medication-naïve schizophrenia. *Schizophr Res.* 2006;82(1):51-64. doi:10.1016/j.schres.2005.09.020

51. Wong NT, Chen EYH. A study of sustained attention impairments in first-episode medication-naive schizophrenic patients. *Schizophr Res.* 2001;49(2)(suppl.):124.

52. Chan SKW, Chiu CPY, Lam MML et al. Relationship of neurocognitive function and impairment of insight in first episode schizophrenia. The 2nd Biennial Schizophrenia International Research Conference, Apr 10–14, 2010, Florence, Italy. *Schizophr Res.* 2010;117(2–3):209. doi:10.1016/j.schres.2010.02.290.

53. Chan SK, Chan KK, Hui CL, et al. Correlates of insight with symptomatology and executive function in patients with first-episode schizophrenia-spectrum disorder: a longitudinal perspective. *Psychiatry Res.* 2014;216(2):177-184. doi:10.1016/j.psychres.2013.11.028

54. Liu KC, Chan RC, Chan KK, et al. Executive function in first-episode schizophrenia: a three-year longitudinal study of an ecologically valid test. *Schizophr Res.* 2011;126(1-3):87-92. doi:10.1016/j.schres.2010.11.023

55. Shallice T, Burgess PW. Deficits in strategy application following frontal lobe damage in man. *Brain.* 1991;114 (Pt 2):727-741. doi:10.1093/brain/114.2.727

56. Chan RC, Chen EY, Cheung EF, Chen RY, Cheung HK. The components of executive functioning in a cohort of patients with chronic schizophrenia: a multiple single-case study design. *Schizophr Res.* 2006;81(2-3):173-189. doi:10.1016/j.schres.2005.08.011

57. Chan KK, Xu JQ, Liu KC, Hui CL, Wong GH, Chen EY. Executive function in first-episode schizophrenia: a three-year prospective study of the Hayling Sentence Completion Test. *Schizophr Res.* 2012;135(1-3):62-67. doi:10.1016/j.schres.2011.12.022

58. Chan RC, Shum D, Toulopoulou T, Chen EY. Assessment of executive functions: review of instruments and identification of critical issues. *Arch Clin Neuropsychol.* 2008;23(2):201-216. doi:10.1016/j.acn.2007.08.010

59. Chan RC, Wang YN, Cao XY, Chen EY. Contribution of working memory components to the performance of the tower of hanoi in schizophrenia. *East Asian Arch Psychiatry.* 2010;20(2):69-75.

60. Chan KK, Chen EY. Theory of mind and paranoia in schizophrenia: a game theoretical investigation framework. *Cogn Neuropsychiatry.* 2011;16(6):505-529. doi:10.1080/13 546805.2011.561576

61. Chan RC, Chen EY. Blink rate does matter: a study of blink rate, sustained attention, and neurological signs in schizophrenia. *J Nerv Ment Dis.* 2004;192(11):781-783. doi:10.1097/01.nmd.0000144697.48042.eb

62. Cheung V, Chen EY, Chen RY, Woo MF, Yee BK. A comparison between schizophrenia patients and healthy controls on the expression of attentional blink in a rapid serial visual presentation (RSVP) paradigm. *Schizophr Bull.* 2002;28(3):443-458. doi:10.1093/ oxfordjournals.schbul.a006952

63. Turken AU, Vuilleumier P, Mathalon DH, Swick D, Ford JM. Are impairments of action monitoring and executive control true dissociative dysfunctions in patients with schizophrenia? *Am J Psychiatry.* 2003;160(10):1881-1883. doi:10.1176/appi.ajp.160.10.1881

64. Law CS, Suen YN, Chang WC, et al. Investigation of motor self-monitoring deficits in schizophrenia with passivity experiences using a novel modified joint position matching paradigm. *Eur Arch Psychiatry Clin Neurosci.* 2022;272(3):509-518. doi:10.1007/ s00406-021-01261-z

65. Li AWY, Viñas-Guasch N, Hui CLM, et al. Verbal working memory in schizophrenia: The role of syntax in facilitating serial recall. *Schizophr Res.* 2018;192:294-299. doi:10.1016/j.schres.2017.04.008

66. Lee TM, Chan MW, Chan CC, Gao J, Wang K, Chen EY. Prose memory deficits associated with schizophrenia. *Schizophr Res.* 2006;81(2-3):199-209. doi:10.1016/j. schres.2005.08.009

67. Wood H, Cupitt C, Lavender T. The experience of cognitive impairment in people with psychosis. *Clin Psychol Psychother.* 2015;22(3):193-207. doi:10.1002/cpp.1878

15

Semantic Dysfunctions: The Central Role of Language Processes in Psychosis

Background

The Semantic Organisation of Language

One of the most important biological functions of the human brain is to enable complex group behaviour (1). Group function is uniquely enabled by the use of language in *Homo sapiens*. Semantics is concerned with the study of language and its meaning. The term was first applied to the psychology of language by the French philologist Michel Bréal in the late nineteenth century (2). The Greek origin of the word σήμα means 'sign, mark, or token' (3). Other related terms are σημαίνω, 'to signify, to indicate' and σημαντικός 'significant' (4). In addition to meaning, linguistic semantics also studies how grammar is related to meaning and its relation to language use and acquisition.

Semantics focuses on the processes involved in understanding the meaning of utterances and how the meaning of words or phrases are represented in the mind. Meaning encompasses not just a literal understanding of words but the way they appear in phrases and sentences and what they reflect about the knowledge of and interaction with the world (5). Language organisation encompasses the levels of syntax, semantics, discourse, phonetics, and lexicon (6). For instance, abnormalities affecting the syntactic level would include deviant grammatical organisation, i.e., the abnormal juxtaposition of verbs, adjectives, and nouns in a sentence, irrespective of their meaning. Failure at the semantic level would result in a failure to organise meaning in a sequential language expression that is otherwise grammatically correct. Similarly, failure may also occur at the discourse level, resulting in an overall compromise in the conveyance of meaning in a longer linguistic expression.

Theories of Language Production

Theories of language production have been concerned with how messages are encoded into linguistic signals. Although it is assumed that there might be some interaction between closely related levels of representation, information processing predominantly occurs in unidirectional ways (7). More recently, Brown and Kuperberg (2015) proposed a hierarchical organised circuit model to better account for retrograde feedback mechanisms from lower to higher levels. This, they argue, allows the speech 'production plan' to be updated in real-time and the monitoring of speech production (7). Mismatches between plan and monitoring may then be addressed by 'conversational repair processes'.

Thought and Language Dysfunction in Psychosis

Language and thought disturbances were described by Kraepelin who identified a sub-group of patients with severe confusion of speech characterised by 'an unusually striking disorder of expression in speech, with relatively little impairment of the remaining psychic activities'. He called this symptom 'schizophasia' (8). Bleuler considered alterations of associations the only basic and primary symptom of schizophrenia (9, 10). Language disturbance is also included in Wernicke's description of endogenous psychosis (11).

Exploring the mechanisms underlying semantic dysfunction, Cameron investigated 'overinclusive thinking' in the 1930s and defined it as an inability to preserve conceptual boundaries thereby making thought processes less precise and more abstract (12, 13). Language disturbances in schizophrenia are now thought to be wide-ranging and include positive language symptoms such as idiosyncratic semantic associations, neologisms, and word approximation, as well as negative language symptoms in the form of poverty of speech and reduced grammatical complexity (14, 15, 16, 17, 18, 19). They have been studied with regard to their specificity, pathogenesis, inheritance, familial patterns, and aetiological implications (16, 20, 21, 22).

There have been several research strands investigating the nature of language abnormalities in psychotic disorders, among them the link between thought disorder and incoherent speech, abnormalities in high-level structure and meaning of sentences and discourse, low-level sensory and perceptual deficits affecting the processing of spoken and written language, and patients' ability to distinguish their own inner speech from external speech in relation to auditory hallucinations (7). Earlier experimental studies of general language-related impairments have focused on the language comprehension system as it is easier to control in experimental settings (23, 24, 25). Language production processes more directly related to clinical language disorganisation were investigated by several research groups sometime later

(26, 27, 28, 29). These studies have highlighted the need to distinguish between studies of a general pattern of language use in schizophrenia and studies addressing the language disorder clinically expressed as formal thought disorder (FTD).

For the latter, it is important to capture the phenomenon traditionally detected by a trained observer in an interview context. This usually involves the use of rating scales that utilise a linguistically relevant framework to capture macroscopic abnormalities in broad psycholinguistic levels (30, 31, 32, 33).

Semantic Function Studies in Psychosis in Hong Kong

The Development of the Clinical Language Disorder Rating Scale

We developed the Clinical Language Disorder Rating Scale (CLANG) to capture levels of dysfunction in language organisation in a more comprehensive linguistic framework (34). This had become necessary as the older instruments such as the Thought, Language and Communication (TLC) disorder scale did not fully incorporate a comprehensive framework of linguistic structure (31, 32). CLANG captures four major domains of language production – syntax, semantics, discourse, and pragmatics – and was shown to have good psychometric properties (34).

The Organisation of Language Dysfunction

It has been established that the positive and negative aspects of language disorders in schizophrenia should be considered separately. Formal thought disorder corresponds to the positive aspect of language disorganisation (35, 36, 37). Negative aspects of language disorganisation are usually considered as part of negative symptoms, i.e., poverty of speech. More broadly, we postulated that there is a hierarchical relationship in the order of discourse, semantics, and syntax. Discourse can be affected by the mildest impact of language disorder, whereas syntax will only be affected in the most severe psychopathology. This hypothesis has been supported by several studies showing that language abnormalities occur at both syntax, i.e., 'grammatical unclarity' and 'vague reference', semantic, i.e. 'weak conceptual boundaries' as well as discourse levels and that involvement was likely to be heterogeneous at different levels (31, 35, 38). It also appears that impairments of global linguistic ability were associated with general intellectual impairment. Clinical language disorganisation may be more specifically related to the semantic processes (26). In addition, Gjerde (1983) and Nuechterlein et al. (1986) argued that effortful and intentional processes are more prone to be affected (39, 40).

We recruited patients with schizophrenia to investigate our hypothesis of a hierarchical structure to language disorganisation. More than half of the subjects had at least one abnormality in syntax, semantics, and discourse. There were asymmetrical relationships between patients having syntactic, semantic, and discourse abnormalities, in the direction consistent with the model of a hierarchical language output system. Patients with a syntactic disorder were more likely to also have discourse and semantic disorders, but not vice versa. We also showed that subjects with normal syntax, semantics, or discourse performed better in tests of attention, executive functioning, and cognitive flexibility than those with anomalies in any of the domains. On average, the best performers were those with normal discourse and the worst ones were those with abnormal syntax. Subjects with abnormal syntax performed the worst in tests of attention, executive functioning, and cognitive flexibility, whereas those with abnormal discourse performed the best.

Our study is suggestive of dysfunctions in semantics and discourse co-occurring and constituting higher levels on the intentional-automatic dimension of speech production. In schizophrenia, intentional cognitive processes appear to be more vulnerable. The relationship between discourse and semantic impairment can be regarded as being embedded in a single dimension of severity, in such a way that a greater impact would result in semantic as well as discourse-level disruption, while a milder impact would affect the discourse level only. This relationship can also be considered in terms of the range of associative relationships. Compared to discourse disorder, a semantic disorder affects linguistic units (words or phrases) in close proximity to one another, typically within a sentence. Discourse failure addresses long-range relationships between sentences, and thus units within a sentence exhibit normal relationships. If a production process involving either attention or executive function is deficient, the longer-range relationship is more vulnerable as it requires resources to remain organised whereas a shorter-range relationship is less resource-demanding and therefore has a higher threshold for disruption. Most people who had crossed the threshold for semantic disorder would also have already crossed the threshold for discourse failure and not vice versa. This interpretation was consistent with the observed co-occurrence pattern, and a greater number of subjects with abnormal discourse compared with those with abnormal semantics. The syntactic level, on the other hand, is thought to be related to the automatic dimension of speech production and is, therefore, more resilient to disruption. However, a hierarchical relationship between syntax and semantic/discourse disorder as had been postulated could not be fully established. Our data suggest that syntax occupies a separate dimension and might be more closely related to and interact with the negative aspects of language disorder such as poverty of speech and other pragmatic and phonetic abnormalities.

Semantic Memory and Semantic Categorisation in Psychotic Disorders

Semantic memory is defined as stored information for use in language and is thought to be related to but distinct from episodic memory. It has been shown that semantic memory is organised into categories and that words will be recognised to be belonging to a particular category more quickly if they have a closer resemblance to the prototype of the category. This is called the semantic-relatedness effect (41, 42, 43). It takes the longest to respond when an item is on the category boundary, i.e., they are sometimes considered to be within the category and sometimes not. With an item clearly outside the category, the response time is shortened (the false-relatedness effect).

Compared to matched controls, schizophrenia patients showed a slower response time when asked to categorise words, particularly when items were outside the category but semantically related, such as in the example 'Is an aircraft a bird?' (24, 42). In contrast, controls took the longest to respond to ambiguous words at the borderline of a category, for example, 'Is a penguin a bird?'. This suggests that the boundary of semantic categories is shifted outwards to include a broader set of borderline items as well as some related items outside the category boundary. The overinclusiveness of semantic concepts appeared to be related to executive dysfunction (25, 44).

Longitudinally, we demonstrated that semantic categorisation abnormalities were worse during first-episode schizophrenia, and subsequently improved and stabilised (45, 46). Interestingly, semantic performance deficits, particularly a diminished typicality effect, correlated with negative symptoms in the initial episode, but not at remission. Medication appears unlikely to affect categorisation abnormalities as both medicated and unmedicated first-episode patients showed these difficulties.

It has been recognised that executive dysfunction is likely to play an important role in language disorganisation. Despite improvements in semantic and syntactic deficits following the resolution of psychotic symptoms, language production often continues to be impaired and seems to be associated with negative symptoms and predicted by attentional difficulties (47).

Theoretical Frameworks of Semantic Memory

Theories of semantic memory propose that memory traces are organised in networks consisting of nodes that correspond to named concepts. These nodes become activated for a short period of time when they are involved in language comprehension or production. Thus, it follows that cognitive representations are not static but rather come into being when they are used (48, 49). Nodes activated in the semantic network in turn serve as a source of activation by 'spreading' to semantically related nodes until passive decay or active inhibition occurs (48, 50, 51, 52, 53, 54). The amount of activation arriving at the recipient node is inversely related to its semantic distance from the source node. When the amount of activation of a node reaches a threshold, retrieval of the corresponding concept occurs. Accordingly, the time required for retrieval is less if the node is already partially activated (55). This provides a theoretical account for the empirically observed semantic priming effect. Semantic priming has been investigated predominantly in patients with chronic schizophrenia and results have been inconsistent (56).

Priming Abnormalities in Psychosis

To elucidate the relationship between priming abnormalities, the course of psychotic illness and medication effects, we recruited 24 medication-naïve and 21 medicated first-episode schizophrenia patients and 53 matched controls (56). We detected heightened semantic facilitation among unmedicated patients that normalised after exposure to antipsychotics. These elevated priming effects may be related to heightened spreading activation and failure of inhibition in untreated first-episode schizophrenia patients, and antipsychotics may suppress abnormal increases in semantic facilitation via their modulatory effects on dopaminergic transmission.

Neurocognitive Theories of Semantic Abnormalities in Psychosis

Two main neurocognitive theories have been postulated to explain semantic abnormalities, namely deficits in accessing semantic knowledge or its storage. Some studies concluded that schizophrenia patients had difficulties retrieving from an intact semantic store, whereas others indicated that the semantic store was degraded (57, 58, 59, 60). We used a repeated verbal fluency task to examine these theories (61). When a semantic fluency task (e.g., animal naming) is repeated the subject will produce new items as well as items that overlap with the previous task. As the repetition proceeds, more overlapping items will be produced. The asymptote of new items versus overlapping items will then allow an estimation of the capacity of the semantic store (e.g., of animal items) in semantic memory. We found that poor verbal fluency was at least partly attributable to a reduction in the semantic store rather than just difficulties with retrieving information.

Network analysis enables novel analysis of words produced in a word association task. Elvevaag, De Deyne and our team proposed an expanded theoretical construct involving a network-based framework to not only account for individual words within semantic categories but also their semantic relations to other words (62, 63, 64). We examined semantic network disruptions using a word association task (61). Compared to matched controls, patients during relapse had networks with higher density, longer 'shortest path length', higher clustering coefficient, and lower modularity. After the resolution of psychotic symptoms, the semantic network was less dense and the clustering coefficient was lower as symptoms and functioning improved.

Dialogical Behaviour in Psychosis

We have also pioneered the study of dialogical behaviour. Considerations of an evolutionary perspective reveal that language is not only a communicative tool in a cooperative situation but is also used in controlling information dissemination. In this context, it is equally important that language can be used smoothly to check information dissemination in a competitive social encounter. We found that patients were inefficient in both situations. They communicated less information in cooperative situations while giving too many details in competitive conditions. They were less flexible in shifting their communication strategy between competitive and cooperative conditions. These difficulties were associated with negative symptoms, specifically anhedonia/asociality, as well as hallucinations and persecutory delusions (65).

Expressive Language Disorder in the Cantonese Language

How expressive language disorder varies in different languages has not been systematically studied. The varying characters of different languages may present distinct challenges to the brain. For example, in the Chinese language, a larger number of words share the same phonemic expressions. There is greater demand placed upon speakers who have to consider the context to disambiguate sounds in order to assess the meaning of utterances. As a result, in the Cantonese language clang associations are more frequent than in English. For example, one of our patients observed that her husband brought her shampoo for use in the hospital and interpreted that he would kill her. Shampoo is semantically associated with hair-washing (*lin tou*, 淋頭), which shares the sound in a metaphor meaning that catastrophe is awaiting (*si dao lintou*, 死到臨頭).

Verbal Fluency and Semantic Function

Verbal fluency tests are one of the most commonly used methods to assess cognitive ability and more specifically frontal lobe functioning. Verbal fluency has been extensively studied in schizophrenia patients (66). Verbal fluency tasks involve participants having to generate words based on certain criteria, such as words starting with a particular letter in alphabet-based languages or being part of a certain semantic category. The latter is also called the semantic fluency test and requires the integrity of executive functions, as well as a well-organised category structure that is related to long-term memory (67). Both letter and semantic fluency have been found to be impaired in schizophrenia, with greater negative effects on semantic fluency (66, 68).

In Hong Kong, the semantic verbal fluency test has been useful in assessing executive functioning; however, the letter fluency test based on the alphabet has had limited utility due to the differing basic structure of the English and Chinese languages (69). Interestingly, normative data showed that healthy participants generated more words in the categories 'food' and 'animal' compared to 'means of transport' and 'furniture'. Also, higher educational attainment and female gender were associated with better performance in the categories of 'food', 'means of transport', and 'furniture', but not 'animal' (70).

In order to gain a more thorough understanding of semantic deficits as familial trait markers among schizophrenia patients and their non-psychotic relatives, we recruited 23 Chinese schizophrenia patients, 21 of their non-psychotic siblings and 26 healthy volunteers, matched for age, sex, and education (71). Siblings had significantly less word output in the verbal fluency test as compared to controls. Given that siblings showed reduced verbal fluency, we believe that the anomaly is a familial trait marker for schizophrenia.

Reflections: The Central Role of Language Functions

Language dysfunction in schizophrenia is a phenomenon important not only for its scientific significance but also for its clinical impact. Yet its observation and description are often inadequate owing to its complexity. One of the challenges is the multiple levels in which utterances are expressed. This has been approached in two main ways, addressing two different linguistic phenomena that produce overlapping anomalous linguistic occurrences. First, there is a generic reduction in the efficiency of language processes. This is considered a language disorder and, among other features, is characterised by a less complex structure and a reduction of referential links, which take place alongside a wide range of cognitive impairments. The second approach concerns the specific clinical phenomenon of FTD, which sometimes occurs in psychotic states and can resolve during remission.

Generic language dysfunction in the presence of other cognitive impairments could be considered a downstream consequence of basic cognitive processes such as attention. This view, however, may under-emphasise linguistic processes that cannot be reduced to more basic non-linguistic processes. There are some suggestions that linguistic function is not just one of the many cognitive abilities available once the human mind has developed sufficient general upstream cognitive capabilities. Indeed, it has been postulated that many of the human cognitive functions have evolved as part of the development of linguistic abilities as a uniquely human tool for complex social interactions. For example, in the study of short-term memory, a conventional cognitive approach often uses a sequential list of unrelated nouns as a stimulus. This addresses general cognitive ability, which has been shown to be impaired in schizophrenia. On top of that, we explored what would happen if, instead of isolated terms, we used phrases that contained verbs in addition to nouns, and when words were arranged in a syntactically correct sequence, i.e., noun-verb-noun in English. We found that while in healthy subjects the syntactic structure facilitated short-term memory, this syntactic facilitation effect was compromised in schizophrenia. This observation is interesting because it reveals that the mind is more than a general information-processing system. It has a predilection for linguistic functions, and this function is affected in psychotic disorders (72).

The phenomenon of FTD is of special importance in understanding psychosis. As one of the clinical signs of psychosis, it has significance for clinicians that has not yet been fully exploited. Firstly, it is a symptom that cannot be fabricated. Secondly, it occurs in schizophrenia and manic episodes, but seldom in other psychiatric or neurological conditions. Intriguingly the presence of FTD in substance-induced psychosis is questionable except in phencyclidine-induced psychosis (73). Although FTD in schizophrenia and manic episodes is described with different characteristic features, it is clinically questionable whether they are distinguishable. If we consider bipolar mania and schizophrenic psychosis together, FTD is one of the few symptoms in psychiatry that is close to being pathognomonic. Clinically, FTD occurs in clear consciousness. The patient talks fluently and appears unaware of the incomprehensibility of their speech. In contrast to nominal dysphasia, in FTD, there is little evidence of attempts to repair and make speech more comprehensible. The fact that formal thought disorder does not occur in amphetamine-induced psychosis suggests that dopamine abnormalities alone may be insufficient to account for FTD.

The extent of disorganisation of thought varies according to the subject matter being expressed. It is worse in more abstract topics, and when other psychotic content is described by the patient. Thought disorganisation in written language can occur separately from that in verbal language. Thought disorder is a clinical sign rather than a symptom. It does not originate from a subjective experience in the patient, but rather is an observation that can be made by different observers, and indeed can be measured instrumentally with computational technology such as latent semantic analysis (74). In contrast to other mental symptoms, FTD cannot be fabricated. One can easily confirm this by trying to mimic disorganised speech. It is extremely difficult for a healthy individual to maintain for any length of time beyond a few seconds because semantic organisation is built into language systems in the brain.

Research has highlighted that a proportion of syntactic and semantic language disorders improve alongside the remission of psychotic symptoms, although more subtle language difficulties remain. These residual difficulties, particularly in discourse and some syntactic functions, are likely to be mediated by persistent executive cognitive difficulties and negative symptoms. The partial reversibility of FTD is important evidence pointing to the existence of an episodic fluctuation in brain state in addition to the dopamine-related processes. We also noticed that there is a narrower form of psychosis with delusions and hallucinations but no formal thought disorder, which could be induced by amphetamine intoxication. Psychosis with thought disorder is likely to involve glutaminergic transmission potentially upstream to dopamine mechanisms, as we have observed above in phencyclidine-induced thought disorder.

Finally, detecting subtle speech abnormalities in clinical high-risk youths may hold specific promise in predicting the onset of psychosis. Bedi et al. (2015) used a novel computerised method combined with machine learning to predict the later onset of psychosis (75). It was shown that semantic coherence and two syntactic markers of speech complexity were associated with the later development of psychosis. If the findings can be replicated, this would open up the possibility not only for early, more accurate identification of those progressing to frank psychosis but also for early intervention, thereby hopefully improving long-term outcomes.

References

1. Dunbar RI. The social brain hypothesis and its implications for social evolution. *Ann Hum Biol.* 2009;36(5):562-572. doi:10.1080/03014460902960289
2. Wilkins AS. *Bréal's Semantics—Semantics: Studies in the Science of Meaning.* By Michel Bréal. Translated by Mrs Henry Cust, with a preface by J. P. Postgate. William Heinemann. 8vo. Pp. lxvi, 342. 7s. 6d. net. *The Classical Review.* 1901;15(2):127-128. doi:10.1017/S0009840X00029759
3. Liddell HG, Scott R. *A Greek-English Lexicon.* Revised and augmented throughout by Sir Henry Stuart Jones. With the assistance of Roderick McKenzie. Clarendon Press; 1940. http://www.perseus.tufts.edu/hopper/text?doc=Perseus%3Atext%3A1999.04.0 057%3Aentry%3D%2393797&redirect=true
4. Liddell HG, Scott R. *An Intermediate Greek-English Lexicon.* Clarendon Press; 1889. http://www.perseus.tufts.edu/hopper/text?doc=Perseus%3Atext%3A1999.04.0058% 3Aentry%3D%2329446&redirect=true
5. Sanford AJ. Semantics in Psychology. In: Brown K, ed. *Encyclopedia of Language & Linguistics.* 2nd ed. Elsevier; 2006: 152-158, doi:10.1016/B0-08-044854-2/01106-8.
6. Crystal D. *The Cambridge Encyclopedia of Language.* Cambridge University Press; 1987.
7. Brown M and Kuperberg GR. A hierarchical generative framework of language processing: linking language perception, interpretation, and production abnormalities in schizophrenia. *Front. Hum. Neurosci.* 2015;9:643. doi: 10.3389/fnhum.2015.00643
8. Kraepelin E, Barclay RM & Robertson GM. *Dementia Praecox.* Chicago Medical Book Co.; 1919.
9. Bleuler E. Dementia praecox oder Gruppe der Schizophrenien. In: von Aschaffenburg G, ed. *Handbuch der Psychiatrie.* Deuticke. 1911:1-420; reprinted by Arts & Boeve. 2001.

10. Maatz A, Hoff P, Angst J. Eugen Bleuler's schizophrenia – a modern perspective. *Dialogues Clin Neurosci.* 2015;17(1):43-49. doi:10.31887/DCNS.2015.17.1/amaatz
11. Wernicke C. *Über die Klassifikation der Psychosen.* Sclettersche Buchhandlung; 1899.
12. Cameron N. A study of thinking in senile deterioration and schizophrenic disorganization. *Amer J. Psychol.* 1938, 51, 650-664.
13. Cameron, N. Deterioration and regression in schizophrenic thinking. *J. Abnorm. Soc. Psychol.,* 1939;34:265-270.
14. Kuperberg GR. Language in schizophrenia Part 2: What can psycholinguistics bring to the study of schizophrenia . . . and vice versa? *Lang Linguist Compass.* 2010;4(8):590-604. doi:10.1111/j.1749-818X.2010.00217.x.
15. Covington MA, He C, Brown C, et al. Schizophrenia and the structure of language: the linguist's view. *Schizophr Res.* 2005;77(1):85-98. doi:10.1016/j.schres.2005.01.016
16. DeLisi LE. Speech disorder in schizophrenia: review of the literature and exploration of its relation to the uniquely human capacity for language. *Schizophr Bull.* 2001;27(3):481-496. doi:10.1093/oxfordjournals.schbul.a006889
17. Ditman T, Kuperberg GR. Building coherence: A framework for exploring the breakdown of links across clause boundaries in schizophrenia. *J Neurolinguistics.* 2010;23(3):254-269. doi:10.1016/j.jneuroling.2009.03.003
18. Fraser WI, King KM, Thomas P, Kendell RE. The diagnosis of schizophrenia by language analysis. *Br J Psychiatry.* 1986;148:275-278. doi:10.1192/bjp.148.3.275
19. Morice R, McNicol D. Language changes in schizophrenia: a limited replication. *Schizophr Bull.* 1986;12(2):239-251. doi:10.1093/schbul/12.2.239
20. Docherty NM, Rhinewine JP, Labhart RP, Gordinier SW. Communication disturbances and family psychiatric history in parents of schizophrenic patients. *J Nerv Ment Dis.* 1998;186(12):761-768. doi:10.1097/00005053-199812000-00004
21. Berrios GE. Falret, Séglas, Morselli, and Masselon, and the "language of the insane": a conceptual history. *Brain Lang.* 1999;69(1):56-75. doi:10.1006/brln.1999.2042
22. Spitzer M. A cognitive neuroscience view of schizophrenic thought disorder. *Schizophr Bull.* 1997;23(1):29-50. doi:10.1093/schbul/23.1.29
23. Paulsen JS, Romero R, Chan A, Davis AV, Heaton RK, Jeste DV. Impairment of the semantic network in schizophrenia. *Psychiatry Res.* 1996;63(2-3):109-121. doi:10.1016/0165-1781(96)02901-0
24. Aloia MS, Gourovitch ML, Weinberger DR, Goldberg TE. An investigation of semantic space in patients with schizophrenia. *J Int Neuropsychol Soc.* 1996;2(4):267-273. doi:10.1017/s1355617700001272
25. Chen EY, Wilkins AJ, McKenna PJ. Semantic memory is both impaired and anomalous in schizophrenia. *Psychol Med.* 1994;24(1):193-202. doi:10.1017/s0033291700026957
26. Rodriguez-Ferrera S, McCarthy RA, McKenna PJ. Language in schizophrenia and its relationship to formal thought disorder. *Psychol Med.* 2001;31(2):197-205. doi:10.1017/s003329170100321x
27. Baltaxe CA, Simmons JQ 3rd. Speech and language disorders in children and adolescents with schizophrenia. *Schizophr Bull.* 1995;21(4):677-692. doi:10.1093/schbul/21.4.677
28. Barch DM, Berenbaum H. Language production and thought disorder in schizophrenia. *J Abnorm Psychol.* 1996;105(1):81-88. doi:10.1037//0021-843x.105.1.81

29. Barch DM, Berenbaum H. The effect of language production manipulations on negative thought disorder and discourse coherence disturbances in schizophrenia. *Psychiatry Res.* 1997;71(2):115-127. doi:10.1016/s0165-1781(97)00045-0

30. Ceccherini-Nelli A, Crow TJ. Disintegration of the components of language as the path to a revision of Bleuler's and Schneider's concepts of schizophrenia. Linguistic disturbances compared with first-rank symptoms in acute psychosis [published correction appears in *Br J Psychiatry.* Jan 2004;184:87]. *Br J Psychiatry.* 2003;182:233-240. doi:10.1192/bjp.182.3.233

31. Liddle PF, Ngan ET, Caissie SL, et al. Thought and Language Index: an instrument for assessing thought and language in schizophrenia. *Br J Psychiatry.* 2002;181:326-330. doi:10.1192/bjp.181.4.326

32. Andreasen NC. Thought, language, and communication disorders. I. Clinical assessment, definition of terms, and evaluation of their reliability. *Arch Gen Psychiatry.* 1979;36(12):1315-1321. doi:10.1001/archpsyc.1979.01780120045006

33. Andreasen NC. Thought, language, and communication disorders. II. Diagnostic significance. *Arch Gen Psychiatry.* 1979;36(12):1325-1330. doi:10.1001/archpsyc.1979.01780120055007

34. Chen EYH, Lam LCW, Kan CS, et al. Language disorganization in schizophrenia: validation and assessment with a new clinical rating instrument. *Hong Kong Journal of Psychiatry.* 1996;6(1):4-13.

35. Gordinier SW, Docherty NM. Factor analysis of the Communication Disturbances Index. *Psychiatry Res.* 2001;101(1):55-62. doi:10.1016/s0165-1781(00)00239-0

36. Peralta V, Cuesta MJ, de Leon J. Formal thought disorder in schizophrenia: a factor analytic study. *Compr Psychiatry.* 1992;33(2):105-110. doi:10.1016/0010-440x(92)90005-b

37. Andreasen NC, Olsen S. Negative v positive schizophrenia. Definition and validation. *Arch Gen Psychiatry.* 1982;39(7):789-794. doi:10.1001/archpsyc.1982.04290070025006

38. Kuperberg GR, McGuire PK, David AS. Sensitivity to linguistic anomalies in spoken sentences: a case study approach to understanding thought disorder in schizophrenia. *Psychol Med.* 2000;30(2):345-357. doi:10.1017/s0033291700001744

39. Gjerde PF. Attentional capacity dysfunction and arousal in schizophrenia. *Psychol Bull.* 1983;93(1):57-72.

40. Nuechterlein KH, Edell WS, Norris M, Dawson ME. Attentional vulnerability indicators, thought disorder, and negative symptoms. *Schizophr Bull.* 1986;12(3):408-426. doi:10.1093/schbul/12.3.408

41. Kintsch W. Semantic memory: a tutorial. In: Nickerson RS, ed. *Attention and Performance,* VIII. Lawrence Erlbaum Associates; 1981:595-620.

42. Baddeley AD. *Human Memory: Theory and Practice.* Erlbaum; 1990.

43. Wilkins AJ. Conjoint frequency, category size and categorization time. *J Verbal Learning and Verbal Behavior.* 1971;10:382-385. doi:10.1016/S0022-5371(71)80036-1.

44. Hui CL, Longenecker J, Wong GH, et al. Longitudinal changes in semantic categorization performance after symptomatic remission from first-episode psychosis: a 3-year follow-up study. *Schizophr Res.* 2012;137(1-3):118-123. doi:10.1016/j.schres.2012.02.010

45. Chan KK, Xu JQ, Liu KC, Hui CL, Wong GH, Chen EY. Executive function in first-episode schizophrenia: a three-year prospective study of the Hayling Sentence Completion Test. *Schizophr Res.* 2012;135(1-3):62-67. doi:10.1016/j.schres.2011.12.022

208 • *Psychosis and Schizophrenia in Hong Kong*

46. Xu JQ, Hui CL, Longenecker J, et al. Executive function as predictors of persistent thought disorder in first-episode schizophrenia: a one-year follow-up study. *Schizophr Res.* 2014;159(2-3):465-470. doi:10.1016/j.schres.2014.08.022

47. Chen EYH, Cheung V, Fung RJ, Lau BST. N400 and P600 event-related potential responses to neutral and affect-laden semantic stimulus in schizophrenic patients. *Schizophr Res.* 2000;41(1):153, doi:10.1016/S0920-9964(00)90671-6.

48. Needly JH. Semantic priming and retrieval from lexical memory: role of inhibitionless spreading activation and limited capacity attention. *J Exp Psychol Gen.* 1977;106(3): 226-254.

49. Quillian MR. Word concepts: a theory and simulation of some basic semantic capabilities. *Behav Sci.* 1967;12(5):410-430. doi:10.1002/bs.3830120511

50. Anderson JR. *Language, memory, and thought.* Lawrence Erlbaum Associates; 1976.

51. Anderson JR, *The architecture of cognition.* Harvard University Press; 1983.

52. Spitzer M, Braun U, Maier S, Hermle L, Maher BA. Indirect semantic priming in schizophrenic patients. *Schizophr Res.* 1993;11(1):71-80.doi:10.1016/0920-9964(93)90040-p

53. Ober BA, Vinogradov S, Shenaut GK. Semantic priming of category relations in schizophrenia. *Neuropsychology.* 1995;9(2):220-228. doi:10.1037/0894-4105.9.2.220

54. McNamara, TP, Altarriba J. Depth of spreading activation revisited: Semantic mediated priming occurs in lexical decisions. *J Memory and Language.* 1988;27:545-559.

55. Doughty OJ, Done DJ. Is semantic memory impaired in schizophrenia? A systematic review and meta-analysis of 91 studies. *Cogn Neuropsychiatry.* 2009;14(6):473-509. doi:10.1080/13546800903073291

56. Wong AW, Chen EY. Semantic memory anomaly in first-episode schizophrenia patients. *Schizophr Res.* 2001;49(2) (suppl. 1):147-148. doi:10.1016/S0920-9964(01)00159-1

57. Allen HA, Liddle PF, Frith CD. Negative features, retrieval processes and verbal fluency in schizophrenia. *Br J Psychiatry.* 1993;163:769-775. doi:10.1192/bjp.163.6.769

58. Doughty OJ, Done DJ, Lawrence VA, Al-Mousawi A, Ashaye K. Semantic memory impairment in schizophrenia – deficit in storage or access of knowledge? *Schizophr Res.* 2008;105(1-3):40-48. doi:10.1016/j.schres.2008.04.039

59. McKay AP, McKenna PJ, Bentham P, Mortimer AM, Holbery A, Hodges JR. Semantic memory is impaired in schizophrenia. *Biol Psychiatry.* 1996;39(11):929-937. doi:10.1016/0006-3223(95)00250-2

60. Rossell SL, David AS. Are semantic deficits in schizophrenia due to problems with access or storage? *Schizophr Res.* 2006;82(2-3):121-134. doi:10.1016/j.schres.2005.11.001

61. Chen RY, Chen EY, Chan CK, Lam LC, Lieh-Mak F. Verbal fluency in schizophrenia: reduction in semantic store. *Aust N Z J Psychiatry.* 2000;34(1):43-48. doi:10.1046/j.1440-1614.2000.00647.x

62. De Deyne S, Elnevåg B, Hui CLM, Poon VWY, Chen EYH. Rich semantic networks applied to schizophrenia: A new framework. *Schizophr Res.* 2016;176(2-3):454-455. doi:10.1016/j.schres.2016.05.016

63. Ko W [高瑋彤]. *Semantic Networks and Their Disruptions in Psychotic Disorders.* Thesis. University of Hong Kong; 2018. https://hub.hku.hk/handle/10722/261463

64. Pintos A, Hui C, De Deyne S, Cheung C, Ko WT, Suen YN, Chan S, Chang WC, Lee E, Lo A, Lo W, Elnevåg B, Chen E. A longitudinal study of semantic networks

in schizophrenia and other psychotic disorders using the word association task. *Schizophrenia Bulletin Open.* 2022;3(1)sgac054. doi:10.1093/schizbullopen/sgac054

65. Xu J. [徐佳琪]. (2013). *Verbal information management in patients with schizophrenia and their healthy siblings: a novel paradigm for conversational analysis.* Thesis. University of Hong Kong. doi:10.5353/th_b5177304

66. Bokat CE, Goldberg TE. Letter and category fluency in schizophrenic patients: a meta-analysis. *Schizophr Res.* 2003;64(1):73-78. doi:10.1016/s0920-9964(02)00282-7

67. Feinstein A, Goldberg TE, Nowlin B, Weinberger DR. Types and characteristics of remote memory impairment in schizophrenia. *Schizophr Res.* 1998;30(2):155-163. doi:10.1016/s0920-9964(97)00129-1

68. Goldberg TE, Aloia MS, Gourovitch ML, Missar D, Pickar D, Weinberger DR. Cognitive substrates of thought disorder, I: the semantic system. *Am J Psychiatry.* 1998;155(12):1671-1676. doi:10.1176/ajp.155.12.1671

69. Chan RCK, Chen EYH. Development of a Chinese verbal fluency test for the Hong Kong psychiatric setting. *Hong Kong J Psychiatry.* 2004;14(2):8-11.

70. Chan RCK, Wong M, Chen EYH, Lam LCW. Semantic categorisation and verbal fluency performance in a community population in Hong Kong: a preliminary report. *East Asian Arch Psychiatry.* 2003;13:14-20.

71. Chen YL, Chen YH, Lieh-Mak F. Semantic verbal fluency deficit as a familial trait marker in schizophrenia. *Psychiatry Res.* 2000;95(2):133-48. doi: 10.1016/s0165-1781(00)00166-9. Erratum in: *Psychiatry Res.* Nov 20, 2000;96(3):281. LiehMF [corrected to Lieh-Mak, F].

72. Li AWY, Viñas-Guasch N, Hui CLM, et al. Verbal working memory in schizophrenia: the role of syntax in facilitating serial recall. *Schizophr Res.* 2018;192:294-299. doi:10.1016/j.schres.2017.04.008

73. Javitt DC, Zukin SR. Recent advances in the phencyclidine model of schizophrenia. *Am J Psychiatry.* 1991;148(10):1301-1308. doi:10.1176/ajp.148.10.1301

74. Elvevåg B, Cohen AS. Translating natural language processing into mainstream schizophrenia assessment. *Schizophr Bull.* 2022;48(5):936-938. doi:10.1093/schbul/sbac087

75. Bedi G, Carrillo F, Cecchi GA, et al. Automated analysis of free speech predicts psychosis onset in high-risk youths. *NPJ Schizophr.* 2015;1:15030. Published Aug 26, 2015. doi:10.1038/npjschz.2015.30

16

Neurological Soft Signs: A Simple Enough Clinical Sign in Psychosis

Background

Definition and Historical Context

Neurological soft signs (NSS) denote subtle non-localisable neurological abnormalities in sensory integration, motor coordination, sequencing of complex motor acts, and primitive reflexes (1, 2). Interest in delineating neurological signs in mental disorders has been longstanding due to the fact that eliciting psychiatric symptoms depends on patient reports and is thus more open to interpretation, whereas clinical signs are considered to be more objective and can be more reliably assessed. Neurological pathology in the form of localised and focal signs is not usually found in psychiatry. However, it has been recognised for a long time that a significant proportion of psychiatric patients present with more subtle sensory and motor signs representing abnormal brain states. The question of whether there might be defined neurological signs in psychiatric disorders struck at the heart of a longstanding debate in the late nineteenth century, namely how one may differentiate psychiatric from neurological disease. Carl Wernicke, Professor of Neurology and Psychiatry in Breslau from 1885 to 1904, proposed the boundary to be drawn at the presence or absence of localising neurological signs in his book *Lehrbuch der Gehirnkrankheiten für Ärzte und Studierende* (3).

Loretta Bender was the first to coin the term 'neurological soft signs' and to describe several of these signs in 100 children with schizophrenia in 1947, although the clinical picture of most of the described cases would nowadays suggest a diagnosis of childhood autism rather than psychosis (4). Nonetheless, Bender's early study paved the way for more systematic investigations of soft non-localising signs in children with a variety of neurodevelopmental difficulties.

Neurological Soft Signs in Psychotic Disorders

With the emergence of neurodevelopmental considerations in the aetiology of schizophrenia neurological soft signs have been increasingly studied since the 1970s. They have been consistently shown at a higher frequency in schizophrenia compared to healthy controls including in medication-naïve patients (5). Torrey (1980) reported a correlation between NSS and more chronic and severe schizophrenia (6), a finding confirmed by Manschreck and Ames (1984) in their cross-sectional study on NSS in schizophrenia (1). Their research and studies undertaken by the Heidelberg group in Germany indicated a significant reduction in NSS as patients were recovering from an acute state or their first episode of schizophrenia and that these improvements were sustained for at least four years (7, 8, 9, 10).

It has been proposed that NSS are an inherent feature of schizophrenia supported by the fact that NSS scores are significantly higher in relatives of schizophrenia patients including unaffected monozygotic twins (11). Bachmann and colleagues (2014) published a meta-analysis of 17 studies on the longitudinal course of NSS in schizophrenia. 787 patients were included in the analysis with follow-up for up to four years. Fourteen studies found a decrease in NSS as psychopathology remitted, but NSS scores remained elevated when compared to healthy controls.

One may conclude that NSS represent both a state and trait characteristic of schizophrenia given that patients have higher scores during remission when compared to healthy controls and NSS increase during acute episodes. Chan and Gottesman (2008) suggested NSS as candidate endophenotypes for schizophrenia and Xu et al. (2016) reported moderately significant heritability in healthy monozygotic Han Chinese twins of schizophrenia patients (12, 13).

Data on the longitudinal course of NSS, neurobiological correlates, and their association with psychopathology are scarce, although some researchers believe that NSS deterioration reflects the progression of brain pathology (14, 15). There is some evidence that atrophy of the precentral gyrus, the cerebellum, the inferior frontal gyrus, and the thalamus is associated with increased severity of NSS (16, 17, 18). Kong et al. (2020) analysed brain network characteristics in patients with schizophrenia and NSS and found alterations in cortical-subcortical-cerebellar circuits, and particular sub-groups of NSS have been shown to be associated with abnormalities in certain brain regions (19).

It has been argued that NSS are a useful predictor of treatment outcomes in schizophrenia. Two recent studies support this notion, i.e., total NSS scores, and motor and cognitive sub-scores at baseline were predictive of a diagnosis of schizophrenia in first-episode psychosis (FEP) patients at 12 months. In addition, non-remitting patients had shown significantly higher NSS scores at baseline (15, 20).

Studies on Neurological Soft Signs in Hong Kong and China

The Measurement of Neurological Soft Signs

In Hong Kong, NSS and their relationship to clinical outcomes have been extensively investigated by our group including Professor Raymond Chan who subsequently led a group in China in addressing this area. Our interest in the subject has been motivated by wishing to elucidate the nature and course of deficits that reflect brain dysfunctions in schizophrenia (21). We developed the Cambridge Neurological Inventory (CNI) to operationalise the study of NSS (22). The CNI is a comprehensive neurological examination and takes approximately 30 to 45 minutes to administer. Typically, localising neurological signs such as plantar reflexes, power, reflexes, dyskinesia, and extrapyramidal signs are first assessed. Neurological soft signs, which include motor coordination, sensory integration, and disinhibition, are elicited thereafter. Catatonic signs are also examined in this integrated neurological examination. The CNI was validated in a patient population and healthy controls and was shown to be a comprehensive assessment tool, reliable and easy to administer.

Neurological Soft Signs and Their Neuroanatomical Correlates

Chan et al. (2006) published a study examining the brain regions involved in several soft sign motor sequencing tasks in healthy volunteers using functional magnetic resonance imaging (fMRI) (23). Subjects were scanned while performing the following tasks: palm tapping (PT), pronation/supination (P/S), and fist-edge palm (FEP). These tasks represent increasingly complex motor movements. It was shown that fist-edge palm led to significant activation in bilateral sensorimotor areas, the supplementary motor area, the left parietal, and the right cerebellum, but no activation in the prefrontal area. Also, signal changes within the left sensorimotor, left thalamus, and right cerebellum were observed indicating an increase in activation with task complexity. These findings suggest that more complex motor sequencing tasks involve wide cortical networks.

The Course of Neurological Soft Signs in Psychosis

Our patients with schizophrenia were found to have significantly more NSS and hard neurological signs, other than pyramidal signs, when compared to healthy controls, and soft signs were more strongly associated with schizophrenia than hard signs. NSS appeared to be stable as the illness progressed, at least during the early stages of the disorder, although tended to increase with age both in patients and healthy controls (24, 25, 26). Also, dyskinesia appeared to be more common in people over 45 years old (27). Motor NSS were particularly high in those who were medication-naïve (25). Prospective studies demonstrated significant increases in motor coordination NSS in stabilised chronic schizophrenia patients over the course of three years, while psychopathology and medication remained largely unchanged (28, 29). Moreover, treatment-resistant patients exhibited progressive worsening of NSS over the course of five years (30).

Neurological Soft Signs and Cognition

NSS were associated with impaired cognition, in particular, prefrontal impairments were correlated with motor coordination signs while sensory integration signs were related to more generalised cognitive impairments. Sustained attention has been shown to be impaired in schizophrenia and this cognitive sub-domain is significantly correlated with motor coordination and disinhibition NSS (31, 32, 33, 34). Verbal and visual memory, as well as blink rate, may also be associated with NSS (34, 35).

Rates of Neurological Soft Signs in Chinese and Caucasian Populations

Rates of NSS in our studies were similar to those found in Caucasian samples (36). To compare rates of NSS in patients and controls coming from different ethnic backgrounds more directly, we compared NSS in 289 Chinese and 132 Caucasian subjects (37). We established that in healthy controls, NSS were significantly correlated with estimates of verbal intelligence and, in the Chinese sample, also with educational attainment. Whereas motor coordination and sensory integration were inversely correlated with verbal intelligence estimates and education level for healthy Chinese subjects, only sensory integration showed a statistically significant association with verbal intelligence in the healthy Caucasian sample. Total NSS scores and the three NSS sub-scores (motor coordination, sensory integration, and disinhibition) of Chinese schizophrenia patients were correlated with age, educational attainment, and verbal intelligence estimates. No gender or ethnicity effect could be established for patients or controls although there was a trend for healthy Caucasians to have more sensory integration signs. Antipsychotic medication appeared to be moderately associated with NSS in Chinese patients, whereas anticholinergic medication was not. When clinical characteristics were examined, we found that negative symptoms in the 'thought' domain were significantly associated with overall NSS scores and in the sub-domains of motor coordination and sensory integration in female patients. There was no correlation between age and NSS in Chinese patients and controls when education level was controlled for. However, illness duration showed a significant association with total NSS and motor coordination signs.

Neurological Soft Signs as State and Trait Characteristics

We were also interested in whether neurological signs represented genetic or familial vulnerability factors (38). Our team recruited 15 Chinese schizophrenia patients, 21 of their non-psychotic siblings and 26 healthy controls and showed that both patients and their siblings had significantly higher global neurological impairments than healthy controls. Impairment of motor coordination of siblings was less pronounced than in schizophrenia patients, but higher than in healthy controls. Disinhibition signs were similar in patients and siblings, and lower in controls, whereas extrapyramidal and sensory integration signs were more severe in patients than in siblings or controls. These findings point towards a heterogeneous picture of NSS possibly underpinned by varying aetiologies in sub-categories. Bolton et al. (1998) also observed significant NSS in individuals with obsessive compulsive disorder (OCD) (39). Although we have not found direct and strong associations between NSS and negative symptoms in our studies, our systematic review of the literature demonstrated a clear link, and also an association with disorganisation symptoms (40). Questions remain regarding the confounding effects of age, education, and intelligence on the nature and frequency of NSS, and although NSS were not specific to schizophrenia, they appear to be both a state and trait variable in the course of the disorder.

Reflections: Neurological Soft Signs as a Proxy Measure of Brain Dysfunction

Despite NSS being easily detectable and occurring more frequently in FEP and schizophrenia patients, they are not routinely assessed in clinical practice. Their presence at illness onset is likely to represent neurodevelopmental processes indicative of vulnerability related to brain maturation. While we have to take into consideration their presence both as a trait and a state marker, our observation of their progression in otherwise stable chronic schizophrenia patients reflects ongoing changes in underlying brain circuitry following the onset of psychotic symptoms. Psychosis may then better be conceptualised as an evolving disorder rather than being the static end result of a neurodevelopmental disorder. We and Professor Chan's team in Beijing have also found several potential correlations between motor coordination and cognitive ability. Based on Wing et al.'s (1973) work on a finger-tapping task, we propose that, like simple motor tasks, digit recall requires an internal timer and the disruption of this internal timer may also underlie reduced efficiency of the phonological working memory loop (41).

More recent research has also shown that NSS are at least partly localisable with abnormalities detectable in the cerebellar-thalamic-prefrontal brain network (16). Evidence is now emerging that NSS are present in unipolar depression and bipolar disorder (42, 43, 44). It remains unclear whether the type or frequency of NSS differs in psychotic and mood disorders. Nonetheless, the presence of NSS may provide an early indication of brain dysfunction in a mental illness and their detection may allow better targeted monitoring and early intervention. Progressive NSS may also indicate a sub-group of patients who are likely to be or become treatment-resistant, and their monitoring may alert the clinician to consider better psychopharmacological options earlier in the course of the disorder.

NSS are simple to examine and are of low burden. An assessment does not require special equipment and can be completed in about ten minutes. They could be used more often as a pragmatic clinic-based proxy marker of neurocognitive dysfunction, and therefore, more extensive evaluation of NSS in clinic settings should be encouraged.

References

1. Manschreck TC, Ames D. Neurologic features and psychopathology in schizophrenic disorders. *Biol Psychiatry*. 1984;19(5):703-719.
2. Bombin I, Arango C, Buchanan RW. Significance and meaning of neurological signs in schizophrenia: two decades later. *Schizophr Bull*. 2005;31(4):962-977. doi:10.1093/schbul/sbi028
3. Wernicke C. *Lehrbuch der Gehirnkrankheiten für Ärzte und Studierende*. Theodor Fischer; 1881.
4. Bender L. Childhood schizophrenia; clinical study on one hundred schizophrenic children. *Am J Orthopsychiatry*. 1947;17(1):40-56. doi:10.1111/j.1939-0025.1947. tb04975.x
5. Rossi A, De Cataldo S, Di Michele V, et al. Neurological soft signs in schizophrenia. *Br J Psychiatry*. 1990;157:735-739. doi:10.1192/bjp.157.5.735
6. Torrey EF. Neurological abnormalities in schizophrenic patients. *Biol Psychiatry*. 1980;15(3):381-388.
7. Schröder J, Niethammer R, Geider FJ, et al. Neurological soft signs in schizophrenia. *Schizophr Res*. 1991;6(1):25-30. doi:10.1016/0920-9964(91)90017-l
8. Schröder J, Tittel A, Stockert A, Karr M. Memory deficits in subsyndromes of chronic schizophrenia. *Schizophr Res*. 1996;21(1):19-26. doi:10.1016/0920-9964(96)00027-8
9. Schröder J, Silvestri S, Bubeck B, et al. D2 dopamine receptor up-regulation, treatment response, neurological soft signs, and extrapyramidal side effects in schizophrenia: a follow-up study with 123I-iodobenzamide single photon emission computed tomography in the drug-naive state and after neuroleptic treatment. *Biol Psychiatry*. 1998;43(9):660-665. doi:10.1016/s0006-3223(97)00442-3
10. Bachmann S, Bottmer C, Schröder J. Neurological soft signs in first-episode schizophrenia: a follow-up study. *Am J Psychiatry*. 2005;162(12):2337-2343. doi:10.1176/appi. ajp.162.12.2337

216 • *Psychosis and Schizophrenia in Hong Kong*

11. Niethammer R, Weisbrod M, Schiesser S, et al. Genetic influence on laterality in schizophrenia? A twin study of neurological soft signs. *Am J Psychiatry.* 2000;157(2):272-274. doi:10.1176/appi.ajp.157.2.272

12. Chan RC, Gottesman II. Neurological soft signs as candidate endophenotypes for schizophrenia: a shooting star or a Northern star? *Neurosci Biobehav Rev.* 2008;32(5):957-971. doi:10.1016/j.neubiorev.2008.01.005

13. Xu T, Wang Y, Li Z, et al. Heritability and familiality of neurological soft signs: evidence from healthy twins, patients with schizophrenia and non-psychotic first-degree relatives. *Psychol Med.* 2016;46(1):117-123. doi:10.1017/S0033291715001580

14. Bachmann S, Degen C, Geider FJ, Schröder J. Neurological soft signs in the clinical course of schizophrenia: results of a meta-analysis. *Front Psychiatry.* 2014;5:185. Published Dec 23, 2014. doi:10.3389/fpsyt.2014.00185

15. Lizano P, Dhaliwal K, Lutz O, et al. Trajectory of neurological examination abnormalities in antipsychotic-naïve first-episode psychosis population: a 1-year follow-up study. *Psychol Med.* 2020;50(12):2057-2065. doi:10.1017/S0033291719002162

16. Zhao Q, Li Z, Huang J, et al. Neurological soft signs are not 'soft' in brain structure and functional networks: evidence from ALE meta-analysis. *Schizophr Bull.* 2014;40(3):626-641. doi:10.1093/schbul/sbt063

17. Cai XL, Wang YM, Wang Y, et al. Neurological soft signs are associated with altered cerebellar-cerebral functional connectivity in schizophrenia. *Schizophr Bull.* 2021;47(5):1452-1462. doi:10.1093/schbul/sbaa200

18. Li Z, Huang J, Hung KSY, et al. Cerebellar hypoactivation is associated with impaired sensory integration in schizophrenia. *J Abnorm Psychol.* 2021;130(1):102-111. doi:10.1037/abn0000636

19. Kong L, Herold CJ, Cheung EFC, Chan RCK, Schröder J. Neurological soft signs and brain network abnormalities in schizophrenia. *Schizophr Bull.* 2020;46(3):562-571. doi:10.1093/schbul/sbz118

20. Ferruccio NP, Tosato S, Lappin JM, et al. Neurological signs at the first psychotic episode as correlates of long-term outcome: results from the AESOP-10 study. *Schizophr Bull.* 2021;47(1):118-127. doi:10.1093/schbul/sbaa089

21. Chen EYH. Neurological signs and cognitive impairments in schizophrenia. *Hong Kong Journal of Psychiatry.* 1997;7(2):14-18.

22. Chen EY, Shapleske J, Luque R, et al. The Cambridge Neurological Inventory: a clinical instrument for assessment of soft neurological signs in psychiatric patients. *Psychiatry Res.* 1995;56(2):183-204. doi:10.1016/0165-1781(95)02535-2

23. Chan RC, Rao H, Chen EE, Ye B, Zhang C. The neural basis of motor sequencing: an fMRI study of healthy subjects. *Neurosci Lett.* 2006;398(3):189-194. doi:10.1016/j.neulet.2006.01.014

24. Chen EY, Lam LC, Chen RY, Nguyen DG. Neurological signs, age, and illness duration in schizophrenia. *J Nerv Ment Dis.* 1996;184(6):339-345. doi:10.1097/00005053-199606000-00002

25. Chen EY, Chan RC, Dunn EL, et al. Motor soft neurological signs in first-episode schizophrenia: a two-year longitudinal study. The 9th International Congress on Schizophrenia Research; Mar 29–Apr 2, 2003; Colorado Springs, CO. *Schizophr Res.* 2003;60(suppl. 1):129. doi:10.1016/S0920-9964(03)80909-X

26. Chen EY, Hui CL, Chan RC, et al. A 3-year prospective study of neurological soft signs in first-episode schizophrenia. *Schizophr Res.* 2005;75(1):45-54. doi:10.1016/j.schres.2004.09.002

27. Lam LCW, Chen EYH, Nguyen DGH, Chen RYL. Differential presentation of soft neurological signs and schizophrenic symptoms in relation to sex and age of onset. The 9th Biennial Winter Workshop on Schizophrenia; Feb 7–13, 1998; Davos, Switzerland. *Schizophr Res.* 1998;29(1-2):182. doi:10.1016/S0920-9964(97)88772-5

28. Chen EY, Kwok CL, Au JW, Chen RY, Lau BS. Progressive deterioration of soft neurological signs in chronic schizophrenic patients. *Acta Psychiatr Scand.* 2000;102(5):342-349. doi:10.1034/j.1600-0447.2000.102005342.x

29. Chen EYH, Lan BST. Deterioration of soft neurological signs in chronic schizophrenia patients: a longitudinal panel study. The 9th Biennial Winter Workshop on Schizophrenia; Feb 7–13, 1998; Davos, Switzerland. *Schizophr Res.* 1998;29(1-2):180. doi:10.1016/S0920-9964(97)88767-1

30. Lui SSY, Yip SSL, Wang Y, et al. Different trajectories of neurological soft signs progression between treatment-responsive and treatment-resistant schizophrenia patients. *J Psychiatr Res.* 2021;138:607-614. doi:10.1016/j.jpsychires.2021.05.018

31. Chen EY, Lam LC, Chen RY, Nguyen DG, Chan CK, Wilkins AJ. Neuropsychological correlates of sustained attention in schizophrenia. *Schizophr Res.* 1997;24(3):299-310. doi:10.1016/s0920-9964(96)00120-x

32. Chen EY, Lam LC, Chen RY, Nguyen DG, Kwok CL, Au JW. Neurological signs and sustained attention impairment in schizophrenia. *Eur Arch Psychiatry Clin Neurosci.* 2001;251(1):1-5. doi:10.1007/s004060170059

33. Chen EYH, Lam LCW, Wilkins A. Soft neurological signs and sustained attention impairment in schizophrenia. The 9th Biennial Winter Workshop on Schizophrenia; Feb 7–13, 1998; Davos, Switzerland. *Schizophr Res.* 1998;29(1-2):180-181. doi:10.1016/S0920-9964(97)88768-3

34. Chan RC, Wang Y, Wang L, et al. Neurological soft signs and their relationships to neurocognitive functions: a re-visit with the structural equation modeling design. *PLoS One.* 2009;4(12):e8469. Published Dec 24, 2009. doi:10.1371/journal.pone.0008469

35. Chan RC, Chen EY. Blink rate does matter: a study of blink rate, sustained attention, and neurological signs in schizophrenia. *J Nerv Ment Dis.* 2004;192(11):781-783. doi:10.1097/01.nmd.0000144697.48042.eb

36. Chan RC, Chen EY. Neurological abnormalities in Chinese schizophrenic patients. *Behav Neurol.* 2007;18(3):171-181. doi:10.1155/2007/451703

37. Chen EYH, Chan RCK. The Cambridge Neurological Inventory: clinical, demographic and ethnic correlates. *Psychiatric Annals.* 2003;33(3):202-210.

38. Chen YL, Chen YH, Mak FL. Soft neurological signs in schizophrenic patients and their nonpsychotic siblings. *J Nerv Ment Dis.* 2000;188(2):84-89. doi:10.1097/00005053-200002000-00004

39. Bolton D, Gibb W, Lees A, et al. Neurological soft signs in obsessive compulsive disorder: standardised assessment and comparison with schizophrenia. *Behav Neurol.* 1998;11(4):197-204. doi:10.1155/1999/639045

40. Hui CL, Wong GH, Chiu CP, Lam MM, Chen EY. Potential endophenotype for schizophrenia: neurological soft signs. *Ann Acad Med Singap.* 2009;38(5):408-6.

218 • *Psychosis and Schizophrenia in Hong Kong*

41. Wing A, Kristofferson A. Response delays and the timing of discrete motor responses. *Attention Perception & Psychophysics.* 1973;14(1):5-12. doi:10.3758/BF03198607
42. Zhao H, Guo W, Niu W, Zhong A, Zhou X. Brain area-related neurological soft signs in depressive patients with different types of childhood maltreatment. *Asia Pac Psychiatry.* 2015;7(3):286-291. doi:10.1111/appy.12172
43. Negash A, Kebede D, Alem A, et al. Neurological soft signs in bipolar I disorder patients. *J Affect Disord.* 2004;80(2-3):221-230. doi:10.1016/S0165-0327(03)00116-2
44. Sagheer TA, Assaad S, Haddad G, Hachem D, Haddad C, Hallit S. Neurological soft signs in bipolar and unipolar disorder: a case-control study. *Psychiatry Res.* 2018;261:253-258. doi:10.1016/j.psychres.2017.12.073

PART V

RECOVERY

17

Ways to Improve Cognition: Beyond Medications

Background

Cognitive impairments are considered a core feature of psychotic disorders. They involve a wide array of social and non-social cognitive domains and are usually detectable in the early stages of the illness. Cognitive disturbance has been shown to persist in the course of psychosis. It has a significant impact on functional outcomes and prognosis (1, 2).

Both social and non-social cognition have been extensively studied in psychotic disorders, and consistent associations with functional outcomes have been replicated across the world, with impairments in social cognition having an even greater effect on outcomes than deficits in non-social cognitive domains (3, 4, 5, 6). Cognitive dysfunction is often already present in the prodromal phase of the illness and progresses further in first-episode psychosis (7, 8). These deficits have been demonstrated in treated and untreated patients and can be a significant subjective experience affecting perceived recovery (9, 10).

Pharmacological and Non-pharmacological Approaches to Improving Cognition

Pharmacological and non-pharmacological interventions have been explored to enhance cognition. Several hypotheses involving diverse neurotransmitter systems, particularly glutamatergic and cholinergic pathways, have been explored. However, despite extensive efforts, pharmacological approaches have at best yielded small effect sizes for cognitive dysfunction (11, 12). Keefe et al. (2007) in their randomised, double-blind multicentre trial involving 400 patients demonstrated modest effects of atypical antipsychotics on neurocognition after 12 and 52 weeks of treatment (13). α-Amino-3-hydroxy-5-methyl-4-isoxazolepropionate (AMPA) receptor agonists and cholinesterase inhibitors showed small to medium effects on working memory in early trials. However, none of these findings have been replicated in larger phase III studies (12). Similarly, several research teams have investigated the effects of oxytocin on social cognition. A recent meta-analysis of 12 studies did not find an overall effect of intranasal oxytocin versus placebo on social cognitive measures, although several studies suggested significant but small positive effects for mentalising tasks (14).

Several non-pharmacological interventions have also been investigated, ranging from repetitive transcranial magnetic stimulation (rTMS), transcranial direct current stimulation (tDCS) therapy, social skills training, and cognitive remediation to exercise. High-frequency rTMS positioned over the dorsolateral prefrontal cortex has been shown to significantly enhance working memory in schizophrenia patients, and improvements appear to have been maintained in the longer term. Language function also appears to benefit from this treatment (15).

A recent meta-analysis revealed robust medium to large improvements in social cognition in the domains of facial affect recognition, mentalising and social perception when participants received social cognitive training (16). Evidence also suggests that social skills training may lead to structural and functional brain changes (17). Interestingly, gains in social cognition were not accompanied by improvements in non-social cognition and vice versa (16, 18). Questions remain as to whether treatment effects are long-lasting and whether they translate into real-world improvements in social interaction (19).

Cognitive remediation has shown significant, moderate gains in cognitive functioning and is associated with structural white and grey matter changes, as well as functional brain changes in prefrontal and thalamic areas (18, 20, 21). However, these gains have not been shown to translate tidily into improved functional outcomes, and it has been recognised that additional interventions are necessary to achieve meaningful changes in psychosocial functioning (22, 23).

The Effects of Aerobic Exercise on Cognitive Functioning

There has been longstanding interest in the effects of aerobic exercise on outcomes in schizophrenia, given the fact that a significant proportion of patients also experience metabolic side effects of prescribed antipsychotic medication affecting both physical morbidity and mortality (24). In addition, schizophrenia patients are known to be less physically active than the general population and have significant difficulties associated with motivation (25). Robust improvements in clinical symptoms as a result of engaging in physical exercise have been reported by Vancampfort et al. (2012) (26). A meta-analysis has also shown that physical exercise can improve global cognition and specific sub-domains in schizophrenia compared to non-aerobic control activities and that greater amounts of exercise lead to larger improvements in cognitive functioning (27). It appears that better aerobic fitness may lead to enhancements in specific cognitive domains, such as short-term memory, and correlates with changes in hippocampal volumes (28).

Pajonk et al. (2010) undertook a study to determine whether aerobic exercise would increase the hippocampal volume of patients with schizophrenia (28). With exercise training, relative hippocampal volumes significantly increased in both patients (12%) and controls (16%), and were correlated with measures of improved aerobic fitness. Also, cognitive performance for short-term memory was correlated with changes in hippocampal volumes (29). Small pilot studies have investigated the combination of cognitive remediation and aerobic exercise and have shown differential improvements in several domains of cognition and psychosocial functioning (29).

Mind-Body Exercises and Their Impact on Symptomatology and Quality of Life

Other forms of exercise such as yoga and Tai chi have been less well studied despite their popularity. Yoga is considered to encompass exercises for the mind and body with a distinctive meditative component. A recent meta-analysis by Govindaraj et al. (2020) suggests that add-on yoga can improve quality of life, cognitive symptoms, and positive and negative symptoms in patients with schizophrenia. These positive changes may be mediated via neurohormonal and functional changes in brain activity (30).

The underlying neurobiological mechanisms of improved cognitive functioning mediated by mind-body exercises remain largely unknown. Several hypotheses have been suggested such as increases in parasympathetic nervous activity and attenuation of sympathetic activity during controlled breathing (31, 32). Yoga practice has been shown to reduce salivary cortisol levels in patients with depressive and anxiety disorders, as well as healthy controls (33, 34, 35). Increases in brain γ-aminobutyric acid (GABA) levels, blood serotonin concentration, and higher serum dopamine levels have also been reported (36, 37, 38). It is thought that with yoga practice a reduction in stress-related physiological parameters leads to improved cognition, particularly in light of the finding that high psychological arousal and stress affect working memory (39, 40, 41).

Studies on Interventions for Cognitive Dysfunction in Hong Kong

In Hong Kong, several studies have examined both pharmacological and non-pharmacological interventions regarding their efficacy in improving neuropsychological functioning, with a particular emphasis on aerobic exercise and yoga practice.

Motivation to Engage in Exercise in Psychosis

To understand how to best promote regular physical activity among psychosis patients, we first surveyed the physical activity states of a representative sample of psychosis patients (42, 43). Within a motivational framework, just over half of our sample had the intention to engage in regular physical exercise, a quarter were in the preparation stage, less than 20% were in the precontemplation stage, and only 6.1% were in the action and maintenance stage. Across the different stages of change, patients exhibited significant differences in self-efficacy. These findings were an important first step to identifying factors affecting patients' motivation to engage in physical exercise and to considering how interventions can be best tailored to encourage maintenance of physical activity among psychosis patients.

Aerobic Exercise, High-Intensity Interval Training, Yoga, and Tai Chi in Psychosis

We investigated the differential effects of aerobic exercise and yoga programmes compared to a waitlist control group with a randomised controlled trial (RCT) (44, 45, 46). Significant improvements in general health, physical functioning, energy, emotional well-being, and depressive symptoms were evident after a 12-week course of three times weekly Hatha yoga sessions lasting 60 minutes each, or thrice weekly supervised walking or cycling exercises (44, 46). Negative symptoms also improved in the yoga group. Verbal acquisition, working memory, and attention were enhanced in the yoga group, and working memory in the aerobic exercise group. Aerobic exercise was associated with an increase in hippocampal grey matter volume, particularly in the left hippocampus. No such changes were found in the yoga group. We also detected increased thickness of the left superior frontal gyrus and right inferior frontal gyrus in the aerobic exercise group, and volume increases in the post-central gyrus and posterior corpus callosum in the yoga group. Changes in the post-central gyrus appeared to correlate well with enhancements in working memory (47). A positive association between the number of sessions attended and changes in working memory was observed. However, no significant difference in physical fitness was found as measured by VO2 max/kg, and changes in fitness were not correlated with changes in cognitive performance (46).

We also reported on the amplitude of low-frequency fluctuations (ALFF) using resting-state functional magnetic resonance imaging (fMRI) (48). ALFF is an indicator reflecting spontaneous neural activity in the brain (49). Studies have shown that intrinsic resting-state activity promotes specific brain circuits to participate in cognitive tasks. Resting activity predicts subsequent task-induced brain responses and behavioural performance (50). ALFF measures brain activity without cognitive load, and brain abnormalities in this state that are associated with cognition might be the basis for cognitive impairments seen in schizophrenia (51). In the yoga group, ALFF changes in the precuneus were significantly correlated with changes in Positive and Negative Syndrome Scale (PANSS) negative scores, especially with blunted affect sub-scores (48).

Having shown the effectiveness of both yoga and aerobic exercise on cognitive ability, we and our collaborator Rainbow Ho were interested in exploring whether another mind-body exercise, Tai chi, could yield similar results. This form of exercise is rooted in Eastern health philosophy, with an emphasis on motor coordination and relaxation (52, 53). We showed that compared to a control group, chronic schizophrenia patients who had engaged in thrice weekly Tai chi practice over three months had significant decreases in motor deficits, and increases in backward digit span and mean cortisol, while the aerobic exercise group displayed significant decreases in motor deficits, negative and depression symptoms, and increases in forward digit span, daily living function, and mean cortisol (53).

Like yoga, Tai chi, and aerobic exercise, high-intensity interval training (HIIT) can also enhance cognitive functioning, with improvements in sleep-dependent procedural memory being more pronounced after 12 weeks (54). This study extended the range of cognitive benefits from hippocampus-based verbal memory to striatum-based procedural memory. It also initiated an important link between exercise and sleep activity. Sleep is disrupted in schizophrenia. Exercise itself has a sleep-promoting effect. The discovery that exercise and cognition can be mediated by sleep-dependent memory consolidation processes suggests a new pathway in which exercise could facilitate cognition.

Motivational Coaching and Exercise

Despite the positive effects of various forms of exercise on physical, emotional, and cognitive well-being, as well as better psychosocial functioning, psychosis patients have disproportionate difficulties with self-motivation and thus find it difficult to sustain physical exercise (55, 56). We have shown that adjunctive motivational coaching in a group setting can be effective in increasing physical activity in patients immediately following an exercise programme and six months thereafter. It appears that younger patients, those who were unmarried, unemployed, and had a longer duration of untreated psychosis benefited the most from motivational coaching (55).

Pharmacological Strategies to Improve Cognition

Nutritional neuroprotective agents may also provide opportunities for cognitive improvements. HT1001, a proprietary North American ginseng extract containing known levels of active ginsenosides, was shown in our RCT to improve visual

Reflections: The Emerging Evidence of Exercise Interventions Supporting Cognitive Recovery

Psychotic disorders are complex illnesses manifesting clinically with psychotic episodes. Yet alongside a psychotic episode, there are many other facets. Psychosis was debilitating before the advent of antipsychotic medication. With psychopharmacology, treatment of psychotic symptoms, and prevention of relapse became possible for a large proportion of patients. When positive psychotic symptoms are well controlled, the outcome in functioning is more determined by other facets of the disorder, such as cognition and negative symptoms. Antipsychotic medication is not particularly effective in alleviating cognitive dysfunction or negative symptoms and there is a pressing need to develop alternative interventions. The neurobiological underpinnings of cognitive dysfunction in psychosis are complex. Apart from the likely involvement of a large number of genes, recent research has implicated an increasingly wide range of factors that could diffusely affect brain systems, such as immune and inflammatory processes, oxidative stress, myelination, and metabolic and inhibitory processes. Accordingly, it would be reasonable to expect interventional efficacy from diverse approaches that are likely to have more diffuse rather than focal effects.

We have focused on physical activity interventions based on the observation that physical inactivity is a particularly prevalent problem for psychosis patients. As physical activity is associated with a wide range of brain and systemic processes, it is reasonable to expect that it could help reverse some of the deterioration in brain functioning and physical health. There is increasing evidence that exercise can improve cognitive, symptomatic, and functional outcomes, as well as improve metabolic parameters. These are areas of concern in the long-term outcome of psychosis. Exercise interventions provide a promising way to address these challenges, which are not only untouched but probably aggravated by antipsychotic medication. One particular difficulty of exercise interventions is sustainability. This is an area where behavioural and cultural factors may be decisive in driving biological processes against deleterious outcomes. This may involve motivational coaching, the creative use of mobile technology and reconceptualising physical exercise as part of daily living activities.

The possibility of improving neuroplasticity and cognitive outcomes with physical exercise, pharmacological augmentation and cognitive strategies is not only an exciting area of research but also an important message to patients to help them come to terms with an often devastating diagnosis and to engage them meaningfully in treatment planning, as well as improving adherence over the long term.

References

1. Rund BR. A review of longitudinal studies of cognitive functions in schizophrenia patients. *Schizophr Bull.* 1998;24(3):425-435. doi:10.1093/oxfordjournals.schbul. a033337
2. Malla AK, Norman RM, Manchanda R, Townsend L. Symptoms, cognition, treatment adherence and functional outcome in first-episode psychosis. *Psychol Med.* 2002;32(6):1109-1119. doi:10.1017/s0033291702006050
3. Green MF. What are the functional consequences of neurocognitive deficits in schizophrenia? *Am J Psychiatry.* 1996;153(3):321-330. doi:10.1176/ajp.153.3.321
4. Green MF, Kern RS, Heaton RK. Longitudinal studies of cognition and functional outcome in schizophrenia: implications for MATRICS. *Schizophr Res.* 2004;72(1):41-51. doi:10.1016/j.schres.2004.09.009
5. Couture SM, Penn DL, Roberts DL. The functional significance of social cognition in schizophrenia: a review. *Schizophr Bull.* 2006;32 Suppl 1(Suppl 1):S44-S63. doi:10.1093/schbul/sbl029
6. Fett AK, Viechtbauer W, Dominguez MD, Penn DL, van Os J, Krabbendam L. The relationship between neurocognition and social cognition with functional outcomes in schizophrenia: a meta-analysis. *Neurosci Biobehav Rev.* 2011;35(3):573-588. doi:10.1016/j.neubiorev.2010.07.001
7. Carrión RE, Goldberg TE, McLaughlin D, Auther AM, Correll CU, Cornblatt BA. Impact of neurocognition on social and role functioning in individuals at clinical high risk for psychosis. *Am J Psychiatry.* 2011;168(8):806-813. doi:10.1176/appi. ajp.2011.10081209
8. Horan WP, Green MF, DeGroot M, et al. Social cognition in schizophrenia, Part 2: 12-month stability and prediction of functional outcome in first-episode patients. *Schizophr Bull.* 2012;38(4):865-872. doi:10.1093/schbul/sbr001
9. Bilder RM, Goldman RS, Robinson D, et al. Neuropsychology of first-episode schizophrenia: initial characterization and clinical correlates. *Am J Psychiatry.* 2000;157(4):549-559. doi:10.1176/appi.ajp.157.4.549
10. Chen EY, Tam DK, Wong JW, Law CW, Chiu CP. Self-administered instrument to measure the patient's experience of recovery after first-episode psychosis: development and validation of the Psychosis Recovery Inventory. *Aust N Z J Psychiatry.* 2005;39(6):493-499. doi:10.1080/j.1440-1614.2005.01609.x
11. Geyer MA, Tamminga CA. Measurement and treatment research to improve cognition in schizophrenia: neuropharmacological aspects. *Psychopharmacology* 2004;174:1-2. doi:10.1007/s00213-004-1846-2
12. Sinkeviciute I, Begemann M, Prikken M, et al. Efficacy of different types of cognitive enhancers for patients with schizophrenia: a meta-analysis. *NPJ Schizophr.* 2018;4(1):22. Published Oct 25, 2018. doi:10.1038/s41537-018-0064-6

228 • *Psychosis and Schizophrenia in Hong Kong*

13. Keefe RS, Sweeney JA, Gu H, et al. Effects of olanzapine, quetiapine, and risperidone on neurocognitive function in early psychosis: a randomized, double-blind 52-week comparison. *Am J Psychiatry.* 2007;164(7):1061-1071. doi:10.1176/ajp.2007.164.7.1061

14. Bürkner PC, Williams DR, Simmons TC, Woolley JD. Intranasal oxytocin may improve high-level social cognition in schizophrenia, but not social cognition or neurocognition in general: a multilevel Bayesian meta-analysis. *Schizophr Bull.* 2017;43(6):1291-1303. doi:10.1093/schbul/sbx053

15. Jiang Y, Guo Z, Xing G, et al. Effects of High-Frequency transcranial magnetic stimulation for cognitive deficit in schizophrenia: a meta-analysis. *Front Psychiatry.* 2019;10:135. Published Mar 29, 2019. doi:10.3389/fpsyt.2019.00135

16. Kurtz MM, Gagen E, Rocha NB, Machado S, Penn DL. Comprehensive treatments for social cognitive deficits in schizophrenia: a critical review and effect-size analysis of controlled studies. *Clin Psychol Rev.* 2016;43:80-89. doi:10.1016/j.cpr.2015.09.003

17. Campos C, Santos S, Gagen E, et al. Neuroplastic changes following social cognition training in schizophrenia: a systematic review. *Neuropsychol Rev.* 2016;26(3):310-328. doi:10.1007/s11065-016-9326-0

18. Prikken M, Konings MJ, Lei WU, Begemann MJH, Sommer IEC. The efficacy of computerized cognitive drill and practice training for patients with a schizophrenia-spectrum disorder: a meta-analysis. *Schizophr Res.* 2019;204:368-374. doi:10.1016/j.schres.2018.07.034

19. Horan WP, Green MF. Treatment of social cognition in schizophrenia: current status and future directions. *Schizophr Res.* 2019;203:3-11. doi:10.1016/j.schres.2017.07.013

20. Best MW, Bowie CR. A review of cognitive remediation approaches for schizophrenia: from top-down to bottom-up, brain training to psychotherapy. *Expert Rev Neurother.* 2017;17(7):713-723. doi:10.1080/14737175.2017.1331128

21. Wykes T, Huddy V, Cellard C, McGurk SR, Czobor P. A meta-analysis of cognitive remediation for schizophrenia: methodology and effect sizes. *Am J Psychiatry.* 2011;168(5):472-485. doi:10.1176/appi.ajp.2010.10060855

22. Penadés R, González-Rodríguez A, Catalán R, Segura B, Bernardo M, Junqué C. Neuroimaging studies of cognitive remediation in schizophrenia: a systematic and critical review. *World J Psychiatry.* 2017;7(1):34-43. Published Mar 22, 2017. doi:10.5498/wjp.v7.i1.34

23. Ran MS, Chen EY. Cognitive enhancement therapy for schizophrenia. *Lancet.* 2004;364(9452):2163-2165. doi:10.1016/S0140-6736(04)17609-5

24. Rotella F, Cassioli E, Calderani E, et al. Long-term metabolic and cardiovascular effects of antipsychotic drugs. A meta-analysis of randomized controlled trials. *Eur Neuropsychopharmacol.* 2020;32:56-65. doi:10.1016/j.euroneuro.2019.12.118

25. Lindamer LA, McKibbin C, Norman GJ, et al. Assessment of physical activity in middle-aged and older adults with schizophrenia. *Schizophr Res.* 2008;104(1-3):294-301. doi:10.1016/j.schres.2008.04.040

26. Vancampfort D, Probst M, Helvik Skjaerven L, et al. Systematic review of the benefits of physical therapy within a multidisciplinary care approach for people with schizophrenia. *Phys Ther.* 2012;92(1):11-23. doi:10.2522/ptj.20110218

Ways to Improve Cognition • 229

27. Firth J, Stubbs B, Rosenbaum S, et al. aerobic exercise improves cognitive functioning in people with schizophrenia: a systematic review and meta-analysis. *Schizophr Bull.* 2017;43(3):546-556. doi:10.1093/schbul/sbw115

28. Pajonk FG, Wobrock T, Gruber O, et al. Hippocampal plasticity in response to exercise in schizophrenia. *Arch Gen Psychiatry.* 2010;67(2):133-143. doi:10.1001/archgenpsychiatry.2009.193

29. Jahshan C, Rassovsky Y, Green MF. Enhancing neuroplasticity to augment cognitive remediation in schizophrenia. *Front Psychiatry.* 2017;8:191. Published Sep 27, 2017. doi:10.3389/fpsyt.2017.00191

30. Govindaraj R, Varambally S, Rao NP, Venkatasubramanian G, Gangadhar BN. Does Yoga Have a Role in Schizophrenia Management? *Curr Psychiatry Rep.* 2020;22(12):78. Published Nov 3, 2020. doi:10.1007/s11920-020-01199-4

31. Innes KE, Bourguignon C, Taylor AG. Risk indices associated with the insulin resistance syndrome, cardiovascular disease, and possible protection with yoga: a systematic review. *J Am Board Fam Pract.* 2005;18(6):491-519. doi:10.3122/jabfm.18.6.491

32. Udupa K, Madanmohan, Bhavanani AB, Vijayalakshmi P, Krishnamurthy N. Effect of pranayam training on cardiac function in normal young volunteers. *Indian J Physiol Pharmacol.* 2003;47(1):27-33.

33. Granath J, Ingvarsson S, von Thiele U, Lundberg U. Stress management: a randomized study of cognitive behavioural therapy and yoga. *Cogn Behav Ther.* 2006;35(1):3-10. doi:10.1080/16506070500401292

34. Michalsen A, Grossman P, Acil A, et al. Rapid stress reduction and anxiolysis among distressed women as a consequence of a three-month intensive yoga program. *Med Sci Monit.* 2005;11(12):CR555-CR561.

35. West J, Otte C, Geher K, Johnson J, Mohr DC. Effects of Hatha yoga and African dance on perceived stress, affect, and salivary cortisol. *Ann Behav Med.* 2004;28(2):114-118. doi:10.1207/s15324796abm2802_6

36. Streeter CC, Jensen JE, Perlmutter RM, et al. Yoga Asana sessions increase brain GABA levels: a pilot study. *J Altern Complement Med.* 2007;13(4):419-426. doi:10.1089/acm.2007.6338

37. Yu X, Fumoto M, Nakatani Y, et al. Activation of the anterior prefrontal cortex and serotonergic system is associated with improvements in mood and EEG changes induced by Zen meditation practice in novices. *Int J Psychophysiol.* 2011;80(2):103-111. doi:10.1016/j.ijpsycho.2011.02.004

38. Jung YH, Kang DH, Jang JH, et al. The effects of mind-body training on stress reduction, positive affect, and plasma catecholamines. *Neurosci Lett.* 2010;479(2):138-142. doi:10.1016/j.neulet.2010.05.048

39. Rocha KK, Ribeiro AM, Rocha KC, et al. Improvement in physiological and psychological parameters after 6 months of yoga practice. *Conscious Cogn.* 2012;21(2):843-850. doi:10.1016/j.concog.2012.01.014

40. Elzinga BM, Roelofs K. Cortisol-induced impairments of working memory require acute sympathetic activation. *Behav Neurosci.* 2005;119(1):98-103. doi:10.1037/0735-7044.119.1.98

41. Buchanan TW, Tranel D. Stress and emotional memory retrieval: effects of sex and cortisol response. *Neurobiol Learn Mem.* 2008;89(2):134-141. doi:10.1016/j.nlm.2007.07.003

42. Lee JTM, Lee EHM, Chan SKW, Chang WC, Chen EYH, Hui CLM. T133 Understanding the physical activity behaviour among patients with psychosis. The 4th Biennial Schizophrenia International Research Conference, Florence, Italy, 5-9 April 2014. In *Schizophr Res.* 2014;153(Suppl. 1): S337. doi:10.1016/S0920-9964(14)70950-8

43. Lee JTM, Law EYL, Lo LLH, et al. Psychosocial factors associated with physical activity behavior among patients with psychosis. *Schizophr Res.* 2018;195:130-135. doi:10.1016/j.schres.2017.09.042

44. Lin J, Lam M, Chiu C, et al. The impacts of yoga and exercise on neuro-cognitive function and symptoms in early psychosis. The 13th International Congress on Schizophrenia Research (ICOSR 2011); Apr 2–6, 2011; Colorado Springs, CO. In *Schizophr Bull.* 2011;37(Suppl. 1):171. doi:10.1093/schbul/sbq173

45. Chen EYH, Lin X, Lam MML, et al. The impacts of yoga and aerobic exercise on neuro-cognition and brain structure in early psychosis: a preliminary analysis of the randomized controlled clinical trial. The 3rd Biennial Schizophrenia International Research Conference (SIRS 2012); Apr 14–18, 2012; Florence, Italy. In *Schizophr Res.* 2012;136(Suppl. 1):S56.

46. Lin J, Chan SK, Lee EH, et al. Aerobic exercise and yoga improve neurocognitive function in women with early psychosis. *NPJ Schizophr.* 2015;1(0):15047. Published Dec 2, 2015. doi:10.1038/npjschz.2015.47

47. Lin, J. [林晶霞]. *The impacts of aerobic exercise and mind-body exercise (yoga) on neuro-cognition and clinical symptoms in early psychosis: a single-blind randomized controlled clinical trial.* (Thesis). Pokfulam, Hong Kong SAR: University of Hong Kong; 2013. doi:10.5353/th_b5177314

48. Lin J, Geng X, Lee EH, et al. Yoga reduces the brain's amplitude of low-frequency fluctuations in patients with early psychosis results of a randomized controlled trial. *Schizophr Res.* 2017;184:141-142. doi:10.1016/j.schres.2016.11.040

49. Wang P, Yang J, Yin Z, et al. Amplitude of low-frequency fluctuation (ALFF) may be associated with cognitive impairment in schizophrenia: a correlation study. *BMC Psychiatry.* 2019;19(1):30. Published Jan 17, 2019. doi:10.1186/s12888-018-1992-4

50. Zou Q, Ross TJ, Gu H, et al. Intrinsic resting-state activity predicts working memory brain activation and behavioral performance. *Hum Brain Mapp.* 2013;34(12):3204-3215. doi:10.1002/hbm.22136

51. Xu Y, Zhuo C, Qin W, Zhu J, Yu C. Altered spontaneous brain activity in schizophrenia: a meta-analysis and a large-sample study. *Biomed Res Int.* 2015;2015:204628. doi:10.1155/2015/204628

52. Ho RT, Wan AH, Au-Yeung FS, et al. The psychophysiological effects of Tai-chi and exercise in residential schizophrenic patients: a 3-arm randomized controlled trial. *BMC Complement Altern Med.* 2014;14:364. Published Sep 27, 2014. doi:10.1186/1472-6882-14-364

53. Ho RT, Fong TC, Wan AH, et al. A randomized controlled trial on the psychophysiological effects of physical exercise and Tai-chi in patients with chronic schizophrenia. *Schizophr Res.* 2016;171(1-3):42-49. doi:10.1016/j.schres.2016.01.038

54. Lo LLH, Lee EHM, Hui CLM, et al. Effect of high-endurance exercise intervention on sleep-dependent procedural memory consolidation in individuals with schizophrenia: a randomized controlled trial [published online ahead of print, Oct 7, 2021]. *Psychol Med.* 2021;1-13. doi:10.1017/S0033291721003196

55. Suen YN, Lo LHL, Lee EH, et al. Motivational coaching augmentation of exercise intervention for early psychotic disorders: A randomised controlled trial. *Aust N Z J Psychiatry.* 2022;56(10):1277-1286. doi:10.1177/00048674211061496

56. Lee EH, Hui CL, Chang WC, et al. Impact of physical activity on functioning of patients with first-episode psychosis – a 6-month prospective longitudinal study. *Schizophr Res.* 2013;150(2-3):538-541. doi:10.1016/j.schres.2013.08.034

57. Chen EY, Hui CL. HT1001, a proprietary North American ginseng extract, improves working memory in schizophrenia: a double-blind, placebo-controlled study. *Phytother Res.* 2012;26(8):1166-1172. doi:10.1002/ptr.3700

18

Remission and Recovery: The Journeys towards Getting Well

Background

The Concepts of Remission and Recovery

Recovery is considered the ultimate goal of treatment in psychosis and focuses on patients regaining functional abilities, and participating in meaningful social and vocational activities (1). Several criteria have been proposed to define recovery; however, a consensus definition has not been achieved to date. Criteria for recovery have included being either symptom-free or achieving a low score on rating scales such as the Positive and Negative Syndrome Scale (PANSS), and maintaining functional improvement for a specified duration such as two or five years (2, 3). Although no clear operational definition has been agreed upon, researchers concur that recovery involves the development of a sense of hope, self-reliance, and awareness of one's strengths and limitations (2, 4).

In contrast, remission has been more clearly defined. The Remission in Schizophrenia Working Group (RSWG) developed a consensus definition of symptomatic remission and proposed criteria for remission based on key symptoms of schizophrenia. It was also specified that symptoms must all have a severity score of mild or less for at least six months (5, 6). In their systematic review of 32 studies examining remission using the RSWG criteria, Lambert et al. (2010) found that 70% of patients achieved remission at some point during the follow-up period (6). Remission rates were reported to increase over time from 24% at six months to 39% at 12 months, 47% at two years and up to 55% at longer follow-up periods. The first episode of psychosis was associated with a higher remission rate compared to several episodes (48% vs. 43%).

The Subjective Experience of Remission and Recovery

Since the introduction of the RSWG criteria, there has been relatively little data on service users' and clinicians' perspectives on remission. In an observational study of 131 patients with schizophrenia, of the 58 patients who had achieved remission according to RSWG criteria, only 39% of patients and 32% of their relatives agreed that this was the case (7). 61% of psychiatrists considered that remission had been achieved, and in only 18% of cases, all three groups agreed in their assessment of patients' remission status. Patients' assessment of their clinical status diverged most from RSWG remission, whereas psychiatrists' assessment showed the best accordance. Interestingly, subjective well-being was considered most important for remission by patients, whereas relatives favoured both subjective well-being and symptom reduction, and psychiatrists also regarded functional improvement as an important goal. These preliminary results point towards the need for a more thorough assessment and consideration of patients' and relatives' experiences of illness, remission, and recovery.

Rates of Recovery in Psychosis

In contrast to remission, recovery is attained less often. Jääskeläinen and colleagues (2013) undertook a meta-analysis of 37 studies comprising approximately 9000 patients with schizophrenia to examine recovery rates. They defined recovery as having made improvements in clinical and social domains, with improvements in at least one domain persisting for at least two years, and current symptoms no worse than mild. They reported a median recovery rate of 13.5% (8). Similarly, the Schizophrenia Outpatients Health Outcomes (SOHO) study, which analysed data from 6,642 patients, showed that 13% achieved long-lasting functional remission during a 3-year follow-up period (9). However, among first-episode psychosis (FEP) patients a more recent systematic review and meta-analysis showed much higher remission and recovery rates of 38%, with recovery rates being stable after the first two years, thereby suggesting that a progressive deteriorating course of illness was not typical (10). Existing remission criteria often do not distinguish between different symptom dimensions. There may be a need to specify the symptom dimension in which remission is anchored. From the perspective that relapse mainly relates to positive symptoms, it may be important to specify criteria for positive symptom remission.

The Personal Recovery Approach

Over the last 15 to 20 years, efforts have focused on the concept of personal recovery, considered by Anthony (1993) as 'a deeply personal, unique process of changing one's attitudes, values, feelings, goals, skills, and/or roles. It is a way of living a satisfying, hopeful, and contributing life even within the limitations caused by illness. Recovery involves the development of new meaning and purpose in one's life as one grows beyond the catastrophic effects of mental illness' (11).

Mental health policy in many countries has adopted a personal recovery approach and several recovery frameworks have been developed, most notably the CHIME framework (12, 13, 14, 15, 16, 17, 18). This framework has emerged from a systematic review and narrative synthesis of recovery and consists of 13 characteristics involving the recovery journey, five recovery processes, and recovery stage descriptions. The recovery processes encompass connectedness, hope and optimism about the future, identity, meaning in life, and empowerment, giving rise to the acronym CHIME (18).

Research into recovery and personal recovery has not only been hampered by the lack of an operationalised definition but also by difficulties in developing comprehensive, reliable, and valid measures to capture this multifaceted concept (19).

Studies on Remission and Recovery in Hong Kong

In Hong Kong, our interest in the concepts of remission and recovery emerged alongside the development of the city-wide early intervention programme in the early 2000s. Although the majority of clinicians regularly addressed the issue of remission and recovery in consultations, most considered there to be major differences in expectations among patients, caregivers and healthcare professionals (20). A significant proportion of clinicians had noticed that patients and their caregivers were more focused on regaining full premorbid functioning rather than on relapse prevention. In addition, we established differences in the way healthcare professionals and patients viewed remission. Clinicians predominantly concentrated on alleviating positive, affective, cognitive, and negative symptoms to help patients achieve remission, whereas patients were less focused on symptom reduction (20, 21). Recovery for clinicians, on the other hand, was defined by attaining independence, meeting their patients' and caregivers' expectations, and improving social interaction and patients' self-esteem (20).

Remission, Functional Outcome, and Subjective Quality of Life

Due to limited data on the concurrent and predictive validity of the RSWG consensus definition of symptomatic remission in the early course of psychosis, Chang et al. (2013) explored its relationship with functional outcomes and subjective quality of life (SQoL) in a cohort of FEP patients aged 18 to 55 years (22). In their sample, almost 60% of patients achieved symptomatic remission after twelve months of treatment. Remitted patients had significantly fewer negative and disorganisation symptoms at initial presentation compared to those who had not attained remission. In addition to fewer positive and negative symptoms, patients in remission also had significantly lower symptom scores in disorganisation and excitement dimensions, superior functional outcomes, and better SQoL than non-remitters. The remission rate increased to over 80% after two years of follow-up and was associated with fewer psychotic and depressive symptoms and with higher levels of functioning and SQoL. However, sustained symptomatic remission rates were found to be below 50% at three years (23). At three years, verbal memory impairment, premorbid functioning, and negative symptom severity independently predicted remission status (23). Remission status appeared to independently predict functional outcomes even when the effects of educational level, baseline functioning, and negative symptom scores were controlled for. From the findings, Chang et al. (2013) concluded that the RSWG's operationally defined criteria for symptomatic remission represented a clinically valid construct that was closely related to concurrent and longitudinal outcomes in psychopathology, functioning, and SQoL in the early stage of psychosis (22).

Remission and Recovery in Youth with First-Episode Psychosis

Chang et al. (2012) found a remission rate of almost 60% in youth presenting with FEP (24). In contrast, only around 17% of young people had attained recovery after three years of intervention, and around half had not achieved symptomatic or functional remission in the last 12 months of follow-up. Less than half of those who achieved sustained symptomatic remission were also in functional remission. Predictors of symptomatic remission in youth with FEP were female sex, older age at onset of psychosis, shorter duration of untreated psychosis (DUP) and early symptom resolution, and possibly better cognitive performance (24, 25). Higher educational attainment, superior baseline occupational status, and shorter DUP were found to be predictive of recovery (24).

Long-term clinical remission was predicted by a shorter DUP. Higher educational levels and a shorter period of unemployment during the initial three years of FEP predicted functional recovery. Complete recovery was associated with a higher educational level and longer employment, in addition to medication discontinuation in the first three years of the illness (26).

We used qualitative interviews to gain a better understanding of how young people view their early symptoms of FEP and their recovery. Several themes around the subjective perception of psychotic experiences, pathways to care, stigma, and perceived recovery were identified (27, 28). Participants seemed to view psychosis or *sijueshitiao* (思覺失調) as more positive with a better outlook compared to schizophrenia or *jingshenfenliezheng* (精神分裂症). One patient attributed their illness to 'unbalanced dopamine levels in the brain'. In contrast to chronic physical illnesses, psychotic disorders were thought to be more mysterious, less understood, and more debilitating. Feelings of loss, uncertainty about the future, and fear associated with the experience of losing touch with reality emerged as sub-themes. Patients' perception of recovery was focused on regaining previous cognitive and social functioning. They believed that participating in meaningful activities that contributed to and introduced them to the world of others would enable them to be less preoccupied with their own inner worlds. Most participants did not think that they had fully recovered because they still needed medication and psychiatric support. Concerns about perceived side effects of medication were significant and recurrent, and the ability to bear children while on medication was also raised. These concerns negatively affected participants' confidence about re-entering the workplace.

In relation to stigma, participants expressed significant anxiety about whether to disclose their diagnosis to friends, family, prospective employers, and colleagues. All of them said that they had concealed the illness from others, except for immediate family members living in the same household. The perceived consequences of disclosure included being rejected, gossiped about, treated differently, and discriminated against in the workplace, as well as having their ability to travel restricted. The subject of stigma experienced by individuals with psychosis is discussed in detail in Chapter 2.

Some of the participants considered their illness life-enhancing. They reported having developed new values and views on life and relationships, slowing down in their pace of life, placing greater emphasis on meaningful relationships, enjoying simple pleasures, supporting others, and being more mature. Patients with FEP also believed that they had made better progress compared to those suffering from chronic ill health (27, 28).

Remission and Recovery in Patients with Chronic Schizophrenia

In contrast, patients with chronic psychotic disorders viewed recovery as an ideal state comprising being medication-free, attaining higher psychosocial functioning, and having meaningful relationships (29). Like young people, they also endorsed cessation of medication as an essential requirement for a full recovery. However, at the same time, they considered medication an important part of their treatment helping with symptom control, improving cognitive symptoms, and preventing relapse. One subject thought of medication as a supplement to prevent degeneration of the brain. Other important considerations were optimal functioning in the domains of work, family relationships, and independent living. Most viewed romantic relationships as desirable. However, most considered a romantic relationship as too stringent a requirement for the concept of recovery. Many subjects were not aware of their diagnosis and were uncertain about their prognosis.

Those suffering from chronic psychosis also experienced little understanding and support from others during their recovery.

It seemed that increasing isolation had led participants to develop polarised views of normality, and they expected those without mental illness to be without difficulties and lead successful lives. Participants viewed the right medication, psychological help, support, and monitoring from family members as important factors to promote their recovery. The clearest theme emerging from the discussion was that recovery was an ideal unattainable state comprising being medication-free, attaining higher psychosocial functioning, and having meaningful relationships. This contrasted with the view of professionals, who considered ongoing medication treatment a part of recovery alongside satisfactory psychosocial functioning and symptom control (29).

Reflections: The Concepts of Remission and Recovery

Our research efforts have confirmed that good remission rates can be achieved in early psychosis with tailored individual treatment in a specialist early intervention service. However, sustained recovery remains a distant treatment goal for most patients. As we review the definitions of remission and recovery and their application to real-life patients, we are confronted with the empirical reality that psychosis is a pervasive disorder. It causes not only psychotic symptoms but also cognitive, motivational, and mood symptoms, which are more often the cause of functional impairments even when psychotic symptoms are well controlled. We also observe that the proportion of patients in recovery would reduce if the criteria require a longer period of symptomatic remission and good functioning. This suggests that the condition tends to fluctuate with time.

It is important to study recovery with a prospective first-episode sample of patients. Studies that investigate established clinic populations tend to be biased by non-attendance over time. Who are the patients who do not come back to the clinic? In one of our follow-up studies, we took note of FEP patients who had participated in one of our research projects, but who stopped receiving treatment and attending clinic appointments. We grouped their mental health status as either being free from psychotic illness or likely still burdened by the consequences of the disorder. We found both types of patients in comparable proportions. We could then use this knowledge to complement our empirical data, which is typically based on a 70% to 80% follow-up rate.

Thus, the overall picture is that while a small proportion of patients can remain well without clinical input, most of our patients require continued support. For these patients, the condition fluctuates with challenges pertaining to either symptom control or functioning, thus preventing prolonged periods of recovery.

Fewer individuals enjoy sustained recovery with treatment, and there is also a small proportion of patients who remain unwell but do not receive treatment.

Several predictive factors for remission and recovery have been identified, such as older age at onset, female gender, higher educational attainment, good cognitive ability, and better premorbid functioning. Among the modifiable parameters were a shorter period of unemployment, a shorter DUP, and the severity of negative symptoms.

Interestingly, patients do not solely base their views on recovery on regaining psychosocial functioning and symptomatic improvement, but consider other factors such as their cognitive abilities and the need for ongoing medication and psychiatric follow-up.

Extensive cognitive assessments are usually not carried out in routine clinical practice due to their time requirements and costs. As a result, many clinicians are unaware of the often subtle cognitive abnormalities experienced by patients with psychosis. This may lead to miscommunication and gaps in the therapeutic relationship, particularly when professionals fail to acknowledge that some patients may have difficulties in regaining previous cognitive abilities. It has been known that cognitive performance can be affected up to 18 months prior to the development of frank psychosis and that patients experience ongoing cognitive difficulties following the resolution of clinical symptoms. Perhaps unsurprisingly, patients often attribute their cognitive difficulties to antipsychotic medication, and this not uncommonly leads to non-adherence increasing the risk of relapse and poorer long-term psychosocial outcomes. However, it is important to note that cognitive symptoms tend to improve over one or two years and to educate patients regarding the nature and course of their cognitive difficulties.

Subjective notions of remission and recovery have been shown to change during the course of psychosis. As patients recover from their first episode, their focus is usually on regaining their previous abilities and getting back to normal as it were. As noted, lingering cognitive dysfunction often leaves patients feeling impaired, and unless carefully managed may lead to a sense of despondency and despair with potentially detrimental effects on their mental state and treatment adherence. During the chronic stage of psychosis, patients' expectations usually adapt to the realities of having to manage a chronic relapsing and remitting illness and having to develop a sense of purpose and meaning when faced with difficult life circumstances. Thus, it is crucial to support patients during their illness journey to develop a realistic understanding of psychosis, foster a sense of agency and adequate coping strategies, offer psychosocial rehabilitation, and address associated cognitive difficulties in addition to antipsychotic treatment.

The complex interplay between the different facets of psychotic disorders and their treatment over time challenges us to confront a fundamental issue: Which is the most important outcome – functioning, symptom control, or subjective well-being? In psychosis, we see a condition that has multiple pathogenic factors converging on an individual during different life stages, leading to a trajectory that evolves into psychotic symptoms. Psychotic symptoms are debilitating if they are not controlled. However, once they are managed, the clinical outcome is still compromised by a wide range of other pathogenic factors. We then see that antipsychotic medication can alleviate psychotic symptoms, but are limited in helping with other facets of the condition. Medication is effective in preventing relapse, but symptoms may re-emerge once it is stopped. As with any long-term medical treatment, adherence is often challenging. Higher doses of medications are associated with metabolic side effects and cognitive impairment, while lower doses are associated with relapse and increasing treatment refractoriness.

Non-pharmacological interventions can be effective, but are resource-intensive and have mostly been studied only in the short term. There is certainly a need for cost-effective and sustainable non-pharmacological interventions to address aspects of the illness not treated by medication, such as cognition and functioning. Exercise programmes have shown initial promise, but further work is required to develop them into sustainable interventions. The participation of the individual patient in their treatment is crucial. However, for some patients, the illness also compromises their core capacity for complex decision-making.

With the multiplicity of possible causative factors, early intervention and personalisation of treatment are of utmost importance in securing the best possible outcomes for the individual patient. The challenges for patients, carers, researchers, and professionals are huge. It is in response to these needs that this book has summarised a snapshot of a body of coherent studies conducted on the same clinical population in a specific clinical context, to present ideas and insights that would otherwise be difficult to articulate in individual study reports and papers.

The prototypical concept of recovery involves the recovery of a loss in health status due to a distinctive illness process. For example, after a fracture, the bone is expected to heal and return to its previous structure and function so that the person can perform all of the former actions without additional support. This corresponds to the prototypical concept of 'complete recovery', i.e., the body is returned to its prior state before the illness. The same idea can be applied to some infections – when the microorganisms are eliminated, the body returns to its previous state. However, this is not always the case in human pathophysiology where pathological processes are gradual and progressive, such as when a person has predisposing vulnerabilities before the onset of discrete pathology. For example, reduced bone density due to a variety of reasons is a common precursor to fractures. In this case the underlying vulnerability, i.e., reduced bone density will need to be addressed in addition to the healing of the fracture. The contributory causes might have been

240 • *Psychosis and Schizophrenia in Hong Kong*

genetic, developmental, or degenerative, and may only be partially reversible with treatment. In these cases, the simple concept of a 'complete recovery' may not apply. Instead, one needs to conceptualise a way to manage the balance of risk and protective factors to prevent a recurrence of the condition.

This framework is familiar in oriental concepts of health, illness, and medical treatment. In the ancient East Asian view, the body is a microcosm of nature, where different forces, such as yin-yang and the five elements, interplay to produce a balanced healthy state, reflecting a dynamical template of interlocked excitatory and inhibitory forces, reflected in the seasons of the year. According to this perspective, illness arises from an imbalance of the natural forces, and recovery can be conceived as redressing the equilibrium by adjusting the strength of each natural element in order to attain a sustained state of balance. This state of health can be attained via a new equipoise of the forces rather than returning to the premorbid old equilibrium, i.e., it is a heterostasis rather than homeostasis. In psychotic disorders, similar to other complex disorders such as hypertension, diabetes, or indeed osteoporosis, the notion of recovery may be enriched by this framework of multiple balancing attunements with numerous naturally occurring forces. This is particularly important to facilitate an awareness of the multifaceted nature of psychotic disorders and the need for combined approaches using pharmacological and non-pharmacological means to address their different aspects. One further important observation is that human beings are not static entities; they are developing continually, whether in disease or health. They are revitalised with new experiences and new possibilities and never return to their previous 'old' state. This way of thinking about healing processes can help patient-carer-clinician systems not to be entrapped in the dilemmas inherent in a simplistic notion of 'complete recovery'.

References

1. Leucht S. Measurements of response, remission, and recovery in schizophrenia and examples for their clinical application. *J Clin Psychiatry*. 2014;75 Suppl 1:8-14. doi:10.4088/JCP.13049su1c.02

2. Liberman RP, Kopelowicz A. Recovery from schizophrenia: a concept in search of research. *Psychiatr Serv*. 2005;56(6):735-742. doi:10.1176/appi.ps.56.6.735

3. Andresen R, Oades L, Caputi P. The experience of recovery from schizophrenia: towards an empirically validated stage model. *Aust N Z J Psychiatry*. 2003;37(5):586-594. doi:10.1046/j.1440-1614.2003.01234.x

4. Lysaker, PH, Buck, KD. Is Recovery from schizophrenia possible? An overview of concepts, evidence, and clinical implications. *Primary Psychiatry*. 2008;15(6): 60-65.

5. Andreasen NC, Carpenter WT Jr, Kane JM, Lasser RA, Marder SR, Weinberger DR. Remission in schizophrenia: proposed criteria and rationale for consensus. *Am J Psychiatry*. 2005;162(3):441-449. doi:10.1176/appi.ajp.162.3.441

6. Lambert M, Karow A, Leucht S, Schimmelmann BG, Naber D. Remission in schizophrenia: validity, frequency, predictors, and patients' perspective 5 years later. *Dialogues Clin Neurosci.* 2010;12(3):393-407. doi:10.31887/DCNS.2010.12.3/mlambert
7. Karow A, Naber D, Lambert M, Moritz S; EGOFORS Initiative. Remission as perceived by people with schizophrenia, family members and psychiatrists. *Eur Psychiatry.* 2012;27(6):426-431. doi:10.1016/j.eurpsy.2011.01.013
8. Jääskeläinen E, Juola P, Hirvonen N, et al. A systematic review and meta-analysis of recovery in schizophrenia. *Schizophr Bull.* 2013;39(6):1296-1306. doi:10.1093/schbul/sbs130
9. Novick D, Haro JM, Suarez D, Vieta E, Naber D. Recovery in the outpatient setting: 36-month results from the Schizophrenia Outpatients Health Outcomes (SOHO) study. *Schizophr Res.* 2009;108(1-3):223-230. doi:10.1016/j.schres.2008.11.007
10. Lally J, Ajnakina O, Stubbs B, et al. Remission and recovery from first-episode psychosis in adults: systematic review and meta-analysis of long-term outcome studies. *Br J Psychiatry.* 2017;211(6):350-358. doi:10.1192/bjp.bp.117.201475
11. Anthony, WA. Recovery from mental illness: the guiding vision of the mental health service system in the 1990s. *Psychosocial Rehabilitation Journal.* 1993;16(4):11-23. https://doi.org/10.1037/h00956552
12. *Fourth National Mental Health Plan: An Agenda for Collaborative Government Action in Mental Health, 2009–2014.* Department of Health and Ageing, Canberra, Australia; 2009.
13. *Changing Directions, Changing Lives: The Mental Health Strategy for Canada.* Mental Health Commission of Canada, Calgary; 2012.
14. *No Health Without Mental Health: Delivering Better Mental Health Outcomes for People of All Ages.* Department of Health, London; 2011.
15. *Blueprint II: How Things Need to Be.* Mental Health Commission, Wellington, New Zealand; 2012.
16. *Achieving the Promise: Transforming Mental Health Care in America.* Pub no SMA-03-3832. Department of Health and Human Services, President's New Freedom Commission on Mental Health, Rockville, Maryland; 2003.
17. Slade M, Adams N, O'Hagan M. Recovery: past progress and future challenges. *Int Rev Psychiatry.* 2012;24(1):1-4. doi:10.3109/09540261.2011.644847
18. Leamy M, Bird V, Le Boutillier C, Williams J, Slade M. Conceptual framework for personal recovery in mental health: systematic review and narrative synthesis. *Br J Psychiatry.* 2011;199(6):445-452. doi:10.1192/bjp.bp.110.083733
19. Shanks V, Williams J, Leamy M, Bird VJ, Le Boutillier C, Slade M. Measures of personal recovery: a systematic review. *Psychiatr Serv.* 2013;64(10):974-980. doi:10.1176/appi.ps.005012012
20. Tsang HW, Chen EY. Perceptions on remission and recovery in schizophrenia. *Psychopathology.* 2007;40(6):469. doi:10.1159/000108128
21. Tang JYM, Chiu CPY, Hui CLM, et al. Poster 229. Clinical and cognitive correlates of perceived extent of recovery in Chinese patients with psychosis. The 2nd Biennial Schizophrenia International Research Conference; Apr 10–14, 2010; Florence, Italy. *Schizophr Res.* 2010;117(2–3):516. doi:10.1016/j.schres.2010.02.990

22. Chang WC, Chan TC, Chen ES, et al. The concurrent and predictive validity of symptomatic remission criteria in first-episode schizophrenia. *Schizophr Res.* 2013;143(1):107-115. doi:10.1016/j.schres.2012.10.016

23. Chang WC, Ming Hui CL, Yan Wong GH, Wa Chan SK, Ming Lee EH, Hai Chen EY. Symptomatic remission and cognitive impairment in first-episode schizophrenia: a prospective 3-year follow-up study. *J Clin Psychiatry.* 2013;74(11):e1046-e1053. doi:10.4088/JCP.13m08355

24. Chang WC, Tang JY, Hui CL, et al. Prediction of remission and recovery in young people presenting with first-episode psychosis in Hong Kong: a 3-year follow-up study. *Aust N Z J Psychiatry.* 2012;46(2):100-108. doi:10.1177/0004867411428015

25. Tso F, Chen EYH, Chan RCK, et al. Treatment response and its correlates with cognitive functions in first-episode psychosis. The 11th Biennial Winter Workshop on Schizophrenia; Feb 24–Mar 1, 2002; Davos, Switzerland. *Schizophr Res.* 2002;53(3) (Suppl. 1):122, abstract A253. doi:10.1016/S0920-9964(01)00381-4

26. Chan SKW, Hui CLM, Chang WC, Lee EHM, Chen EYH. Ten-year follow up of patients with first-episode schizophrenia spectrum disorder from an early intervention service: Predictors of clinical remission and functional recovery. *Schizophr Res.* 2019;204:65-71. doi:10.1016/j.schres.2018.08.022

27. Lam MML, Chan KPM, Law CW, et al. Subjective experience of first episode psychosis in Hong Kong: IPSOS Report. *Early Interv Psychiatry.* 2008;2:A27-A27.

28. Lam MM, Pearson V, Ng RM, Chiu CP, Law CW, Chen EY. What does recovery from psychosis mean? Perceptions of young first-episode patients. *Int J Soc Psychiatry.* 2011;57(6):580-587. doi:10.1177/0020764010374418

29. Ng RM, Pearson V, Lam M, Law CW, Chiu CP, Chen EY. What does recovery from schizophrenia mean? Perceptions of long-term patients. *Int J Soc Psychiatry.* 2008;54(2):118-130. doi:10.1177/0020764007084600

Epilogue

In this book, we have enjoyed a unique opportunity to present data and pose questions about psychotic disorders in an East Asian population, which has received far less attention in contemporary research than their Western counterparts. Our findings suggest that Chinese psychosis patients share similarities but also differ substantially in some aspects from Caucasian subjects. Our observations enable us to make suggestions regarding clinical care and the future direction of research efforts. Advancement of knowledge in a clinical condition as complex as psychosis is a challenging task. It has been suggested that progress in this area is like ascending a helical staircase rather than a ladder. While ascending, one sometimes returns to the same themes after some time. There has been definitive progress in the understanding of the condition, as our wide-ranging reflections have revealed about the work undertaken in Hong Kong and elsewhere over the past decades.

A number of the described themes will be revisited from different angles over the coming years. To enable further research endeavours, it is useful to reflect on and review broader paradigm issues alongside each individual study. There are often additional observations, which emerge during specific research efforts and which do not necessarily constitute typical empirical knowledge, that can help us gain important information about psychosis. These novel perspectives can stimulate the development of interesting hypotheses and influence the direction of clinical developments and research.

We hope that this book has served this purpose for our readers. In our collective endeavour to understand the intricacies of psychotic disorders, we are nowhere near having a complete picture of their aetiology, course, and effective treatment. Yet, we have come a long way from the initial stages of our quest for knowledge and several specific frameworks have emerged over the last three decades, which have been shown to coherently complement each other. From a broader perspective, it is important to note that there are a multitude of facts awaiting discovery, and as a result, several currently favoured paradigms may yet undergo significant revision. We would feel privileged if our book contributes to the debate by providing a broader and more diverse cultural and ethnic perspective based on our research findings over the last 30 years.

For the clinician–researcher, providing interventions cannot be delayed until an illness is completely understood. Each new patient presents a pressing need to make the best possible sense of the currently available information and to pragmatically respond to clinical needs. Many reflections in this work are based on this spirit of responding in a pragmatic manner to emerging evidence. The alarmingly poor outcomes of psychotic disorders suggest that there are still many areas of necessary innovation. From our current reflections, we have identified gaps in knowledge of psychosis and the provision of care. New interventions, when they become available, may help improve outcomes and the quality of life of those suffering from the disorder.

Advancement in knowledge is always steeped within a specific environment, with its unique historical and social, as well as scientific context. Among medical disciplines, this is nowhere as relevant as in psychiatry. Our intention was to provide context to the rich information from the body of work carried out in Hong Kong and summarised in this book. We hope that our commentary will continue to facilitate intellectual debate and creative reflection, which is much needed in this challenging field.

Index

aberrant salience, 162–163

Aetiology and Ethnicity in Schizophrenia and Other Psychoses (AESOP) study, xx, 136

aetiology, 2, 6–7, 36, 41, 45, 66, 126–127, 185, 211; brain development, 6, 185; bullying, 6; cannabis, 6, 98; childhood abuse/trauma, 6; cortisol axis dysfunction, 169; default mode network (DMN), xx, 8, 162, 164; dopamine hypothesis, 7, 186, 205; environmental stressor(s), 163–164, 169; genetic(s), 6–7; inflammatory cytokines, 169; knowledge of, 45; migration, 6; neuroanatomical, 7–8, 162, 212; neurophysiological, 7; obstetric complication(s), 6, 150; psychoactive substances, 6; urban environment, 6

anti-stigma campaign, 45, 69. *See also* public awareness/education campaign(s) and stigma, anti-stigma campaign/ intervention/programme(s)

anxiety disorder, 8, 99, 101, 112, 168, 223

associative learning, 162

at-risk mental state (ARMS), xx, 37, 40, 45, 84, 90–91, 96–102. *See also* clinical high-risk state (CHR); 'basic symptoms', 97; comorbidity, 99; 'first noticed disturbance', 98; functional impairment, 98; gender, 99; hallucinations, 100, 102; non-psychotic disorders, 101, *see also* comorbidity; prodromal symptoms, 99–101; psychosocial treatment, 102; subjective cognitive decline, 98; sub-threshold psychotic symptoms, 97

attention, 8, 25, 54, 97, 162, 183, 184, 187, 188, 199, 200, 203, 213, 224; sustained, 54, 187, 213

attentional blink paradigm, 188

attenuated psychosis syndrome, 39. *See also* at-risk mental state (ARMS) and clinical high-risk (CHR) state

auditory serial recall task, 189

bipolar disorder, 78, 204, 215

Bleuler, Eugen, 76, 183, 197

Bleuler, Manfred, 136

brain anatomy, 7; brain volume, 7, 86, 143, 150, 185; caudate nucleus, 86, 162–163; cerebellar lobes, 163; cortical midline structures (CMS), xx, 163; cortico-striato-pallido-thalamic (CSPT) circuitry, xx, 163; cortical-subcortical-cerebellar circuits, 211; hippocampus/hippocampal, 7, 25–26, 223, 224, 225; mesocorticolimbic areas, 162; dorsolateral prefrontal cortex, 222; thalamus, 163, 211, 212

brain development, 6, 185

brain imaging, 45. *See also* neuroimaging, functional magnetic resonance imaging (fMRI) and Tc-99m HMPAO SPECT

246 • Index

cannabis, 6, 98, 140, 149
carer(s), 2, 9, 20, 28, 66, 68, 78, 111, 114,
128, 136, 138, 239; engagement,
2, 68, 114; experience, 20, 28;
intervention(s), 20, 68; involvement,
9; resilience, 2
case management, 3, 5, 68, 70, 72, 99, 108,
113
Castle Peak Hospital, 3
childhood abuse/trauma, 6
childhood autism, 210
CHIME framework, xx, 234
cholinesterase inhibitors. *See* medication,
cholinesterase inhibitors
clang associations, 202
clinical high-risk (CHR) state, xx, 6, 8, 71,
80, 96–102, 112, 205. *See also* at-risk
mental state (ARMS); basic symptom,
97; 'gaoweiqi' (高危期), 'high-risk
period', 80; 'qianquqi' (前驅期), 'premorbid period', 80; 'fengxianqi' (風險
期), 'risky period', 80; 'sijueguomin'
(思覺過敏), 'sensitivity in thought and
perception', 80; 'yunniangqi' (醞釀期),
'incubation period', 40, 80; 'zaoxianqi'
(早顯期), 'early-manifestation period',
80
clinical sign, 204, 210–215; formal thought
disorder (FTD), 204; neurological soft
sign (NSS), 210–215
clozapine-resistant schizophrenia (CR-
TRS), xx, 151; clozapine augmentation, 151–152
cognition, 10, 28, 84, 139, 153, 183, 184,
186, 213, 223–226, 239; general, 163,
184, 190; mathematical, 26; non-
social, 221–222; self-cognition, 164;
social, 8, 186, 221–222
cognitive decline, 8, 23, 76, 98, 183, 185,
187. *See also* cognitive dysfunction and
impairment, cognitive
cognitive domain, 24, 183–184, 186–88,
213, 221, 223
cognitive dysfunction, 8–9, 23–24, 29, 68,
138–139, 153–155, 183–191, 221,

223–226, 238. *See also* impairment,
cognitive; attentional, 8, 188, 200;
course, 23, 153, 187–188, 190–191,
238; global, 189; historical context,
183; language, 9, 29, 199–200;
memory, 183–185, 188–189, 223,
226; non-pharmacological intervention, 221–227, 239; pharmacological
intervention, 221; processing speed,
184–185, 190; research paradigms,
184; reasoning, 184, 188; semantic,
9, 102, 186–188; specific, 9, 184,
189–190, 223; subjective, 23–24,
29, 68, 139, 190, 221; verbal fluency,
184–185, 201, 203
cognitive flexibility, 53–54, 187, 199
cognitive function/functioning, 9, 23–24,
51, 53–54, 85, 124, 138–139, 153, 184,
185, 188, 190, 222–223; generic, 9,
190; semantic, 9, 187–189, 196–205;
set-shifting, 188; specific, 9, 184–185,
189–90, 222–223; verbal comprehension, 127; visual processing, 188
comorbidity, 99, 173
cortisol, 169, 223, 225
cortisol axis dysfunction. *See* aetiology,
cortisol axis dysfunction
critical period hypothesis, 9, 107
culture, 2, 9, 21, 34–36, 38, 42, 51, 65,
100, 125, 127, 170; Asian, 2, 9, 170;
Chinese, 2, 21, 35, 38, 42, 125, 127;
Western, 2, 35, 38, 65, 100, 125, 170

default mode network (DMN), xx, 8, 162,
164
delusions of reference (DOR), xx, xxi,
159–165
dementia praecox, 76–78, 183
depression, 24, 36, 42, 52, 55, 96, 110, 135,
161, 168, 169, 173, 214, 225; treatment, 67, 101, 102, 110, 169
descriptive psychopathology, 27, 66
dialogical approach, 2, 138
dialogical behaviour, 202
diathesis-stress paradigm, 168

Index · 247

dopamine hypothesis. *See* aetiology, dopamine hypothesis
duration of untreated illness, 84
duration of untreated psychosis (DUP), xx, 8, 10, 42, 52, 56, 65–67, 69–70, 71–72, 84–91, 111–113, 138, 139, 142, 149, 150, 225, 235, 238; brain functioning, 86, 150; cognitive functioning, 84, 85, 86, 139, 238; definition, 84; demographic characteristics, 87; functional outcome, 69–72, 91; help-seeking duration, 8, 84–91; measurement of, 8, 85; long-term outcome(s), 86, 89, 90–91, 112–113, 235; public awareness, 10, 90–91, 112; reduction of, 10, 69, 71–72, 87, 112; relapse, 70, 88, 111, 138, 139, 142; remission, 85, 86, 88–89, 90, 235, 238; symptomatic outcome, 85, 90–91, 235; treatment response, 85; waiting time, 88
Durkheim, Émile, 35

early intervention (EI) in psychosis, xx, 3–5, 8–10, 56, 65–72, 84, 86–88, 90–91, 100–102, 123, 142, 174–175, 205, 234, 237, 239; adolescent onset, 90; adult onset, 70–72, 88, 90, 111–114; aims, 67–69; caseload, 70, 91, 108, 109, 113; case manager, 67, 68, 91, 108, 112; clinical outcomes, 4, 69–70, 151, 239; depressive symptoms, 54, 88, 101, 102; disengagement, 111; Early Assessment Service for Young People (EASY), xx, 67–72, 87, 110, 111, 113, 142, 151, 174–175; effectiveness, 70, 174; extended early intervention, 54, 86–87, 111–112; functional outcomes, 9, 54, 69–72, 101, 107–114, 151; gender, 54, 87, 110, 151; historical context, 66–67; hospitalisation, 70, 72, 110–111, 113, 142; insight, 54, 110, 113; intermediate outcomes, 110–111; Jockey Club Early Psychosis Project (JCEP), xxi, 57, 70, 91, 142–143; long-term

outcomes, 86, 90–91, 107–114, 205; negative symptoms, 54, 69–70, 110, 112, 234; occupational functioning, 54, 113; phase-specific, 10, 67–68, 70–72, 112, 114; premorbid functioning, 109–110, 113, 234, 235, 238; Psychological Intervention Programme in Early Psychosis (PIPE), xxii, 68; public awareness campaign, 67, 69, 89, 91, 112; short-term outcomes, 71–72, 110–111, 114; suicide mortality, 107, 109, 174–175
Early Psychosis Foundation (EPISO), xxi, 39, 69
education attainment/level, 37, 39, 40, 51, 54, 89, 110, 126, 149, 164, 171, 203, 213, 214, 235, 238
Ellis, William Charles, 66
emotion(s): high-expressed, 2, 27
employment, 23, 35, 36, 39, 42, 54, 85, 89, 110, 114, 136, 153, 235. *See also* unemployment
endophenotype, 7, 184, 211; cognitive, 184
environmental stressor(s). *See* aetiology, environmental stressor(s)
executive dysfunction, 8, 153, 184, 187–188, 199–200
exercise intervention(s), 9, 10, 190–191, 222–227, 239; aerobic exercise, 222–223, 224–225; aerobic fitness, 223–224; amplitude of low-frequency fluctuations (ALFF), xx, 224–225; brain volumes, 223–225; cycling, 224; high-intensity interval training (HIIT), xxi, 224–225; hippocampal volume, 223–224; mind-body exercises, 223–225; motivation, 222, 224, 226–227; motivational coaching, 225–226; neurobiological mechanisms, 223; short-term memory, 223; sleep, 225; Tai chi, 223–225; walking, 224; yoga, 223–225

family discord, 2. *See also* emotion(s), high-expressed

248 · Index

family history, 88, 98, 99, 100, 102, 168, 173
five elements, 35, 240
fluency: letter, 202–203; semantic, 186–187, 201, 202–203; verbal, 88, 184, 201, 202–203
functional magnetic resonance imaging (fMRI), xxi, 212, 224. *See also* brain imaging and neuroimaging
functional outcome(s), 9, 51–57, 69–72, 101, 107–114, 139–140, 143, 151, 155, 183, 191, 221, 222, 226, 234–235; amotivation, 9, 53–54, 56; cognitive functioning, 51, 53–54, 56–57, 155, 183, 222, 226; demographic variables, 53–54; functional remission, 54, 57, 110, 235; long-term, 9, 51–53, 107–109, 112–113, 139–140, 143, 226; measurement, 53, 57; modified Wisconsin Card Sorting Test (WCST) performance, 54; negative symptoms, 53–54, 69–70, 110, 112, 226, 234–235; occupational, 52–54, 109, 113–114, 235; psychotic symptoms, 9, 54, 69–71, 107, 110–112, 140, 143, 155, 226, 235; remission, 52, 55, 86, 110–111, 140, 234–235; short-term, 51, 110; subjective quality of life (SQoL), 51–52, 55, 56–57, 235

game theoretical paradigm, 188
gender, 2, 34, 40, 54, 87, 99, 110, 149, 151, 168, 169, 173, 203, 213, 238. *See also* early intervention (EI) in psychosis, gender
genetic(s), 1, 2, 6, 8, 45, 66, 97, 100, 101, 109, 140, 149, 151, 152, 159, 169, 174, 184, 214, 240. *See also* aetiology, genetic(s); genetic polymorphism, 151, 184; genetic predisposition, 159; genetic variants, 2, 184; heritability, 6, 211; polygenic, 6, 151, 190
German Psychiatric Association, 183
ginseng extract HT1001. *See* medication, ginseng extract HT1001
Goffman, Erving, 35

health belief(s), 2, 21, 127
help-seeking, delay in, 8, 37, 84–91
hierarchical language output system, 199
homicide, 40, 135
hopelessness, 78, 168, 170, 173
hospitalisation, 42, 65, 70, 72, 109, 110, 111, 113, 122, 124, 135, 136, 142, 173. *See also* treatment, hospital and treatment, inpatient

ideas and delusions of reference (I/DOR), xxi, 159–165; contextual factors, 165; definition, 159; Ideas of Reference Interview Scale (IRIS), xxi, 161; lifetime prevalence, 160; measurement of, 160; point prevalence, 161; population-level stressors, 163–164
illness course, 1, 4, 6, 8–10, 23, 37, 44, 52, 53, 56–57, 66, 68, 78, 80, 89, 99, 107, 110, 122, 134–136, 140, 142, 153–155, 164, 185–187, 191, 201, 215, 221, 233–234, 238
illness onset, 21, 23, 56, 101, 123, 140, 141, 153, 154, 160, 175, 184, 185, 187, 191, 214, 239; acute, 6, 54, 87; adolescent, 90; adult, 70, 71, 90, 111, 114, 127; age of, 70, 71, 89, 149, 174, 235, 238; insidious, 8, 89, 91; youth, 235
impairment: cognitive, 1, 6, 8, 23–24, 29, 55, 153, 154, 184, 185, 186, 188, 190, 203, 213, 221, 225, 239; functional, 6, 96, 98, 107, 113, 148, 153, 237; intellectual, 198; memory, 235; motivational, 1, 111, 155; neurocognitive, 56, 86; neurological, 214; occupational, 22, 174; prefrontal, 213; semantic, 199, 203; subjective cognitive, 23–24, 28–29, 98, 190; theory of mind (ToM), 162, 186, 188
impulsivity, 173
incidence rates, 1, 2, 95, 143
inflammatory cytokines. *See* aetiology, inflammatory cytokines
'insanity', 66, '*chisin*' (痴線), 80–81

insight, 20, 25, 36, 42, 53, 54, 85, 89, 99, 110, 113, 123, 126, 127, 160, 161, 162, 173, 187, 190
intellectual quotient (IQ), 149, 173, 185
intentional cognitive processes, 199
International Study on Schizophrenia (ISoS) study, xxi, 136
interpersonal functioning, 188
interpersonal theory of suicide, 168–169
intervention. See also treatment; anti-stigma, 37–39; early, see early intervention (EI) in psychosis; exercise, see exercise intervention; medical, 26, 89, 171; phase-specific, see early intervention (EI) in psychosis, phase-specific; non-pharmacological, 128, 221–227, 239; pharmacological, 5, 9, 123–128, 128, 221, 223, 225–226; preventative, 71, 72, 96, 100, 164, 175; psychological, 36, 123, 165, 191; psychopharmacological, 20, 77; psychosocial, 67, 70, 71, 77, 102; therapeutic, 65

Japanese Society of Psychiatry and Neurology (JSPN), xxi, 77
Jaspers, Karl, 20, 159
joint decision-making, 128

Kahn, Eugen, 159
Korean Neuropsychiatric Association, 77
Kraepelin, Emil, 76, 77, 78, 142, 159, 183, 197

language disorder, 198, 199, 202, 203, 204; expressive, 202; nominal dysphasia, 204
language organisation, 196, 198; discourse, 196, 197, 198, 204; lexicon, 196; phonetics; semantics, 196, 198; syntax, 196, 198
latent semantic analysis, 204
learning deficits, 187
life event(s), 99, 163, 168
life expectancy, 107, 174
localising neurological sign, 210, 212

Luria's model of mental processing, 188

Madras study, 136
media reporting, 37, 40, 79, 170
medication. See also treatment; adherence, 20, 24, 27, 36, 110, 111, 125–128, 141, 142, 148, 152, 155, 191, 239. See also non-adherence; amisulpride, 124; 'anti-psyche drug' (抗精神藥物), 126; anticholinergic, 213, antipsychotic(s), 1, 5, 20, 22, 24, 29, 55–56, 67, 69, 84, 85, 121–128, 136, 137–143, 148, 149, 151, 152, 153, 154–155, 165, 174, 185, 190, 222, 226, 238, 239; aripiprazole, 121, 122; attitudes towards, 20, 28–29, 56, 125–127, 141–142; atypical, 121, 221, see also second-generation antipsychotic; benefits, 26, 122, 127, 142; caregiver's perception of relapse, 26–27; cholinesterase inhibitor, 222; clozapine, 121–123, 125, 149–154; discontinuation, 122, 125–126, 137–143, 154–155; dose reduction, 139–140, 142–143; dosing interval, 126; efficacy, 121–122, 124, 152; first-generation antipsychotic(s) (FGA), xxi, 67, 121, 122, 123, 126; first-line treatment, 123, 124; ginseng extract HT1001, 225; grey matter volumes, 124; haloperidol, 122, 124, 125, 152, 153; knowledge of, 41, 126; lamotrigine, 152; long-acting injectable antipsychotic (LAIA), xxi, 124; maintenance, 22, 68, 123, 126, 137–143, 153, 155; -naïve, 187, 212–213; omega-3 polyunsaturated fatty acid EPA, 152; olanzapine, 121, 123–124, 125, 152; optimal duration, 126; perceived relapse risk, 22, 26–27, 126, 141; perphenazine, 152; placebo, 128, 137, 139, 151, 222, 226; poly-pharmacy, 122; prescribing of, 123, 125, 127–128, 138–139, 142, 152; quetiapine, 121, 124, 137; remission and recovery, 235–239; risperidone,

121, 123, 124, 125, 151, 152; second-generation antipsychotic(s) (SGA), xxii, 5, 121, 122; semantic dysfunction, 200–201; side effects, *see* side effects; subjective perception of recovery, 22–23; stigma, 42; sulpiride, 124, 153; thioridazine, 152; typical, 121, *see also* first-generation antipsychotic; valproate, 152; zuclopenthixol, 152

memory, 7, 8, 19, 25, 26, 28, 54, 88, 89, 127, 162, 183, 184, 185, 188, 189, 199, 200, 201, 202, 203, 204, 213, 214, 222, 223, 224, 225, 226, 235; auditory working, 188; deficits, 19, 26, 89, 184, 189; episodic, 26, 199; logical, 88; long-term, 19, 202; meta-memory, 26; procedural, 225; prose, 189; semantic, 199–201; semantic autobiographical, 26; short-term, 203, 204, 223; verbal, 89, 184–185, 213, 225, 235; verbal working, 189; visual, 54, 89, 184–185, 213; visual working, 188, 225–226; working, 127, 162, 185, 188, 214, 222, 224

modified labelling theory, 35

mood disorder, 8, 112, 164, 171, 215

mortality, 107, 109, 122, 125, 151, 170–171, 174, 175, 222

motor memory paradigm, 189

National Federation of Families with Mentally Ill in Japan (NFFMIJ), xxi, 77

network(s): brain, 7, 81, 163, 211, 214; community, 67; cortical, 212; cortical midline structures (CMS), 163; default mode, *see* default mode network; peer, 69; salient, 7; semantic, 200–201; social, 19, 99, 127, 171

network analysis, 169, 201

neurocognitive dysfunction, 6, 153, 215. *See also* cognitive dysfunction and impairment, cognitive

neurocognitive marker(s), 7, 142

neurocognitive tests, 188

neurocognitive theories of semantic abnormalities, 201

neurocomputational frameworks, 185–186

neurodegenerative hypothesis, 150, 185

neurodevelopmental hypothesis, 185

neuroimaging, 152, 153, 154. *See also* brain imaging, functional magnetic resonance imaging (fMRI) and Tc-99m HMPAO SPECT

neurological soft signs (NSS), xxi, 139, 150, 187, 210–215; clinical sign, 210–215; course, 187, 211–215; definition, 210; disinhibition, 212–214; historical context, 210; measurement of, 212; motor coordination, 187, 210, 212–214; neuroanatomical correlates, 212; sensory integration, 187, 210, 212–214

neurotransmitters pathways, 7, 186, 221; cholinergic, 221; dopamine, 7, 86, 124, 141, 149, 154, 155, 162, 186, 201, 204, 205, 223, 235; γ-aminobutyric acid (GABA), xxi, 7, 150, 186, 223; glutamate, 149, 186, 205, 221; N-methyl-D-aspartate (NMDA) receptors, xxi, 149, 186; serotonergic, 124, 149, 223

non-adherence, 25, 125, 126, 127, 136, 139, 149, 153, 190, 238; intentional, 127; non-intentional, 127

non-governmental organisation(s) (NGO(s)), xxi, 3, 67, 68, 69, 70

non-localising neurological signs, 210

Northwick Park Hospital, 67, 183

obstetric complication(s). *See* aetiology, obstetric complication(s)

optimism bias, 25

OPUS project, 108, 113

oxytocin, 222

pathogenesis, 4, 86, 107, 150, 190, 197. *See also* aetiology

pathophysiology, 2, 239

perception of self, 141

phenomenology, 27, 95, 96, 160, 186

Index · 251

physical exercise, 10, 222, 224, 225, 226. *See also* intervention(s), exercise

physical health, 52, 152, 171, 172, 226

physical illness, 153, 174, 175, 235–236

polygenic and multifactorial pathogenesis model of psychosis, 190

population(s): adult, 40, 171; adult-onset, 71, 72; Caucasian, 213; Chinese, 42, 65, 124; city, 2; clinical, 239; diversity, 1–2, 10; Danish, 149; Dutch, 140; East Asian, 2, 243; European, 1–2; Finnish, 121, 122; general, 36, 37, 38, 40, 56, 77, 78, 80, 81, 89, 95, 100, 102, 126, 128, 164, 222; homeless, 35; Hong Kong, 2, 4, 38, 40, 42, 45, 65, 102, 140, 170; local, 71; non-Western, 2; North American, 1–2; patient, 125, 127, 140, 212; prison, 35; urban, 4; Western, 8, 169; youth, 171

population-level stressors, 163–164

premorbid personality, 20

prepsychotic state, 39, 100. *See also* at-risk mental state (ARMS) and clinical high-risk (CHR) state

problem-solving skills, 172, 188

prodromal period, 96, 185. *See also* at-risk mental state (ARMS) and clinical high-risk (CHR) state

prodromal states, 4, 84, 100, 101. *See also* at-risk mental state (ARMS) and clinical high-risk (CHR) state

prodromal symptoms, 90, 97, 99. *See also* at-risk mental state (ARMS) and clinical high-risk (CHR) state

prognosis, 25, 67, 81, 84, 91, 138, 159, 165, 221, 236

psychoeducation, 20, 22, 28, 38, 39, 68, 71, 72, 81, 90, 141, 142, 152, 174

psychopathology, 9, 19, 27, 51, 53, 66, 96, 97, 98, 102, 119, 127, 163, 198, 211, 213, 235

psychosis. *See also* psychotic disorders: dimensions of, 5, 7–8, 53–54, 103, 155, 233; first-episode (FEP), 3, 21, 22, 23, 42, 51, 67, 72, 86, 87, 110, 122, 123, 126, 128, 136–37, 138, 139, 148, 173, 185, 211, 221, 233, 235–236; naming of, 76–82; neurodevelopmental theory, 6; risk factors, 6, 100, 102, 139, 173, 175; '*sijuegongnengzhangai*' (思覺功能障礙), 'thought-perceptual functional impairment', 81; '*sijueshitiao*' (思覺失調), 'dysregulation of thoughts and perception', 41, 69, 78–81, 235; '*sijuezhangai*' (思覺障礙), 'thought and perceptual impairment', 81; treatment-refractory, *see* schizophrenia, treatment refractory & treatment resistance; '*Wode Sijueshitiao*' ('我的思覺失調', 'My Psychosis'), 79; '*yanzhong jingshenbing*' (嚴重精神病), 'serious mental illness', 77; '*zhongxing jingshenbing*' (重性精神病), 'severe mental disorder', 40

psychosis proneness-persistence-impairment model, 95–96

Psychosis Studies, 70–71

Psychosis Study and Intervention (PSI) Team, xxii, 9

psychosocial functioning, 22, 24, 35, 51, 53, 54, 55–56, 57, 68, 96, 99, 110, 111, 114, 150, 191, 222, 223, 225, 236, 237, 238. *See also* functional outcome

psychosocial stress/stressors, 35, 56, 102

psychotic disorder(s): boundary of, 5, 7–8; diagnostic concepts, 5

psychotic disorder symptoms: anhedonia, 53, 202; auditory hallucinations, 96, 100, 152, 153, 161, 184, 197; delusions, 1, 19, 26, 79, 100, 153, 160, 184, 202, 205; disordered thinking, 1; formal thought disorder (FTD), xxi, 198, 203–205; negative symptoms, 6, 19, 22, 24, 42, 53, 54, 56, 67, 69, 70, 84, 85, 88, 89, 98, 110, 112, 135, 149, 150, 153, 154, 162, 186, 188, 190, 198, 200, 202, 204, 214, 223, 224, 226, 234, 235, 238; passivity phenomena, 189; positive symptoms, 22, 24, 28, 37, 54, 56, 69, 70, 78, 84, 85, 89, 96, 97, 110,

252 • Index

111, 121, 124, 127, 135, 137, 140, 150,
162, 187, 188, 223, 226, 233, 234, 235;
poverty of speech; residual, 107, 140;
visual hallucinations, 153
psychotic episode, 20, 23, 24, 25, 28, 44,
110, 134, 138, 149, 155, 226
psychotic-like experiences (PLEs), xxii,
95–96, 100–102, 164; affective
response, 96; assessment of, 96;
conversion rates, 100–101; definition,
95; epidemiological studies, 100, 102;
persistent, 95–96, 101; prevalence, 95,
100, 102; transient, 102
public awareness/education campaign(s),
10, 40, 67, 69, 89, 91, 112. *See also*
anti-stigma campaign and stigma,
anti-stigma campaign/intervention/
programme(s); school-based
programmes, 169

quality of life, 37, 42, 51, 85, 124, 148, 223,
244; definition, 51

rating instrument(s)/scale(s), 20, 21, 100,
114, 123, 135, 148, 160, 198, 232;
Bonn Scale for the Assessment of
Basic Symptoms, 97; Brief Psychiatric
Rating Scale (BPRS), xx, 135, 153;
Cambridge Neurological Inventory
(CNI), xx, 212; Capacity to report
subjective Quality of Life (CapQOL)
screening tool, xx, 55; Clinical Global
Impressions (CGI), xx, 135; Clinical
Language Disorder Rating Scale
(CLANG), xx, 198; Comprehensive
Assessment of 'At-Risk Mental State'
(CAARMS), xx, 97, 98; Global
Assessment of Functioning, 98;
Hayling Sentence Completion Test
(HSCT), xxi, 187; High Royds
Evaluation of Negativity Scale, 153,
186; Ideas of Reference Interview
Scale (IRIS), xxi, 161; Leibowitz
Social Anxiety Scale (LSAS),
xxi, 161–162; Life Functioning

Assessment Inventory (L-FAI), xxi, 53,
56; Medical Outcomes Study Short
Form 12-Item Health Survey (SF-12),
xxii, 124; Modified Six Elements Test
(MSET), xxi, 187; Nottingham Onset
Schedule (NOS), xxi, 85; Positive and
Negative Syndrome Scale (PANSS),
xxii, 98, 123, 135, 173, 225, 232;
Psychosis Recovery Inventory (PRI),
xxii, 21–22; Retrospective Assessment
of the Onset of Schizophrenia
(IRAOS), xxi, 85; Scale for the
Assessment of Positive Symptoms,
161; Schizotypal Personality
Questionnaire, 161; Stigma Scale,
Chinese version of, 42; Structural
Interview for Schizotypy, 160;
Structured Interview for Psychosis
Risk Syndromes (SIPS), xxii, 97;
Subjective Cognitive Impairment
Scale, 24; Thought, Language and
Communication (TLC) disorder scale,
198
receptors, 124, 154, 155, 186;
α-amino-3-hydroxy-5-methyl-4-
isoxazolepropionate (AMPA), xx, 222.
See also cognitive dysfunction, AMPA
receptor agonists; dopamine D2/3
receptor(s), 124, 154, 155; N-methyl-
D-aspartate (NMDA), 186; 5-HT7A
receptor, 124
recovery, 232–240; criteria, 22, 232, 237;
definition, 232, 234, 237; functional,
21, 57, 68, 123, 235; 'fuyuan' (復元),
21; 'houfaan' (好番), 21; personal
recovery approach, 233–234;
predictors, 235; rates, 233; 'sealing
over' style, 25; subjective experience,
see subjective experience, perceived
recovery
relapse, 134–143; assessment of, 135;
definition, 134–135; Johnstone type
I, 134–135, 137, 140; Johnstone type
II, 134–135, 140; predictors, 135–136,
139, 142; prevention, 9, 10, 20, 23,

139, 142–143, 226, 234; rates, 70, 71, 111, 135, 142; re-hospitalisation, 111, 135; ReMind, 139; response to treatment, 134; risk of, 21, 22, 24–27, 68, 123, 125, 126, 136–141; subjective experience of, *see* subjective experience, risk of relapse; symptom threshold, 135

relationship(s): close/romantic, 36, 236; family, 1, 9, 126, 236; long-term/stable, 134, 170; meaningful, 57, 237; quality of, 2; social, 1, 53, 76; stressors, 171; therapeutic, 20, 24, 78, 126, 127, 191, 238

remission, 232–240; clinical, 57, 137, 154, 235; criteria, 89, 135, 232, 233, 235, 237; definition, 134, 135, 232, 234–235, 237; first-episode psychosis, 53, 148, 232, 233, 235–236; functional, 54, 57, 110, 233, 235; predictors, 54, 110, 141, 235; symptomatic, 22, 52, 88, 89, 111, 232, 234, 235, 237; subjective experience, *see* subjective experience, remission; youth, 235–236

Remission in Schizophrenia Working Group (RSWG), xxii, 232–233, 234–235

resilience, 2, 164, 169

risk factors, 6–7, 27, 96, 97, 100, 102, 139, 168–175; adverse life experiences, 6; aetiological, 6–7, *see also* aetiology; discrimination, 6; environmental, 6; ethnic minority, 6

schizoid/schizotypal traits, 54, 88, 139

'schizophasia', 197

schizophrenia, 5, 69, 153; aetiological risk factors, 6–7; antipsychotic medication, 121–122, 124–125; caregiver's perspective, 26–27; chronic, 26, 52, 201, 211, 213, 214, 225, 236–237; cognitive dysfunction, 8, 183–184, 186–189; duration of untreated psychosis (DUP), 86; first-episode, 25, 67, 137, 148, 187, 200, 201; genetics, 2; ideas and delusions of reference (I/DOR), 160–164; improving cognition, 222–226; '*jeongshin-bunyeol-byung*' (精神分裂病), 'mind splitting disorder', 77; '*jingshenfenlie*' (精神分裂), '*jingshenfenliezheng*' (精神分裂症), 'mental split mind disorder', 41, 77, 79, 80, 235; '*johyun-byung*' (調絃病), 'attunement disorder', 77; neurological soft sign (NSS), 210–214; primary symptom, 197; recovery, 233, 235–237; relapse, 135–137, 139; remission, 135, 232–233, 235–237; renaming, 76–82; '*seishin bunretsu byo*' (精神分裂病), 'mind split disease', 77; semantic dysfunctions, 197–204; stigma, 36, 39, 40, 42; subjective experience of, 23; subjective quality of life (SQoL), *see* subjective quality of life (SQoL), schizophrenia; suicide, 168, 173; '*togo shitcho sho*' (統合失調症), 'integration disorder', 77, 81; treatment-refractory, 122, 148, *see also* treatment resistant schizophrenia (TRS)

Schizophrenia Outpatients Health Outcomes (SOHO) study, xxii, 233

schizophrenia spectrum disorder, 88, 125, 138, 151, 161, 172

schizotypal disorder/spectrum, 7, 101

schizotypal traits, 54, 88, 139, 164

Schneider, Kurt, 159

self-cognition, 164

self-esteem, 35, 128, 160, 169, 234

self-harm, 67, 173

self-referential gaze perception (SRGP), xxii, 163

self-referential ideas, 160, 164, 165. See *also* ideas and delusions of reference (I/DOR)

semantic dysfunction, 102, 196–205; negative language symptoms, 197; positive language symptoms, 197; semantic categorisation, 199–200; semantic fluency, 186–187, 201, 202, 203;

254 • Index

semantic inhibition, 188; semantic memory, *see* memory, semantic

semantics, 196, 198, 199; grammar, 196; meaning, 196; semantic fluency task, 201; semantic network, *see* network, semantic; semantic priming effect, 201; semantic-relatedness effect, 200; theoretical frameworks of semantic memory, 200–201

sensitiver Beziehungswahn, sensitive delusion of reference, 159

services: accident and emergency department (AED), xx, 3, 44, 65; community, 3, 135; community psychiatric, 35, 70; early intervention (EI), *see* early intervention (EI) in psychosis; generic, 108, 112, 114, *see also* standard care; medical, 3; mental health, 2, 3, 4, 67, 87, 90, 169, 170; outpatient, 3, 24, 65, 68; psychiatric, 35, 65, 67, 68, 86, 108, 114, 172; public, 5, 69, 72; social, 3

sexual abuse, 168

side effects, 23–24, 43, 52, 56, 67, 121–122, 123–125, 127–128, 138–139, 141, 143, 152, 153, 175, 185, 222, 236, 239; agranulocytosis, 121–122, 152; anticholinergic, 185; dystonia, 125; endocrinological, 124; extrapyramidal, 23, 52, 56, 121–122, 124, 153, 185, 226; metabolic, 23, 121–122, 124, 125, 139, 222, 239; monitoring of, 23, 125, 152; sexual dysfunction, 124, 125; tardive dyskinesia, 125, 150; weight gain, 23, 121

social anxiety/social anxiety disorder (SAD), xxii, 52, 56, 160, 161–162, 164

social cognitive training, 222

social functioning, 22, 52, 54, 84, 85, 99, 141, 173, 236. *See also* functional outcome

social isolation, 2, 35, 165

social skills training, 222

spontaneous blink rate, 139

standard care, xxii, 9, 23, 69, 70, 108, 109, 111, 112, 113, 114, 151, 174

stigma, 34–45; aetiological attribution, 41; affiliate, 42; anti-stigma campaign/intervention/programme(s), 5, 37–39, 45, 69; attitudes towards mental illness, 9, 38–39, 89; clinical high-risk states, 80; dangerousness, 40–41; disengagement, 37; 'face concern', 42; familial, 2; historical context, 34–35; internalised, 36–37, 42, 45, 143, *see also* self-stigma; knowledge of mental disorders, 20, 38–39; media, 37, 38, 40, 44, 69, 79; 'Mindshift programme', 45; personal, 36, 38, *see also* self-stigma; prejudice, 36, 37, 40, 41, 128; public, 38–42; public awareness, 5, 40, 67, 69, 89; quality of life, 37, 42; self-esteem, 35; self-stigma, 36–37, 38, 42, 45, 89; social, 35; social distance, 36, 38–39; sociodemographic factors, 40, 45; stereotyping, 35–36, 39; structural, 36; suicidality, 37; 'The School Tour', 39; transition to psychosis, 37; types of, 35–37

stress-vulnerability model, 7

subjective experience, 10, 19–29, 68, 97, 127, 139, 204, 221, 233; carer(s), *see* carer(s), experience; cognitive abilities, 23–24, 238; cognitive dysfunction, 23–24, 29, 68, 139, 221, *see also* cognitive dysfunction, subjective; help-seeking, 21; illness onset, 21; perceived recovery, 20–23, 221, 235; remission and recovery, 233; risk of relapse, perception of, 22, 24–27

subjective quality of life (SQoL), xxii, 51–53, 55–57, 88, 99, 128, 234–235; anxiety symptoms, 52–53, 56; attitudes towards medication, 56; capacity, 55; cognitive impairment, 55, 56; coping style, 56, 57; depressive symptoms, 52, 56, 88, 99, 235; duration of untreated psychosis (DUP), 56,

88; functional outcome, 51–52, 55–57, 234–235, *see also* functional outcome, subjective quality of life; measurement of, 55, 57; remission, 52–53, 55–56, 234–235; schizophrenia, 52, 55; side effects, 52, 56; social anxiety, 52–53, 56; stigma, 56, 57

substance use, 2, 6, 8, 98, 126, 136, 140, 149, 152, 153, 168, 171, 173, 185; alcohol, 36, 168, 171, 173; amphetamine, 98, 204, 205; cannabis, 6, 98, 140, 149; ecstasy, 98; inhalants, 171; ketamine, 98; opiates, 98; rates, 2; smoking/tobacco, 139, 173, 185; solvents, 98

suicidal behaviour, 168–170, 173, 175

suicidal ideation, 99, 110, 168–171, 173

suicide, 9, 10, 42, 67, 70, 107, 110, 113, 124, 134, 135, 136, 138, 140, 168–175; attempted, 109, 124, 136, 168–175; charcoal burning, 170, 171, 172; completed, 113; jumping from a height, 171, 172, 173; mortality, 107; 109, 168–175; protective factors, 169; prevention, 10, 169, 170, 175; psychological autopsy studies, 42, 171–172; in psychotic disorders, 173, 175; rates, 9, 109, 110, 135, 169, 170, 171, 173, 174; risk factors, 168–175; sub-types, 172

supervisory attentional system, 188

support: family, 99, 141; psychiatric, 236; psychological, 68, 152; psychosocial, 151; social, 99, 141, 189

syntax, 189, 196, 198, 199, 200, 204, 205

Tc-99m HMPAO SPECT, 153

theories of language production, 197

theory of mind (ToM), xxii, 162, 163, 186, 188

Tower of Hanoi task, 188

transcranial direct current stimulation therapy (tDCS). *See* treatment, transcranial direct current stimulation therapy (tDCS)

treatment: adherence, 168, 173, 175; antipsychotic, 1, 84, 85, 141–142, 152, 154, 174, 185, 221–222, 238; approach, 4; attitudes toward, 20, 21, 28; cognitive behaviour therapy for psychosis (CBTp), xx, 68, 70, 123; caregiver's perception, 26–27; cognitive remediation, 9, 57, 190, 191, 222, 223; community, 35; counselling, 152; culturally sensitive, 2, 21; delay in, 8, 51, 67, 71, 72, 84, 90, 107, 122, 150; disengagement, 25, 37, 111; duration of untreated psychosis (DUP), 84, 85–91; early intervention (EI), 65–72; extended, 54; electroconvulsive therapy, 152; family therapy, 123; goal, 19, 57, 114, 232, 237; hospital, 85, *see also* inpatient; individualised, 20, 57, 111, 114, 128, 141; inpatient, 4, 65, 127; knowledge of, 40, 41; maintenance, 123, 126, 137, 138–139, 141–143; medical, 3; medication, 41, 237; non-adherence, 190; non-pharmacological, 109; outcome, 51, 71, 107, 109–114, 211; pharmacological, 109, 121–128, 152, 169, 226, *see also* treatment, psychopharmacological; phase, 19, 21, 138; phase-specific, 71; physical, 34; planning, 227; psychiatric, 87, 88, 172; psychological, 169; psychopharmacological, 22, 57, 67, 142, 143; psychosocial, 101, 142; refractoriness, 112, 122, 140, 153–155, 239; rehabilitation, 5, 21, 69, 110, 152, 238; relapse, 134, 137–139, 140–143; -related factors, 52; remission and recovery, 234, 236–240; renaming schizophrenia, 76–77, 81; repetitive transcranial magnetic stimulation (rTMS); response, 2, 66, 85, 123, 134, 149, 151; risk states, 95, 97, 101–102; stigma, 36, 37, 39, 40–41, 42–44; subjective experience, 23–24, 28; transcranial direct current stimulation therapy (tDCS), xxii, 222, variables, 53

256 • Index

treatment refractory psychosis, 9, 121,
122, 140, 143, 148–155; case study,
153–154; management of, 152,
154–155
treatment resistance, 86, 148–155;
definition, 148; neurobiological
mechanisms, 149–150, 154; predictive factors, 149; prevalence, 148;
sub-types, 150
treatment resistant schizophrenia (TRS),
xxii, 148–152
Treatment Response and Resistance in
Psychosis (TRRIP) Working Group,
xxii, 148

ultra-high-risk state (UHR), xxii, 97. *See
also* at-risk mental state (ARMS) and
clinical high-risk (CHR) state
unemployment, 54, 100, 148, 171, 172, 235,
238. *See also* employment

Wernicke, Carl, 197, 210
word association task, 201
World Health Organization International
Pilot Study of Schizophrenia (IPSS),
xxi, 161

yin-yang, 240